Update on Incidental Cross-sectional Imaging Findings

Editors

DOUGLAS S. KATZ
JOHN J. HINES JR

RADIOLOGIC CLINICS OF NORTH AMERICA

www.radiologic.theclinics.com

Consulting Editor
FRANK H. MILLER

July 2021 • Volume 59 • Number 4

ELSEVIER

1600 John F. Kennedy Boulevard • Suite 1800 • Philadelphia, Pennsylvania, 19103-2899

http://www.theclinics.com

RADIOLOGIC CLINICS OF NORTH AMERICA Volume 59, Number 4
July 2021 ISSN 0033-8389, ISBN 13: 978-0-323-79648-4

Editor: John Vassallo (j.vassallo@elsevier.com)
Developmental Editor: Karen Solomon

Radiologic Clinics of North America (ISSN 0033-8389) is published bimonthly by Elsevier Inc., 360 Park Avenue South, New York, NY 10010-1710. Months of issue are January, March, May, July, September, and November. Periodicals postage paid at New York, NY and additional mailing offices. Subscription prices are USD 518 per year for US individuals, USD 1309 per year for US institutions, USD 100 per year for US students and residents, USD 611 per year for Canadian individuals, USD 1368 per year for Canadian institutions, USD 703 per year for international individuals, USD 1368 per year for international institutions, USD 100 per year for Canadian students/residents, and USD 315 per year for international students/residents. To receive student and resident rate, orders must be accompanied by name of affiliated institution, date of term and the signature of program/residency coordinatior on institution letterhead. Orders will be billed at individual rate until proof of status is received. Foreign air speed delivery is included in all *Clinics* subscription prices. All prices are subject to change without notice. **POSTMASTER:** Send address changes to *Radiologic Clinics of North America*, Elsevier Health Sciences Division, Subscription Customer Service, 3251 Riverport Lane, Maryland Heights, MO63043. **Customer Service: Telephone: 1-800-654-2452** (U.S. and Canada); **1-314-447-8871** (outside U.S. and Canada). **Fax: 1-314-447-8029. E-mail: journalscustomerservice-usa@elsevier.com (for print support); journalsonlinesupport-usa@elsevier.com (for online support).**

Reprints. For copies of 100 or more of articles in this publication, please contact the Commercial Reprints Department, Elsevier Inc., 360 Park Avenue South, New York, New York 10010-1710. Tel.: +1-212-633-3874; Fax: +1-212-633-3820; E-mail: reprints@elsevier.com.

Radiologic Clinics of North America also published in Greek Paschalidis Medical Publications, Athens, Greece.

Radiologic Clinics of North America is covered in *MEDLINE/PubMed (Index Medicus), EMBASE/Excerpta Medica, Current Contents/Life Sciences, Current Contents/Clinical Medicine, RSNA Index to Imaging Literature, BIOSIS, Science Citation Index,* and *ISI/BIOMED.*

Printed in the United States of America.

Contributors

CONSULTING EDITOR

FRANK H. MILLER, MD, FACR
Lee F. Rogers MD Professor of Medical
Education, Chief, Body Imaging Section and
Fellowship Program, Medical Director, MRI,
Department of Radiology, Northwestern
Memorial Hospital, Northwestern University,
Feinberg School of Medicine, Chicago, Illinois,
USA

EDITORS

DOUGLAS S. KATZ, MD, FACR, FASER, FSAR
Vice Chair for Research, Department of
Radiology, NYU Langone Hospital–Long
Island, Professor of Radiology, NYU Long
Island School of Medicine (Scholar Track),
Mineola, New York, USA

JOHN J. HINES Jr, MD, FACR
Chief of Radiology, Huntington Hospital,
Northwell Health, Associate Professor of
Radiology, Donald and Barbara Zucker School
of Medicine at Hofstra/Northwell, Huntington,
New York, USA

AUTHORS

LEJLA AGANOVIC, MD
Department of Radiology, University of
California, San Diego, UC San Diego
Medical Center, San Diego, California,
USA

MOSTAFA ALABOUSI, MD
Resident Physician, Department of Radiology,
McMaster University, Hamilton, Ontario,
Canada

RAYEH KASHEF AL-GHETAA, MPS
MSc Candidate, Institute of Health Policy,
Management and Evaluation, University of
Toronto, Toronto, Ontario, Canada

JEFFREY B. ALPERT, MD
Associate Professor of Radiology, Department
of Radiology, NYU Grossman School of
Medicine, NYU Langone Health, Center for
Biomedical Imaging, New York, New York,
USA

DANIELLA ASCH, MD
Assistant Professor, Department of Radiology
and Biomedical Imaging, Yale School of
Medicine, New Haven, Connecticut, USA

LEA AZOUR, MD
Clinical Assistant Professor of Radiology,
Department of Radiology, NYU Grossman
School of Medicine, NYU Langone Health,
Center for Biomedical Imaging, New York, New
York, USA

GERALDINE BRUSCA-AUGELLO, DO
Clinical Associate Professor of Radiology,
Department of Radiology, NYU Grossman
School of Medicine, NYU Langone Health,
Center for Biomedical Imaging, New York, New
York, USA

ANDY CHOY, MD
Assistant Professor, Department of Radiology,
Northwell Health, Donald and Barbara Zucker

School of Medicine at Hofstra/Northwell, North Shore University Hospital, Manhasset, New York, USA

MICHAEL T. CORWIN, MD
Associate Professor, Department of Radiology, University of California, Davis, Sacramento, California, USA

GRACE DEWITT, MD
Resident, Department of Radiology and Biomedical Imaging, Yale School of Medicine, New Haven, Connecticut, USA

KATHERINE EACOBACCI, BS
Donald and Barbara Zucker School of Medicine at Hofstra/Northwell, Hempstead, New York, USA

DANIEL I. GLAZER, MD
Assistant Professor, Department of Radiology, Brigham and Women's Hospital, Harvard Medical School, Boston, Massachusetts, USA

MICHAEL GOTTESMAN, MD
Chief Resident, Department of Radiology, Jacobi Medical Center, Bronx, New York, USA

RIYA GOYAL, MD
Department of Radiology, Donald and Barbara Zucker School of Medicine at Hofstra/ Northwell, Hempstead, New York, USA

JOHN J. HINES Jr, MD, FACR
Chief of Radiology, Huntington Hospital, Northwell Health, Associate Professor of Radiology, Donald and Barbara Zucker School of Medicine at Hofstra/Northwell, Huntington, New York, USA

REGINA HOOLEY, MD
Professor, Department of Radiology and Biomedical Imaging, Yale School of Medicine, New Haven, Connecticut, USA

DOUGLAS S. KATZ, MD, FACR, FASER, FSAR
Vice Chair for Research, Department of Radiology, NYU Langone Hospital–Long Island, Professor of Radiology, NYU Long Island School of Medicine (Scholar Track), Mineola, New York, USA

JANE P. KO, MD
Professor of Radiology, Department of Radiology, NYU Grossman School of Medicine, NYU Langone Health, Center for Biomedical Imaging, New York, New York, USA

RAMIT LAMBA, MD, FSAR
Professor, Department of Radiology, University of California, Davis, Sacramento, California, USA

AMELIA LANIER, MD
Department of Radiology, NYU Grossman School of Medicine, NYU Langone Health, Center for Biomedical Imaging, New York, New York, USA

KAREN S. LEE, MD
Assistant Professor in Radiology, Harvard Medical School, Department of Radiology, Beth Israel Deaconess Medical Center, Boston, Massachusetts, USA

MARK E. LOCKHART, MD, MPH
Department of Radiology, The University of Alabama at Birmingham, Birmingham, Alabama, USA

WILLIAM W. MAYO-SMITH, MD
Department of Radiology, Brigham and Women's Hospital, Harvard Medical School, Boston, Massachusetts, USA

MARK A. MIKHITARIAN, DO
Department of Radiology, Northwell Health, Donald and Barbara Zucker School of Medicine at Hofstra/Northwell, North Shore University Hospital, Manhasset, New York, USA

WILLIAM H. MOORE, MD
Professor of Radiology, Department of Radiology, NYU Grossman School of Medicine, NYU Langone Health, Center for Biomedical Imaging, New York, New York, USA

MARIAM MOSHIRI, MD, FSAR, FSRU
Professor, Department of Radiology, University of Washington Medical Center, Seattle, Washington, USA

SHANNON M. NAVARRO, MD, MPH
Assistant Professor, Department of Radiology, University of California, Davis, Sacramento, California, USA

A. ORLANDO ORTIZ, MD, MBA
Professor of Radiology, Albert Einstein College of Medicine, Chairman of Radiology, Jacobi Medical Center, Bronx, New York, USA

GREGORY PARNES, MD
Assistant Professor of Radiology, Albert Einstein College of Medicine, Bronx, New York, USA

RITESH PATEL, MD
Department of Radiology, Northwell Health, Donald and Barbara Zucker School of Medicine at Hofstra/Northwell, North Shore University Hospital, Manhasset, New York, USA

ROSHNI R. PATEL, DO
Chief Neuroradiology Fellow, Department of Radiology, Beth Israel Deaconess Medical Center, Harvard Medical School, Boston, Massachusetts, USA

MICHAEL N. PATLAS, MD, FRCPC, FASER, FCAR, FSAR
Professor, Staff Radiologist, Department of Radiology, McMaster University, Hamilton General Hospital, Hamilton, Ontario, Canada

MARGARITA V. REVZIN, MD, MS, FSRU, FAIUM
Associate Professor of Diagnostic Radiology, Department of Radiology and Biomedical Imaging, Abdominal Imaging and Emergency Radiology, Yale School of Medicine, New Haven, Connecticut, USA

ANNE SAILER, MD
Department of Radiology and Biomedical Imaging, Abdominal Imaging and Emergency Radiology, Yale School of Medicine, New Haven, Connecticut, USA

CYNTHIA S. SANTILLAN, MD
Department of Radiology, University of California, San Diego, UC San Diego Medical Center, San Diego, California, USA

ADAM C. SEARLEMAN, MD, PhD
Department of Radiology, University of California, San Diego, UC San Diego Medical Center, San Diego, California, USA

KEDAR G. SHARBIDRE, MD
Department of Radiology, The University of Alabama at Birmingham, Birmingham, Alabama, USA

BETTINA SIEWERT, MD
Associate Professor in Radiology, Harvard Medical School, Department of Radiology, Beth Israel Deaconess Medical Center, Boston, Massachusetts, USA

FRANKLIN N. TESSLER, MD, CM
Department of Radiology, The University of Alabama at Birmingham, Birmingham, Alabama, USA

SOPHIE L. WASHER, MD
Department of Radiology, NYU Grossman School of Medicine, NYU Langone Health, Center for Biomedical Imaging, New York, New York, USA

PEI-KANG WEI, MD
Instructor in Radiology, Harvard Medical School, Department of Radiology, Beth Israel Deaconess Medical Center, Boston, Massachusetts, USA

EVAN WILSON, MD
Resident Physician, Department of Radiology, McMaster University, Hamilton, Ontario, Canada

Contents

Pulmonary nodules are the most common incidental finding in the chest, particularly on computed tomographs that include a portion or all of the chest, and may be encountered more frequently with increasing utilization of cross-sectional imaging. Established guidelines address the reporting and management of incidental pulmonary nodules, both solid and subsolid, synthesizing nodule and patient features to distinguish benign nodules from those of potential clinical consequence. Standard nodule assessment is essential for the accurate reporting of nodule size, attenuation, and morphology, all features with varying risk implications and thus management recommendations.

Computed tomography (CT) and magnetic resonance (MR) imaging may demonstrate a wide variety of incidental findings in the breast, including primary breast carcinoma, the second most common cancer in women. It important to recognize the spectrum of pathologic conditions in order to properly assess the need for further workup. Some findings may be diagnosed as benign on the basis of CT/ MR imaging and clinical history alone, whereas others will require evaluation with dedicated breast imaging and possibly biopsy. This article serves to guide radiologists' management of the wide spectrum of incidental breast findings encountered on cross-sectional imaging.

Hepatic incidental findings often are seen on cross-sectional imaging examinations of the chest, spine, pelvis, or other nondedicated hepatic imaging. Radiologists are tasked with appropriately triaging, which requires further evaluation, even in the setting of an otherwise limited evaluation. This article reviews common benign entities encountered on ultrasound, computed tomography, or magnetic resonance imaging, along with their characteristic imaging features. Imaging features that are suspicious for malignancy or suggest the need for further evaluation also are discussed. Two algorithms are proposed to guide radiologists in their recommendations based on patient risk factors, focal hepatic abnormality size, and available imaging features.

Incidentally detected adrenal nodules are common, and prevalence increases with patient age. Although most are benign, it is important for the radiologist to be able to accurately determine which nodules require further testing and which are safely left alone. The American College of Radiology incidental adrenal White Paper provides a structured algorithm based on expert consensus for management of incidental adrenal nodules. If further diagnostic testing is indicated, adrenal computed tomography is the most appropriate test in patients for nodules less than 4 cm. In addition to imaging, biochemical testing and endocrinology referral is warranted to exclude a functioning mass.

Incidental splenic focal findings are commonly encountered in clinical practice and frequently represent a diagnostic dilemma due to nonspecific imaging features. Most are benign, particularly in patients without a history of malignancy and without symptoms of fever, weight loss, or left upper quadrant or epigastric pain. Incidental malignant splenic processes are exceedingly rare. This article reviews imaging characteristics of incidental focal splenic findings, and proposes a practical approach for management of such findings, which can prevent unnecessary workup and its related drawbacks in clinical practice.

Incidental pancreatic cysts are commonly encountered in radiology practice. Although some of these are benign, mucinous varieties have a potential to undergo malignant transformation. Characterization of some incidental pancreatic cysts based on imaging alone is limited, and given that some pancreatic cysts have a malignant potential, various societies have created guidelines for the management and follow-up of incidental pancreatic cysts. This article reviews the imaging findings and work-up of pancreatic cysts and gives an overview of the societal guidelines for the management and follow-up of incidental pancreatic cysts.

Renal masses are commonly encountered on cross-sectional imaging examinations performed for nonrenal indications. Although most can be dismissed as benign cysts, a subset will be either indeterminate or suspicious; in many cases, imaging cannot be used to reliably differentiate between benign and malignant masses. On-going research in defining characteristics of common renal masses on advanced imaging shows promise in offering solutions to this issue. A recent update of the Bosniak classification (used to categorize cystic renal masses) was proposed with the goals of decreasing imaging follow-up in likely benign cystic masses, and therefore avoiding unnecessary surgical resection of such masses.

A wide spectrum of incidental bowel findings can be seen on CT, including but not limited to, pneumatosis intestinalis, diverticular disease, non-obstructive bowel dilatation, transient small bowel intussusception, and submucosal fat. Radiologists should be aware that such findings are almost always benign and of little clinical significance in the absence of associated symptoms. Conversely, vigilance must be maintained when evaluating the bowel, because malignant neoplasms occasionally come to clinical attention as incidental imaging findings. When suspicious incidental bowel wall thickening is detected, the radiologist can alert the clinical team to the finding prior to the patient becoming symptomatic, potentially leading to definitive management at an early, more curable stage.

Margarita V. Revzin, Anne Sailer, and Mariam Moshiri

Incidental adnexal masses and uterine findings occur with a high frequency on cross-sectional imaging examinations, particularly in postmenopausal women in whom imaging is performed for a different reason. These incidentalomas encompass a gamut of potential pelvic gynecologic disorders. Most are benign ovarian cysts; however, other less commonly encountered disorders and improperly positioned gynecologic devices may be seen. A knowledge of the management recommendations for such pelvic incidental findings is critical to avoid unnecessary imaging and surgical interventions, as well as to avoid failure in diagnosis and management of some of these conditions.

PROGRAM OBJECTIVE

The objective of the *Radiologic Clinics of North America* is to keep practicing radiologists and radiology residents up to date with current clinical practice in radiology by providing timely articles reviewing the state of the art in patient care.

TARGET AUDIENCE

Practicing radiologists, radiology residents, and other healthcare professionals who provide patient care utilizing radiologic findings.

LEARNING OBJECTIVES

Upon completion of this activity, participants will be able to:

1. Describe the most common "incidentalomas" encountered in medical imaging.
2. Discuss the latest literature and guidelines on how to handle incidental findings on cross-sectional imaging examinations.
3. Recognize the challenges associated with identifying and reporting incidental findings, as well as addressing and managing patients' concerns.

ACCREDITATION

The Elsevier Office of Continuing Medical Education (EOCME) is accredited by the Accreditation Council for Continuing Medical Education (ACCME) to provide continuing medical education for physicians.

The EOCME designates this journal-based CME activity for a maximum of 12 *AMA PRA Category 1 Credit*(s)™. Physicians should claim only the credit commensurate with the extent of their participation in the activity.

All other healthcare professionals requesting continuing education credit for this enduring material will be issued a certificate of participation.

DISCLOSURE OF CONFLICTS OF INTEREST

The EOCME assesses conflict of interest with its instructors, faculty, planners, and other individuals who are in a position to control the content of CME activities. All relevant conflicts of interest that are identified are thoroughly vetted by EOCME for fair balance, scientific objectivity, and patient care recommendations. EOCME is committed to providing its learners with CME activities that promote improvements or quality in healthcare and not a specific proprietary business or a commercial interest.

The planning committee, staff, authors and editors listed below have identified no financial relationships or relationships to products or devices they or their spouse/life partner have with commercial interest related to the content of this CME activity:

Lejla Aganovic, MD; Mostafa Alabousi, MD; Rayeh Kashef Al-Ghetaa, MPS; Jeffrey B. Alpert, MD; Daniella Asch, MD; Lea Azour, MD; Geraldine Brusca-Augello, DO; Regina Chavous-Gibson, MSN, RN; Andy Choy, MD; Michael T. Corwin, MD; Grace DeWitt, MD; Katherine Eacobacci, BS; Daniel I. Glazer, MD; Michael Gottesman, MD; Riya Goyal, MD; John J. Hines Jr, MD, FACR; Douglas S. Katz, MD, FACR, FASER, FSAR; Jane P. Ko, MD; Pradeep Kuttysankaran; Ramit Lamba, MD, FSAR; Amelia Lanier, MD; Karen S. Lee, MD; Mark E. Lockhart, MD, MPH; William W. Mayo-Smith, MD; Mark A. Mikhitarian, DO; William H. Moore, MD; Mariam Moshiri, MD, FSAR, FSRU; Shannon M. Navarro, MD, MPH; A. Orlando Ortiz, MD, MBA; Gregory Parnes, MD; Ritesh Patel, MD; Roshni R. Patel, DO; Margarita V. Revzin, MD, MS, FSRU, FAIUM; Anne Sailer, MD; Cynthia S. Santillan, MD; Adam C. Searleman, MD, PhD; Kedar G. Sharbidre, MD; Bettina Siewert, MD; Franklin N. Tessler, MD, CM; John Vassallo; Sophie L. Washer, MD; Pei-Kang Wei, MD; Evan Wilson, MD.

The planning committee, staff, authors and editors listed below have identified financial relationships or relationships to products or devices they or their spouse/life partner have with commercial interest related to the content of this CME activity:

Regina Hooley, MD: Consultant/advisor: Hologic, Inc

Michael N. Patlas, MD, FRCPC, FASER, FCAR, FSAR: Honorarium: Springer

UNAPPROVED/OFF-LABEL USE DISCLOSURE

The EOCME requires CME faculty to disclose to the participants:

1. When products or procedures being discussed are off-label, unlabelled, experimental, and/or investigational (not US Food and Drug Administration [FDA] approved); and
2. Any limitations on the information presented, such as data that are preliminary or that represent ongoing research, interim analyses, and/or unsupported opinions. Faculty may discuss information about pharmaceutical agents that is outside of FDA-approved labelling. This information is intended solely for CME and is not intended to promote off-label use of these medications. If you have any questions, contact the medical affairs department of the manufacturer for the most recent prescribing information.

TO ENROLL

To enroll in the *Radiologic Clinics of North America* Continuing Medical Education program, call customer service at 1-800-654-2452 or sign up online at http://www.theclinics.com/home/cme. The CME program is available to subscribers for an additional annual fee of USD 356.00.

METHOD OF PARTICIPATION

In order to claim credit, participants must complete the following:

1. Complete enrolment as indicated above.
2. Read the activity.
3. Complete the CME Test and Evaluation. Participants must achieve a score of 70% on the test. All CME Tests and Evaluations must be completed online.

CME INQUIRIES/SPECIAL NEEDS

For all CME inquiries or special needs, please contact elsevierCME@elsevier.com.

RADIOLOGIC CLINICS OF NORTH AMERICA

Preface

How Do You Solve a Problem like Incidentalomas (version 2.0)?

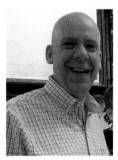 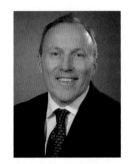

Douglas S. Katz, MD, FACR, FASER, FSAR   John J. Hines Jr, MD, FACR

Editors

It has been a decade since Dr Alec Megibow, a colleague at the same institution across town for one of us, a former attending during fellowship for the other of us, and a mentor to both of us, organized and edited an issue on the major problem of "incidentalomas" in medical imaging. In our clinical practices, regardless of what this encompasses for the individual radiologist, and for our referring practitioners, it seems literally every hour of every day we are faced with incidental findings. These are either truly asymptomatic and frequently are previously unknown, or in some patients, aren't really incidental but are unexpected findings. It may be difficult to determine what truly is "incidental" in a particular patient. In addition, if we are neuroradiologists, for example, we have to identify and sort out lung, kidney, and other findings, which usually do not correspond to our areas of expertise. If we are generalists or emergency radiologists, any cross-sectional imaging examination of any part of the human body can contain one, and sometimes more, incidental findings. The vast majority of these incidental findings are benign and are and will be of no consequence to most patients, but unfortunately a nontrivial minority do have implications and cannot be ignored. Sorting these out prospectively can be problematic and challenging in some patients.

Incidentalomas identified on cross-sectional imaging examinations present us with on-going challenges: how to report them, how to keep up with the increasing and evolving societal guidelines on handling them, what follow-up to recommend if any, how to counsel referring clinicians, and, increasingly, how to direct patient concerns. With portals and apps, many patients in various parts of the world, including those patients with incidental findings, now have immediate access to their imaging reports. Patients read and examine them, sometimes before the health care practitioners, frequently generating agita for everyone involved. Incidental findings pose other substantive challenges that the radiologist and the clinician have to tackle: ethical, economic, and medical-legal, among others. And to add to these challenges, there is the on-going COVID-19 pandemic, with medical and imaging resources still stretched thinly in some places of the world. How do we categorize such findings and keep everyone, patients, referrers, and ourselves, out of trouble? How do we reduce risk and anxiety, while simultaneously avoiding unnecessary imaging and other subsequent procedures, some of which can be quite invasive? What have we learned and what has changed since the initial series of guidelines the American College of Radiology (ACR) and other societies and expert panels have published?

We have assembled a team of experts from North America who present their take on the latest literature and guidelines on how to handle incidental findings on cross-sectional imaging examinations, combined with case material from their own practices, and insights from their own

Radiol Clin N Am 59 (2021) xv–xvi
https://doi.org/10.1016/j.rcl.2021.04.001
0033-8389/21/© 2021 Published by Elsevier Inc.

experiences. These radiologists have frequently been the leaders behind the ACR and other national and international societal guidelines and White Papers on incidental findings and have been leaders behind the various ACR "RADS" and in their own areas of related research. They cover multiple organs and organ systems and provide us with knowledge and reassurance. We hope that this issue builds on the previous work of Dr Megibow and colleagues and will be of utility and interest to many of us in clinical practice, regardless of our specific areas of concentration.

We thank everyone for their efforts, and particularly during this challenging time, where completing any task seems more difficult than usual. It has been an honor and a privilege to be given the responsibility of overseeing this project. We cannot cover every scenario and every body part and imaging modality, but we have tried to include some of the most common situations encountered in actual practice, some of them common and some less common. We hope this issue of the *Radiologic Clinics of North America* will also be helpful for our referring clinicians, who wrestle with these incidentalomas as much as we do now, if not even more so, as they have to counsel patients and to direct their further management.

We would also like to thank Dr Frank Miller, *Radiologic Clinics of North America* Series Editor, as well as the Elsevier staff, particularly John Vassallo and Karen Solomon, for their assistance, their guidance, and particularly, their patience.

Douglas S. Katz, MD, FACR, FASER, FSAR
NYU Langone Hospital–Long Island
259 First Street
Mineola, NY 11501, USA

John J. Hines Jr, MD, FACR
Donald and Barbara Zucker School of Medicine
at Hofstra/Northwell
270 Park Avenue
Huntington, NY 11743, USA

E-mail addresses:
douglasscottkatzmd@gmail.com (D.S. Katz)
jhinesmd@gmail.com (J.J. Hines Jr)

General Review on the Current Management of Incidental Findings on Cross-Sectional Imaging
What Guidelines to Use, How to Follow Them, and Management and Medical-Legal Considerations

Mostafa Alabousi, MD[a],*, Evan Wilson, MD[a],
Rayeh Kashef Al-Ghetaa, MPS[b],
Michael N. Patlas, MD, FRCPC, FASER, FCAR, FSAR[c]

KEYWORDS

- Incidental findings • Guidelines • Diagnostic imaging • Tomography • X-Ray computed
- Multidetector computed tomography • Magnetic resonance imaging

KEY POINTS

- "Incidentalomas" are common part of daily practice for radiologists, and knowledge of appropriate management guidelines ensures no potentially clinically relevant findings are lost to follow-up.
- Awareness of appropriate guidelines, how to follow them, as well as management and medical-legal considerations, is the ideal approach for incidentalomas in daily practice.
- Management guidelines are available for incidentalomas of the brain, thyroid, lungs, liver, adrenals, spleen, pancreas, kidneys, and ovaries, on cross-sectional imaging.
- No established management guidelines are presently available for incidentalomas of the spine, breast, or bowel, to our knowledge.

INTRODUCTION

Incidental imaging findings identified in a patient who is asymptomatic or undergoing diagnostic testing for unrelated reasons, termed "incidentalomas," have become commonplace in a radiologist's daily practice, regardless of what part(s) of the body the imaging that they interpret includes.[1,2] The demand for additional imaging of initially detected incidentalomas continues to grow, and this can result in substantial patient anxiety, particularly when there is clinical uncertainty regarding the best approach for management.[3] As a result of this, in addition to detection and diagnosis, radiologists should take an active role in management recommendations of these incidentalomas. This practice can ensure that concerning findings are not lost to follow-up, and that completely benign findings are not overinvestigated.[1] However, keeping up to date with the

[a] Department of Radiology, McMaster University, 1280 Main St W, Hamilton, ON L8S 4L8, Canada; [b] Institute of Health Policy, Management and Evaluation, University of Toronto, 155 College St 4th Floor, Toronto, ON M5T 3M6, Canada; [c] Department of Radiology, McMaster University, Hamilton General Hospital, 237 Barton St E, Hamilton, ON L8L 2X2, Canada
* Corresponding author.
E-mail address: mostafa.alabousi@medportal.ca

Radiol Clin N Am 59 (2021) 501–509
https://doi.org/10.1016/j.rcl.2021.03.002
0033-8389/21/© 2021 Elsevier Inc. All rights reserved.

latest guidelines for every type of incidentaloma in each organ system can be an increasingly daunting task for any radiologist. The purpose of this chapter is to provide a general review on the current management of incidental findings on cross-sectional imaging, including what guidelines to use and how to follow them, as well as management and medical-legal considerations. Incidental findings of the brain, spine, thyroid, lungs, breasts, liver, adrenals, spleen, pancreas, kidneys, bowel, ovaries, and uterus are discussed, with the greatest focus on the current American College of Radiology (ACR) White Papers relevant to each organ system. This introductory article sets the stage for the multiple articles that follow, and that cover incidentalomas in specific organ systems and scenarios in greater detail.

INCIDENTAL FINDINGS ON COMPUTED TOMOGRAPHY AND MR IMAGING OF THE BRAIN
What Guidelines to Use and How to Follow Them

In terms of incidental findings of the brain, we focus on the pituitary, with the ACR White Paper entitled "Management of Incidental Pituitary Findings on CT, MR imaging, and 18 F-Fluorodeoxyglucose PET."[4] The most common incidental pituitary findings are Rathke cleft cysts and pituitary adenomas, with less common incidentals (or unexpected findings) including epidermoid cysts, metastases, infarctions, or hemorrhage.[4] When large enough, suprasellar or parasellar masses, such as craniopharyngiomas or meningiomas, can mimic primary pituitary masses.[4] The main factors that will affect the need for further imaging of a pituitary incidentaloma include the imaging characteristics, its size, any mass effect, and endocrine function.[4] In terms of imaging characteristics on computed tomography (CT) and MR imaging, if the finding is that of a simple cyst, no further imaging follow-up is required, as this is most likely a Rathke cleft cyst.[4] Meanwhile, a solid or mixed-solid cystic pituitary mass most likely represents a pituitary adenoma. A solid or mixed-solid cystic focus measuring 10 mm or smaller also does not require imaging follow-up.[4] However, any solid or mixed-solid cystic mass measuring larger than 10 mm should have a follow-up pituitary MR imaging in 6 to 12 months.[4] Otherwise, any solid or mixed cystic solid mass should undergo endocrine workup, whereas pituitary masses of any composition causing mass effect or invasion of surrounding structures requires neurosurgical and/or endocrine consultation.[4]

Management and Medical-Legal Considerations

The main considerations for follow-up imaging of incidental pituitary findings are related to growth and hemorrhage (pituitary apoplexy), which are predominantly seen in solid or mixed-solid cystic masses >10 mm.[4,5] Clinical implications of growth or hemorrhage include the risk of hypopituitarism, visual field deficits, or ophthalmoplegia.[4] Although a small portion of pituitary microadenomas (≤10 mm) have been found to have microhemorrhage (3%), this was much lower than the rate in pituitary macroadenomas (>10 mm, 20%).[6] Furthermore, patients with pituitary apoplexy resulting in compressive symptoms all had underlying pituitary macroadenomas, whereas patients with pituitary microadenomas who underwent hemorrhage were asymptomatic.[6] Otherwise, the reported prevalence of incidental neoplasms on brain MR imagings in general was 0.7%.[7,8] The prevalence of non-neoplastic findings was 2.0%, most commonly arachnoid cysts (0.5%) and aneurysms (0.35%).[7–9] Established guidelines exist for the management of intracranial aneurysms, published by the American Heart Association, the American Stroke Association, and the European Stroke Organization, which are beyond the scope of this article.[10,11]

INCIDENTAL SPINE FINDINGS ON COMPUTED TOMOGRAPHY AND MR IMAGING

There are no well-established guidelines that radiologists may follow for incidental findings of the spine on CT and MR imaging, to our knowledge. A review of incidentalomas in spinal cord imaging reported on the following potential incidental findings of the spinal cord and nerve roots: syringohydromyelia, ventriculus terminalis, lipoma of the filum terminale, perineural cysts, cerebrospinal fluid flow artifacts, and enhancement of radicular vein and vein of the filum terminale.[12] In addition, the following incidentalomas of the vertebral body and posterior arch were also reported on: vertebral hemangioma, butterfly vertebra, block vertebra, benign notochord cell tumor, bone island/enostosis, and incomplete vertebral fusion/cleft of C1.[12] The development of management guidelines for potentially clinically relevant spine incidentalomas is warranted. For example, in rare cases of ventriculus terminalis, notochord cell tumors, and vertebral hemangiomas, underlying malignancy or aggressive/malignant features should be excluded, and an intravenous (IV) contrast-enhanced examination may be warranted.[12] A prevalence of upward of 22% has been reported for incidentalomas detected on MR imaging of the spine, although this included extraspinal findings.[1]

IMAGING OF INCIDENTAL THYROID NODULES
What Guidelines to Use and How to Follow Them

For imaging and management guidelines of incidental thyroid nodules, use of the ACR White Paper entitled "ACR Thyroid Imaging, Reporting, and Data System (TI-RADS)"[13] is recommended, along with a dedicated explanation for the lexicon,[14] as well as a user's guide from the TI-RADS committee.[15] This guideline is applied for incidental thyroid abnormalities identified in head and neck imaging of asymptomatic adults without risk factors for thyroid cancer.[16] Both CT and MR imaging examinations are limited in determining whether a thyroid nodule is benign or malignant.[16] As such, management of incidental thyroid nodules is divided into assessment with dedicated thyroid ultrasound versus no dedicated follow-up.[13] If an incidental thyroid finding is identified on CT or MR imaging, any of the following criteria warrant further assessment with a dedicated ultrasound: suspicious imaging features (local invasion, abnormal lymph nodes); patient younger than 35 years and size $\geq$1.0 cm; or patient age $\geq$35 years and size $\geq$1.5 cm.[16] Based on the dedicated thyroid ultrasound findings, a TI-RADS score is assigned, which in combination with size of the abdominality, determines whether further ultrasound follow-up or a fine-needle aspiration (FNA) is needed.[13] The TI-RADS score ranges from TR1 (benign) to TR5 (high suspicion of malignancy), and it is based on size, echogenicity, shape, margin, and the presence of echogenic foci.[13]

Management and Medical-Legal Considerations

Incidental thyroid nodules in adults are quite common, and are reportedly seen in up to 16% to 18% of CT and MR imaging examinations of the head and neck.[17] The estimated rate of thyroid incidentalomas found to be malignant ranges from 19% to 28%.[1] However, failure to diagnose thyroid malignancies smaller than 2 cm is unlikely to affect morbidity and mortality.[16] A study of 401 patients with incidental thyroid nodules on CT or MR imaging found that thyroid nodules were mentioned in the radiology reports of 375 patients (94%), and in the impression section of the reports in 138 patients (37%).[17] In total, 26 (19%) of 138 patients received additional workup, and

patients with the findings mentioned in the impression were 14 times more likely to have further assessment.[17] Only one papillary thyroid cancer was missed to the authors' knowledge in this study.[17]

INCIDENTAL LUNG NODULES ON COMPUTED TOMOGRAPHY: CURRENT FLEISCHNER SOCIETY AND OTHER GUIDELINES
What Guidelines to Use and How to Follow Them

The Fleischner Society guidelines are recommended for the management of incidental lung nodules on CT,[18–21] the most recent of which is the "Guidelines for Management of Incidental Pulmonary Nodules Detected on CT Images: From the Fleischner Society."[18] These recommendations apply to incidental pulmonary nodules seen on CT in patients $\geq$35 years old, and importantly they do NOT apply to patients undergoing lung cancer screening, those with immunosuppression, or those with known primary lung cancer.[18] Management recommendations are dependent on nodule type, size, and stability over time. Furthermore, risk factors for malignancy also influence management, with patients clinically stratified into low-risk or high-risk groups based on smoking history, age, and upper lobar location of the nodules.[18] Guideline recommendations include chest CT follow-up intervals at 3 to 6 months and 6 to 12 months, as well as an optional 12-month follow-up.[18] Concerning nodules may warrant recommendations for PET/CT and/or tissue sampling, whereas nodules smaller than 6 mm in low-risk patients do not require any further follow-up.[18]

Management and Medical-Legal Considerations

Incidental lung nodules are common, with reported prevalence rates of 8.5% in a study of 248 trauma patients undergoing thoracic CT assessment,[22] whereas screening chest CT examinations in older patients with a smoking history had reported lung nodule prevalence rates of 23%, of which 2.7% were malignant.[21] Meanwhile, a study of 243 patients undergoing abdominal CT demonstrated incidental lung nodules in 39% of patients, of which only 8.4% were mentioned in the final patient report.[23] Of note, in populations at high risk of lung cancer, the prevalence of cancer was 0.1% to 1.0% for smaller than 5 mm, 1% to 30% for 5 to 10 mm, and 30% to 80% for larger than 10 mm CT-detected nodules.[24] Furthermore, multiple trials have demonstrated a statistically significant mortality benefit for low-dose screening chest CT in patients at higher risk for lung cancer.[25–27]

INCIDENTAL BREAST FINDINGS ON COMPUTED TOMOGRAPHY AND MR IMAGING

There are no well-established consensus guidelines for incidental findings of the breasts on CT and MR imaging. A practical guide proposes a management algorithm for commonly encountered incidental findings in the breasts on CT in patients without previous mammographic evaluation.[28] Macrocalcifications and macroscopic fat were defined as benign findings, skin thickening, and rounded masses were defined as indeterminate findings, and masses with irregular shape or spiculated margins, masslike enhancement, and axillary adenopathy were defined as highly suspicious features.[28] For definitively benign findings, no further workup is recommended, while suspicious features warrant diagnostic breast imaging.[28] If indeterminate findings are present without suspicious features, correlation with prior relevant imaging examinations, if available, is recommended.[28] If there is documented stability for a period of at least 2 years, no further workup is recommended.[28] Otherwise, further diagnostic breast imaging is recommended.[28] Of note, when breast malignancy is suspected, the presence of skin thickening, nipple retraction, local invasion, and axillary adenopathy may be better assessed on CT than mammography.[28] A study of 11,462 women undergoing liver MR imaging identified breast incidentalomas in 292 patients (3%), and dedicated breast imaging was recommended for 192 of these patients (66%).[29] A total 10 incidental breast malignancies (3% of all breast incidentalomas) were identified.[29]

INCIDENTAL LIVER FINDINGS ON CROSS-SECTIONAL IMAGING
What Guidelines to Use and How to Follow Them

Multiple guidelines are available for assessment of liver findings on cross-sectional imaging. In asymptomatic adult patients for whom a CT was requested for an unrelated reason, the ACR White Paper titled "Management of Incidental Liver Lesions on CT" is recommended for use.[30,31] Guideline recommendations include no further workup, a follow-up hepatic MR imaging in 3 to 6 months, a hepatic MRI examination now, or immediate biopsy.[30,31] Management options are based on size of the identified abnormality, imaging features, and patient risk for hepatic malignancy (eg, cirrhosis, known malignancy, hepatic dysfunction).[30,31] However, these guidelines should not be applied for imaging examinations

to evaluate a known or suspected liver nodule or mass or other hepatic abnormality.[30,31] The Liver Imaging Reporting and Data System (LI-RADS) may be applied in the context of the diagnosis of hepatocellular carcinoma (HCC) with CT or MR imaging in patients with or at high risk for HCC.[32–34] The LI-RADS guidelines should specifically be applied in patients with cirrhosis, chronic hepatitis B virus, or current or prior HCC.[32–34] The LI-RADS scores range from LR-1 (definitely benign) to LR-5 (definitely HCC), as well as LR-TIV (malignancy with tumor in vein) and LR-M (probably or definitely malignant, not HCC-specific).[32–34]

Management and Medical-Legal Considerations

For incidentalomas in asymptomatic patients undergoing liver CT for different reasons, a nodule smaller than 1 cm in a low-risk patient is considered benign and does not require further follow-up, whereas 3-month to 6-month follow-up with MR imaging is recommended in high-risk patients.[30,31] For any other focal liver findings with benign features, no further workup. For those with suspicious features, generally, prompt MR imaging is recommended in low-risk patients, whereas prompt MR imaging or biopsy may be recommended in high-risk patients.[30,31] Flash-filling nodules larger than 1.5 cm in low-risk patients and larger than 1.0 cm in high-risk patients warrant further assessment with MR imaging.[30,31] In the context of the LI-RADS, the prevalence of malignancy by category was reported as 14% in LR-2, 40% in LR-3, 80% in LR-4, 97% in LR-5, 92% in LR-TIV, and 93% for LR-M.[35]

INCIDENTAL ADRENAL FINDINGS ON COMPUTED TOMOGRAPHY
What Guidelines to Use and How to Follow Them

Use of the ACR White Paper titled "Management of Incidental Adrenal Masses" is recommended for management of incidental adrenal masses on CT or MR imaging.[36] Management of adrenal incidentalomas is divided into benign nodules/masses that do not require follow-up, and intermediate nodules/masses requiring further workup.[36] Management recommendations are guided by size, density, and imaging features, such as the presence of fat and calcifications.[36] Further workup options include imaging follow-up with a dedicated adrenal CT (and in limited cases, MR imaging) protocol, PET/CT, biopsy, or resection. This is based on size, growth on follow-up, history of malignancy, and imaging features (including density on nonenhanced CT and washout characteristics on adrenal protocol CT[36]).

Management and Medical-Legal Considerations

Incidental adrenal masses are common, reported in up to 3% to 7% of adults.[36] Malignancy has been reported in up to 0.5% of adrenal incidentalomas.[1] A study of 1149 patients diagnosed with adrenal incidentalomas found that most (68%) were nonfunctional.[37] Adrenal protocol CT demonstrated a sensitivity of 100% and specificity of 95% in differentiating benign from malignant adrenal nodules.[37] In general, an incidental adrenal nodule measuring smaller than 1 cm in the short axis, or one with benign features, including macroscopic fat, hemorrhage, a cyst, or features consistent with adenoma, do not require further imaging follow-up.[36] For incidental adrenal masses that are larger than 4 cm with indeterminate features or are new/growing compared with previous imaging, resection should be considered if there is no cancer history, whereas biopsy or PET/CT is recommended if there is known cancer.[36] Incidental adrenal nodules/masses that show ≥1 year stability are considered benign and do not require follow-up.[36] Incidental adrenal nodules/masses with indeterminate imaging features measuring 1 to 2 cm are likely benign and may have a follow-up adrenal CT in 12 months, whereas an adrenal incidentaloma measuring ≥2 cm and smaller than 4 cm should undergo an adrenal protocol CT.[36]

INCIDENTAL SPLENIC FINDINGS ON CROSS-SECTIONAL IMAGING
What Guidelines to Use and How to Follow Them

For the management of incidental splenic findings, the ACR White Paper titled "Managing Incidental Findings on Abdominal and Pelvic CT and MR imaging, Part 3" is recommended.[38] Recommendations are based on imaging characteristics, clinical history, and findings on prior imaging.[38] Management categories include no further workup, follow-up imaging, evaluation with PET/CT, MR imaging, and/or biopsy.[38] No follow-up imaging is needed if an incidental finding or findings demonstrates benign features or 1-year stability.[38] Follow-up imaging, specifically an MR imaging in 6 months, is recommended for a finding with indeterminate imaging features with no history of cancer, or for a nodule smaller than 1 cm in a patient with a history of cancer.[38] Further evaluation with PET/CT, MR imaging, and/or biopsy is recommended if it demonstrates suspicious features, growth over time, or one that measures ≥1 cm in a patient with history of

cancer.[38] Suspicious imaging features include heterogeneity, enhancement, irregular margins, necrosis, parenchymal/vascular invasion, and growth over time.[38] Benign imaging includes findings of a simple cyst, hemangioma, or a nodule/mass that otherwise appears homogeneous, measuring less than 20 Hounsfield units in density, with smooth margins.[38]

Management and Medical-Legal Considerations

Most incidentally discovered splenic masses are benign and of no clinical significance.[38] Biopsy of splenic masses is rarely recommended, usually in cases of suspected angiosarcoma or in a patient with history of known malignancy with concern for metastasis or lymphoma.[38] A study assessed 379 patients with splenic incidentalomas divided into 3 groups: patients with known malignancy (145 patients), patients with constitutional symptoms and/or abdominal pain (29 patients), and asymptomatic patients (205 patients).[39] The incidence of malignant splenic masses was 49 (34%) of 145 patients with known malignancy, 8 (28%) of 29 of patients with constitutional symptoms and/or abdominal pain, and 2 (1%) of 205 in asymptomatic patients.[39]

INCIDENTAL PANCREATIC CYSTS ON CROSS-SECTIONAL IMAGING
What Guidelines to Use and How to Follow Them

Use of the ACR White Paper titled "Management of Incidental Pancreatic Cysts" is recommended for guideline recommendations of cystic pancreatic incidentalomas.[40] The most commonly seen pancreatic cystic tumors/masses include intraductal papillary mucinous neoplasms, serous and mucinous cystadenomas, solid pseudopapillary epithelial neoplasms, and pseudocysts.[40] Management options include no further workup, 1-year follow-up, 2-year follow-up, endoscopic ultrasound with FNA, and surgical consultation. Management recommendations are based on multiple factors, including size, interval growth, and imaging features, as well as patient age and clinical history (eg, pancreatitis).[40]

Management and Medical-Legal Considerations

Prevalence rates of cysts within the pancreas of 1.0% to 2.6% on CT and 13.5% to 15.9% on MR imaging have been reported.[41] In a study of 1038 patients, radiologists recommended follow-up imaging in 13.5% of cases of incidental pancreatic cysts identified on CT and MR imaging.[41] Radiologists appropriately adhered to the ACR guidance principles in 47.4% of the cases, and there was significant variation in recommendations across different radiologists.[41] MR imaging was the most frequently recommended imaging modality for follow-up.[41] Moreover, most incidental pancreatic cysts were smaller than 2 cm (72.6%), whereas only 9.1% measured larger than 3 cm.[41]

INCIDENTAL RENAL FINDINGS ON CROSS-SECTIONAL IMAGING
What Guidelines to Use and How to Follow Them

Utilization of the ACR White Paper titled "Management of the Incidental Renal Mass on CT" is recommended for incidental renal masses in asymptomatic adult patients without conditions that predispose them to renal neoplasms, or a primary malignancy that may metastasize to the kidneys.[42,43] Management recommendations include no further workup, further assessment with CT or MR imaging, or urologic consultation for management and/or biopsy.[42,43] The recommendations are based on size, attenuation, enhancement, heterogeneity, growth, morphologic change, and the complexity of cystic masses, incorporating the Bosniak classification system.[42–45] Multiple management pathways are provided for the following scenarios for incidental renal masses: noncontrast CT, IV contrast-enhanced CT, cystic renal mass (Bosniak classification), solid renal mass or too small to characterize, and renal mass containing fat.[42,43]

Management and Medical-Legal Considerations

Most incidental renal masses are benign cysts, for which the prevalence increases with age.[42] Benign renal cysts may be seen in up to 40% of patients undergoing an abdominal CT.[42] In a study of 5383 patients in the emergency department undergoing CT for renal colic, a prevalence rate of 3.1% was reported for "significant" incidental renal findings, defined as findings for which the radiologist explicitly stated follow-up imaging was required.[46] This study also confirmed the positive correlation between patient age and the prevalence of significant incidental findings; 80-year-old patients were 4 times more likely than patients aged 18 to 30 to have significant incidental findings.[46]

INCIDENTAL BOWEL FINDINGS ON COMPUTED TOMOGRAPHY

There are no well-established consensus guidelines for bowel incidentalomas on CT, to our knowledge. A previous systematic review of incidental findings in imaging diagnostic tests reported a prevalence of 25% for incidental findings of the gastrointestinal and genitourinary systems seen on diagnostic imaging examination.[47] Incidental findings within the gastrointestinal system were classified as "major", "moderate", or "minor" depending on their clinical significance.[47] A variety of incidentalomas related to the bowel were reported, including but not limited to diverticular disease, hernias, intestinal polyps, and bowel wall thickening.[47] Although a more standardized approach for follow-up is warranted, the systematic review found up to 64% of incidental findings within the gastrointestinal and genitourinary systems had some form of clinical follow-up or clinical confirmation of the diagnosis.[47]

INCIDENTAL ADNEXAL FINDINGS ON CROSS-SECTIONAL IMAGING
What Guidelines to Use and How to Follow Them

For management guidelines of adnexal findings on cross-sectional imaging, use of the ACR White Paper titled "Management of Incidental Adnexal Findings on CT and MR imaging" is recommended, which is an update of the ACR White Paper titled "Managing Incidental Findings on Abdominal and Pelvic CT and MR imaging, Part 1.[48,49] These management guidelines apply to incidental adnexal masses measuring larger than 1 cm in asymptomatic postmenarchal women.[48,49] The guidelines do not apply in women at high genetic risk for ovarian cancer, in women who develop related symptoms, or in findings that are stable for ≥2 years, as this excludes malignancy.[48,49] Adnexal incidentalomas may be placed into 1 of the following 3 categories: (1) simple-appearing cyst smaller than 10 cm, (2) uncertain diagnosis or simple cyst larger than 10 cm, or (3) features characteristic of other diagnosis.[48,49] A simple-appearing cyst smaller than 10 cm may have recommendations for no further follow-up, further characterization with ultrasound, or follow-up imaging with ultrasound depending on cyst size, imaging features, and menopausal status.[48,49] For an uncertain diagnosis or simple cyst larger than 10 cm, an ultrasound or MR imaging is recommended for further characterization.[48,49] Features characteristic of a specific diagnosis, such as a hemorrhagic cyst, fibroma, leiomyoma, hydrosalpinx, peritoneal inclusion cyst, or suspected malignancy, often require further assessment with ultrasound, MR imaging, or gynecologic assessment, with few exceptions.[48,49]

Management and Medical-Legal Considerations

Although it is understood that incidental adnexal simple cysts have a very low risk of malignancy, there are justifications for some adnexal cysts warranting short-interval follow-up in asymptomatic patients.[48,49] One is the risk of incorrect characterization of the incidental finding as a simple cyst, whereas the second is that some simple adnexal cysts may represent slow-growing benign ovarian neoplasms (cystadenomas).[48,49] A study conducted in 2869 women older than 50 years undergoing CT colonography screening identified indeterminate adnexal findings in 118 women (4.1%), with a mean size of 4.1 cm.[50] A total of 80 women underwent further imaging workup, and final surgical pathology of excised masses included 14 cystadenomas, 3 teratomas, 2 endometriomas, 2 cases of hydrosalpinx, and 1 fibroma.[48,49] No ovarian malignancies had been detected based on further imaging workup and surgical excision.[48,49]

SUMMARY

Incidentalomas are common part of daily practice for radiologists, and knowledge of appropriate management guidelines is important in ensuring no potentially clinically important or relevant findings are missed or lost to follow-up in asymptomatic patients. Although familiarization with the latest guideline recommendations for every type of incidentaloma throughout the body may be an increasingly daunting task for any radiologist, awareness of the guidelines available, how to follow them, and where to access them, may be the ideal approach. Hopefully this article, and the more focused articles that follow, will also provide the practicing radiologist with a useful update on a multitude of scenarios that incidental findings are detected on cross-sectional imaging examinations of multiple organ systems in the human body.

CLINICS CARE POINTS

- Incidental imaging findings, or "incidentalomas", may vary from benign findings with no follow-up required to more clinically significant findings for which require additional imaging and/or intervention.
- Radiologists play an important role in making recommendations for the appropriate management of incidentalomas seen on diagnostic imaging.
- Utilization of the most up to date guidelines for management of incidentalomas is key to ensuring clinically significant incidental findings receive the appropriate follow-up, and

completely benign findings are not over-investigated.
- This chapter provides a general review of on the current management of incidental findings on cross-sectional imaging, including what guidelines to use and how to follow them, as well as management and medical-legal considerations.

DISCLOSURE

Dr M.N. Patlas receives an honorarium from Springer. The remaining coauthors have nothing to disclose.

REFERENCES

1. O'Sullivan JW, Muntinga T, Grigg S, et al. Prevalence and outcomes of incidental imaging findings: umbrella review. BMJ 2018;361:k2387.
2. Hitzeman N, Cotton E. Incidentalomas: initial management. Am Fam Physician 2014;90(11):784–9.
3. Powell DK. Patient explanation guidelines for incidentalomas: helping patients not to fear the delayed surveillance. Am J Roentgenol 2014. https://doi.org/10.2214/AJR.13.12337.
4. Hoang JK, Hoffman AR, González RG, et al. Management of incidental pituitary findings on CT, MRI, and 18F-Fluorodeoxyglucose PET: a white paper of the ACR incidental findings committee. J Am Coll Radiol 2018;15(7):966–72.
5. Freda PU, Beckers AM, Katznelson L, et al. Pituitary incidentaloma: an endocrine society clinical practice guideline. J Clin Endocrinol Metab 2011;96(4): 894–904.
6. Sarwar KN, Huda MSB, Van de Velde V, et al. The prevalence and natural history of pituitary hemorrhage in prolactinoma. J Clin Endocrinol Metab 2013;98(6):2362–7.
7. Morris Z, Whiteley WN, Longstreth WT, et al. Incidental findings on brain magnetic resonance imaging: Systematic review and meta-analysis. BMJ 2009;339(7720):547–50.
8. Vernooij MW, Ikram MA, Tanghe HL, et al. Incidental findings on brain MRI in the general population. N Engl J Med 2007;357(18):1821–8.
9. Gibson LM, Paul L, Chappell FM, et al. Potentially serious incidental findings on brain and body magnetic resonance imaging of apparently asymptomatic adults: systematic review and meta-analysis. BMJ 2018;363:k4577.
10. Thompson BG, Brown RD, Amin-Hanjani S, et al. Guidelines for the management of patients with unruptured intracranial aneurysms: a guideline for healthcare professionals from the American Heart Association/American Stroke Association. Stroke 2015;46(8):2368–400.

11. Steiner T, Juvela S, Unterberg A, et al. European stroke organization guidelines for the management of intracranial aneurysms and subarachnoid hae-morrhage. Cerebrovasc Dis 2013;93–112.

12. Hiremath SB, Boto J, Regnaud A, et al. Incidentalomas in spine and spinal cord imaging. Clin Neuroradiol 2019. https://doi.org/10.1007/s00062-019-00773-5.

13. Tessler FN, Middleton WD, Grant EG, et al. ACR Thyroid Imaging, Reporting and Data System (TI-RADS): white paper of the ACR TI-RADS Committee. J Am Coll Radiol 2017;14(5):587–95.

14. Grant EG, Tessler FN, Hoang JK, et al. Thyroid ultrasound reporting lexicon: White paper of the ACR thyroid imaging, reporting and data system (TI-RADS) committee. J Am Coll Radiol 2015;12(12):1272–9.

15. Tessler FN, Middleton WD, Grant EG. Thyroid imaging reporting and data system (TI-RADS): a user's guide. Radiology 2018;287(1):29–36.

16. Hoang JK, Langer JE, Middleton WD, et al. Managing incidental thyroid nodules detected on imaging: white paper of the ACR incidental thyroid findings committee. J Am Coll Radiol 2015;12(2):143–50.

17. Tanpitukpongse TP, Grady AT, Sosa JA, et al. Incidental thyroid nodules on CT or MRI: discordance between what we report and what receives workup. Am J Roentgenol 2015;205(6):1281–7.

18. MacMahon H, Naidich DP, Goo JM, et al. Guidelines for management of incidental pulmonary nodules detected on CT images: from the Fleischner Society 2017. Radiology 2017;228–43.

19. Naidich DP, Bankier AA, MacMahon H, et al. Recommendations for the management of subsolid pulmonary nodules detected at CT: a statement from the Fleischner Society. Radiology 2013;304–17.

20. Bankier AA, MacMahon H, Goo JM, et al. Recommendations for measuring pulmonary nodules at CT: a statement from the Fleischner society. Radiology 2017;285(2):584–600.

21. MacMahon H, Austin JHM, Gamsu G, et al. Guidelines for management of small pulmonary nodules detected on CT scans: a statement from the Fleischner Society. Radiology 2005;395–400.

22. Hammerschlag G, Cao J, Gumm K, et al. Prevalence of incidental pulmonary nodules on computed tomography of the thorax in trauma patients. Intern Med J 2015;45(6):630–3.

23. Rinaldi MF, Bartalena T, Giannelli G, et al. Incidental lung nodules on CT examinations of the abdomen: prevalence and reporting rates in the PACS era. Eur J Radiol 2010;74(3).

24. Aberle DR, Gamsu G, Henschke CI, et al. A consensus statement of the Society of Thoracic Radiology: screening for lung cancer with helical computed tomography. J Thorac Imaging 2001;16(1):65–8.

25. De Koning HJ, Van Der Aalst CM, De Jong PA, et al. Reduced lung-cancer mortality with volume CT screening in a randomized trial. N Engl J Med 2020;382(6):503–13.

26. Aberle DR, Adams AM, Berg CD, et al. Reduced lung-cancer mortality with low-dose computed tomographic screening. N Engl J Med 2011;365(5):395–409.

27. Church TR, Black WC, Aberle DR, et al. Results of initial low-dose computed tomographic screening for lung cancer. N Engl J Med 2013;368(21):1980–91.

28. Al-katib S, Gupta G, Brudvik A, et al. A practical guide to managing CT findings in the breast. Clin Imaging 2020;274–82.

29. Prabhu V, Chhor CM, Ego-Osuala IO, et al. Frequency and outcomes of incidental breast lesions detected on abdominal MRI over a 7-year period. Am J Roentgenol 2017;208(1):107–13.

30. Gore RM, Pickhardt PJ, Mortele KJ, et al. Management of incidental liver lesions on CT: a white paper of the ACR incidental findings committee. J Am Coll Radiol 2017;14(11):1429–37.

31. Bird JR, Brahm GL, Fung C, et al. Recommendations for the management of incidental hepatobiliary findings in adults: endorsement and adaptation of the 2017 and 2013 ACR Incidental Findings Committee White Papers by the Canadian Association of Radiologists Incidental Findings Working Group. Can Assoc Radiol J 2020. https://doi.org/10.1177/0846537120928349.

32. Elsayes KM, Hooker JC, Agrons MM, et al. 2017 version of LI-RADS for CT and MR imaging: an update. Radiographics 2017;37(7):1994–2017.

33. Chernyak V, Fowler KJ, Kamaya A, et al. Liver Imaging Reporting and Data System (LI-RADS) Version 2018: imaging of hepatocellular carcinoma in at-risk patients. Radiology 2018;289(3):816–30.

34. Bashir MR, Chernyak V, Do RK, et al. CT/MRI LI-RADS v2018. American College of Radiology. Available at: https://www.acr.org/Clinical-Resources/Reporting-and-Data-Systems/LI-RADS/CT-MRI-LI-RADS-v2018. Accessed August 26, 2020.

35. van der Pol CB, Lim CS, Sirlin CB, et al. Accuracy of the liver imaging reporting and data system in computed tomography and magnetic resonance image analysis of hepatocellular carcinoma or overall malignancy—a systematic review. Gastroenterology 2019;156(4):976–86.

36. Mayo-Smith WW, Song JH, Boland GL, et al. Management of incidental adrenal masses: a white paper of the ACR Incidental Findings Committee. J Am Coll Radiol 2017;14(8):1038–44.

37. Hong AR, Kim JH, Park KS, et al. Optimal follow-up strategies for adrenal incidentalomas: reappraisal of the 2016 ESE-ENSAT guidelines in real clinical practice. Eur J Endocrinol 2017;177(6):475–83.

38. Heller MT, Harisinghani M, Neitlich JD, et al. Managing incidental findings on abdominal and pelvic CT and MRI, part 3: White paper of the ACR incidental findings committee II on splenic and nodal findings. J Am Coll Radiol 2013;10(11):833–9.

39. Siewert B, Millo NZ, Sahi K, et al. The incidental splenic mass at CT: does it need further work-up? An observational study. Radiology 2018;287(1):156–66.

40. Megibow AJ, Baker ME, Morgan DE, et al. Management of incidental pancreatic cysts: a white paper of the ACR Incidental Findings Committee. J Am Coll Radiol 2017;14(7):911–23.

41. Bobbin MD, Ip IK, Sahni VA, et al. Focal cystic pancreatic lesion follow-up recommendations after publication of ACR white paper on managing incidental findings. J Am Coll Radiol 2017;14(6):757–64.

42. Herts BR, Silverman SG, Hindman NM, et al. Management of the incidental renal mass on CT: a white paper of the ACR Incidental Findings Committee. J Am Coll Radiol 2018;15(2):264–73.

43. Kirkpatrick IDC, Brahm GL, Mnatzakanian GN, et al. Recommendations for the management of the incidental renal mass in adults: endorsement and adaptation of the 2017 ACR Incidental Findings Committee White Paper by the Canadian Association of Radiologists Incidental Findings Working Group. Can Assoc Radiol J 2019;125–33.

44. Bosniak MA. The Bosniak renal cyst classification: 25 years later. Radiology 2012;262(3):781–5.

45. Silverman SG, Pedrosa I, Ellis JH, et al. Bosniak classification of cystic renal masses, version 2019: an update proposal and needs assessment. Radiology 2019;292(2):475–88.

46. Samim M, Goss S, Luty S, et al. Incidental findings on CT for suspected renal colic in emergency department patients: prevalence and types in 5,383 consecutive examinations. J Am Coll Radiol 2015;12(1):63–9.

47. Lumbreras B, Donat L, Hernández-Aguado I. Incidental findings in imaging diagnostic tests: A systematic review. Br J Radiol 2010;83(988):276–89.

48. Patel MD, Ascher SM, Horrow MM, et al. Management of incidental adnexal findings on CT and MRI: a white paper of the ACR Incidental Findings Committee. J Am Coll Radiol 2020;17(2):248–54.

49. Patel MD, Ascher SM, Paspulati RM, et al. Managing incidental findings on abdominal and pelvic CT and MRI, Part 1: white paper of the ACR Incidental Findings Committee II on adnexal findings. J Am Coll Radiol 2013;10(9):675–81.

50. Pickhardt PJ, Hanson ME. Incidental adnexal masses detected at low-dose unenhanced CT in asymptomatic women age 50 and older: implications for clinical management and ovarian cancer screening. Radiology 2010;257(1):144–50.

Preparing for the Unexpected
A Review of Incidental Extraspinal Findings on Computed Tomography/Magnetic Resonance Imaging of the Spine

Michael Gottesman, MD[a],*, Roshni R. Patel, DO[b], Gregory Parnes, MD[c], A. Orlando Ortiz, MD, MBA[d]

KEYWORDS

- Incidental finding • Extraspinal • Magnetic resonance imaging • Computed tomography
- Spine imaging • Cervical spine • Thoracic spine • Lumbar spine

KEY POINTS

- Important components of image acquisition on computed tomography (CT) and magnetic resonance (MR) imaging examinations of the spine affect subsequent search patterns for not only spinal findings but for relevant and incidental and/or unexpected extraspinal findings.
- The CT scout images and MR scout localizers are a potential source of limited but useful diagnostic information, and should be included as part of the image review.
- Spine CT examinations should be reviewed in multiple window settings in addition to bone algorithm (soft tissue and lung windows).
- Incidental extraspinal findings, as have been shown in the literature, occur with sufficient frequency as to merit consideration when reviewing cross-sectional spine imaging examinations.
- Use of a spine segment–specific checklist (cervical, thoracic, and/or lumbar), combined with a knowledge of the commonly encountered extraspinal findings at these levels, assists the interpreting radiologist in the detection and evaluation of extraspinal incidentalomas.

INTRODUCTION

Radiologists, regardless of subspecialty, are responsible for all findings on the images provided for interpretation. Even when a finding that explains or potentially explains the patient's presenting symptoms is detected, it is still important to report potentially clinically relevant incidental findings. An incidental finding is a finding that is detected on an imaging examination that is performed for an unrelated reason. In a retrospective study, extraspinal incidental findings were present on 29.2%, 32.3%, and 35.5% of cervical, thoracic, and lumbar spine magnetic resonance (MR) examinations, respectively.[1] An increase in these incidental findings, also referred to as incidentalomas, is directly related to an increase in the use of cross-sectional imaging in recent years, and increased volume of the image datasets. These systems-based constraints introduce

[a] Department of Radiology, Jacobi Medical Center, 1400 Pelham Parkway South Building #1, Room #4N15, Bronx, NY 10461, USA; [b] Department of Radiology, Beth Israel Deaconess Medical Center, Harvard Medical School, 330 Brookline Avenue, Sherman 231, Boston, MA 02215, USA; [c] Albert Einstein College of Medicine, 1400 Pelham Parkway South Building #1, Room #4N15, Bronx, NY 10461, USA; [d] Albert Einstein College of Medicine, Jacobi Medical Center, 1400 Pelham Parkway South Building #1, Room #4N15, Bronx, NY 10461, USA
* Corresponding author.
E-mail address: gottesmm1@nychhc.org

Radiol Clin N Am 59 (2021) 511–523
https://doi.org/10.1016/j.rcl.2021.03.003
0033-8389/21/Published by Elsevier Inc.

time pressure as well as visual and mental fatigue, all of which can divert the interpreting radiologist's attention away from the extraspinal structures. By their very nature, spine imaging examinations are prime areas for the occurrence of incidentalomas, because the fields of view, on the scout images and on the various other sequences, include more than just the spine, although the spine itself is the focus of the interpreting radiologist. However, some incidental findings are not reported because they are deemed by the interpreting radiologist as not clinically relevant. Other incidentalomas may go undetected on computed tomography (CT) or MR examinations of the spine. In addition to systems-based errors, cognitive biases such as framing, anchoring, or satisfaction of search are possible contributing factors in the latter case.[2] This article helps familiarize radiologists who interpret spine imaging examinations with the commonly encountered incidental extraspinal findings with potential clinical relevance, and helps them use this information to recommend an extraspinal search pattern.

IMAGING TECHNIQUE

As part of a CT examination, so-called scout images are routinely obtained, usually in both the frontal and lateral projections. The purpose of the scout images is to localize the area of interest for the subsequent protocoled CT acquisitions. The scout images yield a broader field of view than the protocoled CT examination, and have the potential to harbor findings that are not within the field of view of the remaining spine examination, and these findings can be completely overlooked, even when obvious, if the scout images are not routinely reviewed by the interpreting radiologist. A retrospective study (n=100) found that 14% of spine examinations had abnormalities identifiable only on the scout images, and not on the acquired CT image dataset.[3] In these cases, the reason the finding was only detectable on the scout views was because it was beyond the field of view of CT acquisition. Although most of the scout findings were located within the spine segments above or below the level of CT acquisition, there were other reported potentially important extraspinal abnormalities in this study, including porcelain gallbladder, an appendicolith, and subcutaneous emphysema.[3] The MR imaging correlate to a CT scout image is the localizer sequence performed at the commencement of an imaging examination to aid in selecting the target area to be imaged. It too incorporates a larger field of view than the rest of the examination itself, and can thus reveal

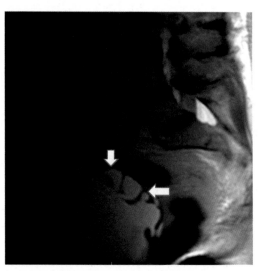

Fig. 1. Sagittal localizer from MR imaging of the lumbar spine in an 88-year-old woman being evaluated for cauda equina compression shows multiple bladder diverticula (*arrows*).

findings that are not detected on the regular sequences (**Figs. 1** and **2**).

With multidetector CT, CT spine examinations can either be performed as isolated examinations of a given spine segment (cervical, thoracic, lumbar, or sacral) or as part of a whole-body CT acquisition or pan-scan, as may be seen in patients with trauma. Axial sections are obtained and are often supplemented with coronal and sagittal

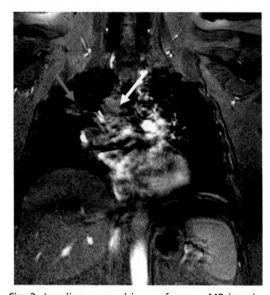

Fig. 2. Localizer coronal image from an MR imaging thoracic spine examination performed for the evaluation of upper motor neuron injury in a 54-year-old man shows a right hilar mass (*white arrow*) with right upper lobe obstructive atelectasis (*red arrow*).

reformations. Although CT of the spine is excellent for evaluating osseous structures, review of images should be performed with multiple windows and levels (bone, soft tissue, and lung window algorithms) settings to accentuate bone, soft tissue, or lung components. Evaluation of the cervical spine and craniocervical junction requires thin-section acquisition. CT of the cervical spine should have a maximum scan width of 3 mm. Thoracic and lumbar spine image acquisition can be a little thicker, as long as a 5-mm scan width is not exceeded. In order to improve spatial resolution, the field of view should be as small as clinically appropriate.[4] The sectioning planes and the window/level settings influence what the radiologist may or may not see in terms of extraspinal findings.

Although MR imaging protocols vary by facility and clinical indication, there are minimum sequences recommended for the routine evaluation of a given spine segment. These sequences include sagittal T1-weighted and T2-weighted sequences, followed by a T2-weighted (or fluid-sensitive) axial acquisition. In the cervical and thoracic spines, an axial gradient-echo sequence is often obtained. For routine examinations, the maximal slice thickness recommended for sagittal and axial sequences is 3 mm in the cervical spine, and 4 mm in the thoracic and lumbar spine. Spinal cord disorder is best evaluated with 2-mm slice thickness. The anatomic region scanned during an MR imaging examination varies based on clinical indication. A routine cervical spine MR imaging includes sagittal images that extend from skull base to the T1 vertebra, and that extend laterally to include the bilateral neural foramina of the entire cervical spine. Axial images are either obtained at the disc space levels or at a predetermined section of the cervical spine. If coronal sequences are performed, they may include the proximal brachial plexus. If the thoracic spine is to be imaged, sagittal images should be obtained from C7 to L1. As in the cervical spine, the images should extend laterally to include the bilateral neural foramina. If an area of interest is selected, axial images should be obtained through that level. Otherwise, axial images could cover the entire thoracic spine. If coronal imaging is performed, the exiting nerves in the region of interest and proximal ribs should be included. Lumbar spine sagittal sequences should include the entire lumbar spine, spanning from T12 to S1, and extend laterally to include the bilateral neural foramina and adjacent paraspinal soft tissues. At a minimum, contiguous axial slices should be obtained from L3-L4 through L5-S1, but may extend cranially to include L1-L2 and L2-L3.[5] As is seen with CT examinations, the area of coverage and the sectioning planes

influence the detection of extraspinal findings on MR imaging spine examinations.

IMAGING FINDINGS
Cervical Spine

In order to arrive at an appropriate search strategy for the detection of incidental findings on cross-sectional spine examinations, it is helpful to understand what are the common incidental extraspinal findings that may be encountered at a given spinal segment. One study on incidental findings detected on CT of the cervical spine performed in patients with trauma (n=1,256) showed that 18.3% of patients had at least 1 incidental finding.[6] Although incidental findings in this study were broadly defined as any finding not representing a C1 to C7 fracture, a range of findings were reported. The most common location for incidental findings was the lung (6.7%). The most common pulmonary incidental finding - within the study's broad definition of incidental - was pneumothorax (1.7%), but nontraumatic incidental findings, particularly lung masses or nodules (0.4%), were reported as well.[6] A subsequent study also reviewed 357 cervical spine CT scans performed in the trauma setting.[7] However, for the purposes of this study, only soft tissue incidental findings not related in any way to the presenting trauma were defined as incidental. In addition, these findings were classified into 1 of 3 categories based on

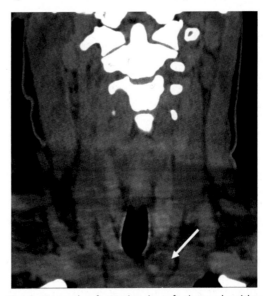

Fig. 3. Coronal reformation in soft tissue algorithm from a nonenhanced CT of the cervical spine performed for trauma evaluation in a 21-year-old woman shows a round soft tissue mass (*arrow*) with central hypoattenuation just inferior to the left lobe of the thyroid. This finding was suspicious for a parathyroid adenoma, and further work-up was recommended.

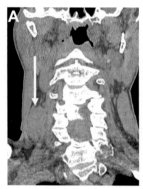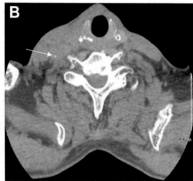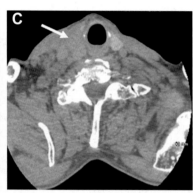

Fig. 4. Coronal (*A*) and axial (*B, C*) images from a nonenhanced CT of the cervical spine in a 52-year-old man performed for a fall shows bulky right internal jugular chain adenopathy, including 1 lymph node (*large arrow in A*), which measured up to 3 cm in craniocaudal dimension, and another lymph node that showed subtle calcification (*small arrow in B*). Low attenuation is seen within the superior aspect of the right thyroid (*arrow in C*). Further work-up to evaluate for papillary thyroid cancer was recommended, but patient was lost to follow-up.

clinical significance: category 1 for findings with no clinical importance, category 2 for findings with possible clinical importance and a need for further investigation, and category 3 for findings with obvious clinical importance. Thyroid abnormality was the most frequently encountered category 3 finding, seen in 24.9% of patients. The second most frequent category 3 abnormality was carotid artery calcification, seen in 22.9% of patients. Two scans revealed a parathyroid mass (0.9%), both inferior to the thyroid, and 1 of these was a known parathyroid adenoma (**Fig. 3**). Category 3 lymph nodes (>1 cm) were not detected in any of the CT examinations (**Fig. 4**).[7] A recent study focused on coronavirus imaging findings that may be present in the lung apices visualized on CT of the cervical spine or neck.[8] Fifty-nine percent of patients with unknown Covid-19 (coronavirus disease 2019) status at the time of their scans (n=17) had neck and cervical spine CT examinations that showed apical findings that were highly consistent with Covid-19 pneumonia. These findings included ground-glass opacities, alveolar consolidation, and so-called crazy paving. Similarly, a recent case report of an 83-year-old patient who underwent cervical spine CT after experiencing a fall showed peripheral ground-glass opacities in the lung apices. This patient subsequently underwent laboratory testing that confirmed positive Covid-19 status (**Fig. 5**).[9]

A retrospective review of 1106 MR imaging examinations of the spine for detection of extraspinal findings included 237 cervical MR imaging scans.[10] Among the cervical MR imaging examinations, there was a 25.7% incidence of extraspinal disorder. The most common finding was thyroid nodules, which were present on 17.3% of all cervical spine MR imaging examinations. The second most frequently encountered extraspinal finding in the cervical spine was paranasal sinus mucosal thickening. Another retrospective review of 192 cervical spine MR scans found an incidence rate of 29.2% for incidental extraspinal findings.[1] The most commonly detected abnormality was paranasal sinus mucosal thickening. Thyroid nodules were also some of the more commonly encountered findings. Although less frequent, there were several instances of cervical adenopathy, and there was also a case in which a thyroglossal duct cyst was discovered (**Fig. 6**).

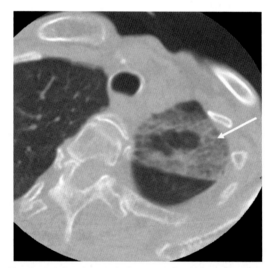

Fig. 5. Axial CT image in lung window algorithm from nonenhanced CT of the cervical spine in a 95-year-old woman who had fallen down shows ground-glass opacity within the left lung apex (*arrow*). The patient was confirmed to be Covid-19 positive on laboratory testing.

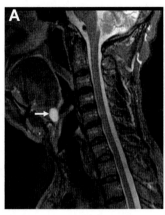 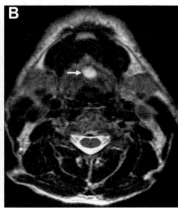

Fig. 6. Sagittal short tau inversion recovery (STIR) (*A*) and T2-weighted axial (*B*) images from a cervical spine MR imaging examination performed for the evaluation of C6-C7 radiculopathy in a 63-year-old man shows a hyperintense round cyst (*arrows*) at the base of the tongue in the midline, which is highly consistent with a thyroglossal duct cyst.

Although the thyroid and lung apices are often included as part of a radiologist's search strategy in the evaluation of cervical spine examinations, other anatomic regions should also be included (**Box 1**). One study in patients undergoing cervical spine CT examinations showed that incidental findings, including Thornwaldt cysts, thyroglossal duct cysts, carotid artery stenosis greater than 70%, laryngoceles, pharyngoceles, and aberrant right subclavian arteries, were all underreported (**Fig. 7**).[11] Only 2.9% of these incidentalomas were documented in the official report for the CT examinations included in this study, despite 28.3% of the patients having at least 1 of these incidental findings. The investigators acknowledged that some of the underreporting may not have been a result of underdetection but may have been caused by radiologists deeming some of these findings as not clinically significant. However, the investigators suggested adding these incidental findings to a standard template when reporting cervical spine CT.[11]

In light of the frequency and potential importance of incidental findings in the thyroid and lung apices, the authors recommend that these sites be routinely reviewed in cervical spine cross-sectional imaging examinations. In addition, although incidentally detected clinically relevant cervical lymphadenopathy is admittedly rare, because of the serious underlying disease that it could represent, we suggest radiologists include the nodal stations in the cervical spine search pattern. The parotids are often included in the field of view for cervical spine CT and MR imaging. Although there are limited data on the frequency and severity of incidental findings in the parotids, to our knowledge, T2-weighted images relatively frequently depict intraparotid lymph nodes or intraparotid cysts.[7] Similarly, the visualized portions of the paranasal sinuses, nasopharynx, oropharynx, and hypopharynx should be examined for any obvious mass, because detecting these findings early could have a substantial impact on the management and outcome for the patient. In addition, the vasculature should be assessed for calcification, stenosis, and aberrancies.

Thoracic Spine

Although not many, if any, studies have been performed to evaluate the incidence of extraspinal findings on CT examinations of the thoracic spine, to our knowledge, there have been several studying this phenomenon on thoracic spine MR imaging. The only incidental extraspinal finding

---

Box 1
Extraspinal checklist for the cervical spine

- Thyroid
  - Search for nodules
- Lung apices
  - Masses/nodules
  - Air-space and/or interstitial disease
- Lymph nodes
  - Search for lymphadenopathy, which may represent infection or neoplasm
- Pharynx and paranasal sinuses
  - Search for masses and inflammatory disorder
- Parotids
- Vasculature
  - Search for calcification, stenosis, or aberrancies

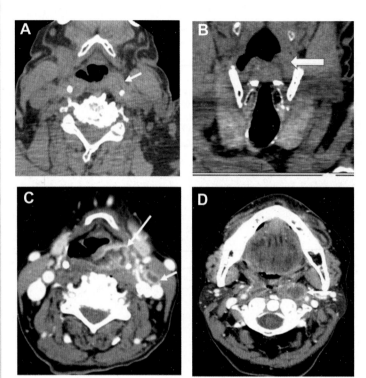

Fig. 7. Axial (*A*) and coronal (*B*) non-enhanced CT images in soft tissue algorithm from a CT scan of the cervical spine performed for trauma in a 62-year-old woman shows a soft tissue mass within the left pyriform sinus (*arrows*). This mass was not detected at the time of the examination. Axial intravenous contrast-enhanced CT of the neck (*C, D*) performed 7 months later after a laryngeal mass was discovered on endoscopy performed for dysphagia evaluation shows a heterogeneously enhancing mass with elements of necrosis in the left pyriform sinus (*large arrow in C*) with associated necrotic nodes (*small arrow in C*), including a large left retropharyngeal node (*arrow in D*). These findings were pathologically proved to represent squamous cell carcinoma.

detected in a review of 19 thoracic MR imaging examinations was thyroid nodules in the lower portions of the gland, with a frequency of 10.5% (**Fig. 8**).[10] In another study, 31 thoracic spine MR imaging scans were reviewed and there was a 32.3% rate of incidental findings.[1] The most frequent finding was pleural effusion, but hepatic masses and para-aortic adenopathy were reported as well (**Fig. 9**). In a prospective review of 120 thoracic spine MR imaging scans, 13.3% of patients (16) showed extraspinal findings.[12] Of the incidental findings detected, 37.5% were considered to be potentially clinically relevant, which included thyroid goiters, a liver mass, and hydronephrosis. Among incidental findings that were not considered clinically relevant were pleural effusions and renal cysts. A list of the more frequently encountered extraspinal findings on thoracic MR imaging includes pulmonary abnormalities such as consolidation, in addition to pulmonary masses and pleural effusions.[13]

When adopting a search pattern for incidental findings on a cross-sectional thoracic spine examination, the radiologist has to consider the anatomy included in the field of view and the frequently encountered findings in the region, as

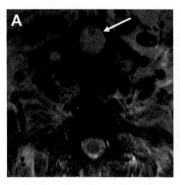
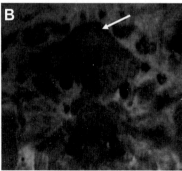
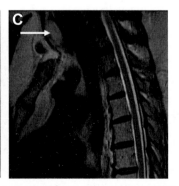

Fig. 8. T1-weighted (*A*), T2-weighted axial (*B*), and T2-weighted sagittal (*C*) sequences from a thoracic spine MR imaging in a 62-year-old woman with pulmonary malignancy showed multiple thyroid nodules, including a 2.6 × 1.4 × 2-cm isthmic nodule (*arrows*). Recommended fine-needle aspirations have not yet been performed.

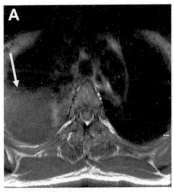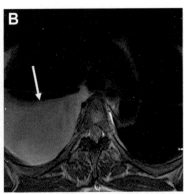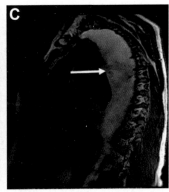

Fig. 9. T1-weighted (*A*) and T2-weighted (*B*) axial and sagittal STIR (*C*) sequences from an MR scan of the thoracic spine in a 43-year-old woman presenting with 5 months of back pain and hyperreflexia show an incidental large right pleural effusion (*arrows*), with T2/STIR hyperintensity and mild T1 hypointensity, representing recurrence of the patient's thoracic endometriosis.

well as those rare findings that may be of clinical relevance (**Box 2**). Although there is much general literature about incidentally detected pulmonary nodules, there are no known dedicated studies of thoracic spine imaging that detail the incidence of incidentally detected nodules, to our knowledge. Nonetheless, a lung nodule could represent a potential malignancy and should therefore be included in the radiologist's search pattern on thoracic spine imaging examinations (**Figs. 10 and 11**). Other pulmonary findings, including pneumonia, pulmonary fibrosis, and pleural effusions, should also be considered. In addition, radiologists should remember that all parts of the mediastinum, including the heart and great vessels, lower portions of the thyroid, mediastinal nodal stations, and esophagus, are potentially included in the field of view, and should be assessed for abnormalities (**Fig. 12**). In addition, the radiologist should assess the visualized upper abdominal and retroperitoneal organs (ie, the liver, spleen, pancreas, adrenals, and kidneys) before completing a review of the imaging examination.

Box 2
Extraspinal checklist for the thoracic spine

- Lungs
  - Nodules/masses
  - Pleural effusion
  - Air-space and/or interstitial disease
- Mediastinum
  - Cardiac masses
  - Vasculature
    - Pulmonary emboli
    - Aneurysms
    - Dissection
  - Lymphadenopathy
  - Esophageal wall thickening/mass
  - Thyroid nodules
- Upper abdomen
  - Liver
  - Spleen
  - Kidneys
  - Adrenals
  - Pancreas

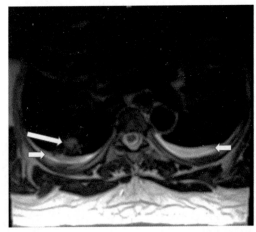

Fig. 10. Axial T2-weighted image from a thoracic spine MR scan in a 50-year-old man shows bilateral small pleural effusions (*short arrows*) as well as a small T2-hyperintense irregular nodule (*long arrow*) that was not detected on this examination. The nodule was subsequently evaluated, and was confirmed to represent carcinoma.

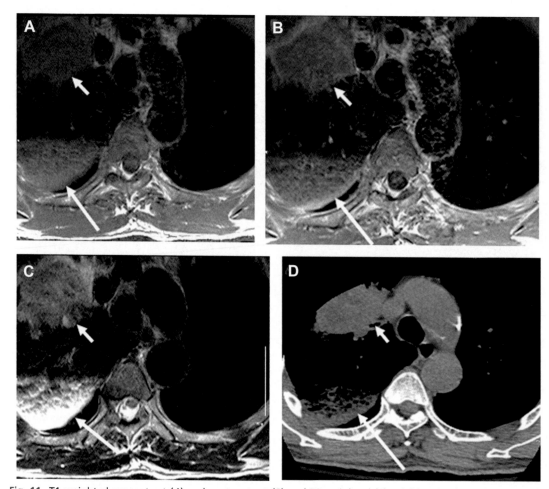

Fig. 11. T1-weighted precontrast (*A*) and postcontrast (*B*) and T2-weighted (*C*) axial images from thoracic spine MR imaging performed for suspected spinal cord compression in a 63-year-old man. MR imaging showed a posterior right upper lobe consolidation (*large arrow*), as well as an anterior right upper lobe mass (*small arrow*) that was characterized by T1 hypointensity, T2 intermediate intensity, and mild enhancement. The mass and consolidation were also detected on nonenhanced CT of the thoracic spine (*D*) performed the same day. The patient was subsequently diagnosed with lung adenocarcinoma.

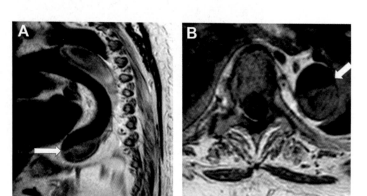

Fig. 12. Sagittal (*A*) and axial (*B*) T1-weighted images from a thoracic spine MR scan performed to evaluate suspected osteomyelitis in an 81-year-old woman show an aortic dissection (*arrows*).

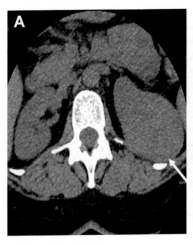
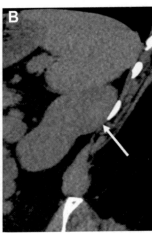

Fig. 13. Axial (*A*) and sagittal (*B*) images in soft tissue algorithm from nonenhanced lumbar spine CT performed in a 32-year-old woman with back pain after a fall shows a large left upper pole renal mass (*arrows*). The patient underwent a partial nephrectomy, and pathology showed an angiomyolipoma.

Lumbar Spine

Although there is limited literature dedicated to incidental extraspinal findings on thoracic spine CT and MR imaging, to our knowledge, there is more robust literature regarding lumbar spine imaging. A prospective review of incidental findings in 400 CT scans of the lumbar spine classified the incidental findings by potential clinical relevance, using a model that had previously been developed for classifying findings on CT colonography (CT Colonography Reporting and Data System [C-rads]).[14] Incidental extraspinal findings were present on 40.5% (162) of the examinations. In addition to studying the dedicated lumbar spine images, the investigators also studied the reconstructed full field of view images of the entire abdomen, which allowed full assessment for extraspinal findings. Despite this exhaustive search pattern, in the entire cohort of 400 patients, only 4.3% (17 patients) had incidental findings that were considered clinically relevant and that therefore warranted further work-up and communication with a clinician (category E4 findings). The most frequent such finding was that of an abdominal aortic aneurysm larger than 3 cm. The most clinically important finding in the study was a solid

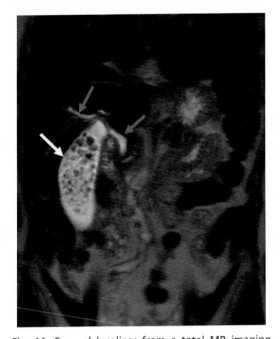

Fig. 14. Coronal localizer from a total MR imaging spine examination performed in a 59-year-old woman to evaluate a suspected cerebrospinal fluid leak shows marked distention of the gallbladder with innumerable gallstones (*white arrow*). There was dilatation of the common bile duct (*red arrow*), as well as of of the central intrahepatic biliary system (*blue arrow*). Patient was subsequently managed for the biliary findings.

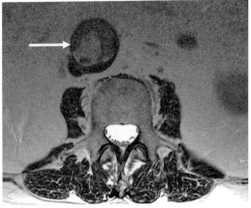

Fig. 15. T2-weighted axial image from a lumbar spine MR scan in a 73-year-old man shows a 4.1 × 3.6-cm partially thrombosed infrarenal abdominal aortic aneurysm (*arrow*).

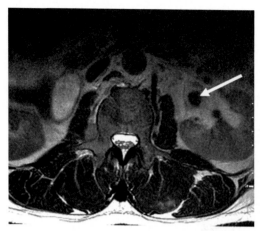

Fig. 16. T2-weighted axial image from a lumbar spine MR scan performed in a 65-year-old man with lower extremity weakness in the setting of metastatic neuroendocrine cancer shows a large round hypointense left ureteropelvic junction calculus (*arrow*).

renal mass that turned out to be a renal cell cancer. In the study, 14.8% of patients were deemed to have category E3 incidental extraspinal findings, a category including findings that were indeterminate but of probable benignity, and for which further work-up could be pursued if indicated. The most frequent finding in this category was an indeterminate renal mass (**Fig. 13**). Some other findings included in this category were a dilated common bile duct, mesenteric stranding and lymph nodes, and aortic ectasia (**Fig. 14**).[14]

A retrospective study that included 850 lumbar spine MR imaging scans showed an incidental extraspinal finding in 14.2% of the examinations.[10] The most common extraspinal finding in this retrospective series was a renal cyst. The second most frequent finding was uterine myoma. Rarer but more clinically concerning findings, including hepatic masses, hydronephrosis, a recurrent renal cell carcinoma, and abdominal aortic aneurysms, were also detected (**Fig. 15**). Another review of 592 lumbar spine MR imaging scans reported a 35.5% rate of incidental findings.[1] In general, the kidney was the organ most affected by incidental findings, with renal cysts being the most commonly encountered finding, and other less common abnormalities included renal stones, hydronephrosis, or a renal mass (**Fig. 16**). A few hepatic masses, para-aortic lymphadenopathy, and an ovarian mass comprised the other incidental findings (**Fig. 17**).

In a large retrospective review of 3000 lumbar spine MR imaging scans, incidental extraspinal findings were detected in 68.3% of the examinations.[15] However, only 17.6% of patients were considered to have clinically indeterminate or clinically significant findings. The most prevalent clinically indeterminate finding was the presence of abdominopelvic fluid, with an incidence rate of 9.9%. Enlarged lymphadenopathy, with an incidence rate of 1.8%, was the most prevalent clinically relevant finding. Another retrospective analysis reviewed 1278 lumbar spine MR imaging

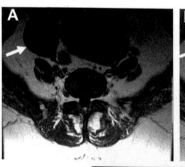
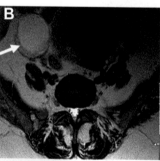
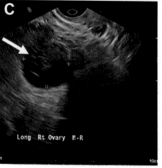

Fig. 17. T1-weighted (*A*) and T2-weighted (*B*) axial images from an MR imaging examination of the lumbar spine performed in a 46-year-old woman for evaluation of radiculopathy shows a T1-hypointense and T2-hyperintense right adnexal cyst (*arrows*). Subsequent transvaginal ultrasonography (*C*) shows this to be an ovarian cyst with internal echoes (*arrow*), suggesting that it likely represents a hemorrhagic ovarian cyst.

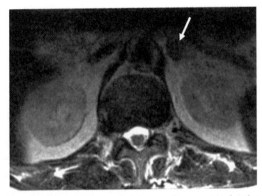

Fig. 18. T2-weighted axial image from a total spine MR examination performed to evaluate possible spinal cord compression shows a left adrenal mass (*arrow*). The 70-year-old man had a known history of lung cancer, and the adrenal mass was suspected to represent a site of metastasis.

Box 3
Extraspinal checklist for the lumbar spine

- Abdominopelvic visceral organs
  - Hepatobiliary system, pancreas, spleen, adrenals, kidneys, colon, bladder
  - Uterus/adnexal regions in women
  - Prostate in men
- Vasculature
  - Abdominal aortic aneurysms
- Adenopathy
  - Mesenteric and/or retroperitoneal
- Fluid collections
  - Free fluid
- Hematomas or abscesses in peritoneal and retroperitoneal cavities

---

scans, and found incidental extraspinal findings in 18.8%.[16] The kidney was the most frequently affected organ, with renal cysts being the most prevalent finding. Interestingly, there were 11 cases in which an adrenal mass was detected, an incidence rate of 0.86% (**Fig. 18**). Of these, only 4 had been documented in the original radiology report. Other clinically important findings reported in this study included hydronephrosis, aortic aneurysms, renal masses, and lymphadenopathy. A third large retrospective study analyzed 3024 lumbar spine MR imaging scans, for which there was a 22% rate of incidental findings.[17] Although 73% of these findings were deemed clinically insignificant, 22% were considered likely unimportant but incompletely characterized, and 5% were considered of potential importance. Again, as in the previously mentioned studies, the kidney was the organ that harbored the most incidental findings, because 70% of the incidental findings that were reported in this study were located within the kidney. Included among the incompletely characterized findings were hydronephrosis, complex renal cysts, and hepatic and ovarian cysts. The most frequent potentially important finding was abdominal aortic aneurysms, with renal/hepatic/adrenal masses, lymphadenopathy, and retroperitoneal abscess/mass among some of the other findings in this category. Of the potentially important findings, 38.6% had not been included in the official report by the reading radiologist at the time of initial MR examination.

These large retrospective lumbar spine MR imaging reviews show variable rates of incidentaloma detection ranging from 14.2% to 68.3%. This variability reflects the operational definition of incidental extraspinal findings in each of these studies. Nonetheless, as is evident on review of the literature, incidental extraspinal findings are common on cross-sectional imaging of the lumbar spine. Although most of the incidental findings are of little to no clinical significance, such as simple renal cysts, there are the occasional clinically impactful findings that radiologists must strive to detect and report. Because lumbar spine imaging includes the retroperitoneum and portions of the abdomen and pelvis, interpreting radiologists should make sure to examine all the visceral organs in these regions (**Box 3**), including the imaged portions of the liver, biliary tract, pancreas, spleen, adrenals, kidneys, colon, bladder, and uterus/adnexal regions in women, and the prostate in men. In addition, because abdominal aortic aneurysms are among the most common clinically relevant incidental findings, the vasculature should be included in the search pattern. The radiologist should also search for both mesenteric and retroperitoneal adenopathy. In addition, any abnormal fluid collections (free fluid or organized collections) should be commented on.

SUMMARY

Before learning how to properly proceed on the discovery of incidental extraspinal findings, the radiologist must first detect these findings. This article introduces the types of incidental findings that have been reported in the literature, and proposes an extraspinal search pattern for each section of the spine. Regardless of the segment of the spine, the scout/localizer should always be assessed for any abnormalities that may not be included in the field of view of the rest of the examination. Familiarity with the common incidentalomas that are encountered within each segment of the spinal axis increases the awareness of these extraspinal findings by the interpreting radiologist. The increased awareness of these extraspinal diagnostic possibilities in turn increases the likelihood of their consideration by the interpreting radiologist at the time of image review. It is imperative that radiologists familiarize themselves with the extraspinal compartments and structures that must be examined, and ensure these are incorporated into their search patterns. With these 2 concepts in mind, radiologists may be assisted with a checklist that they can incorporate into their standardized report templates as a reminder to always look for any extraspinal findings. This practice should help to mitigate some of the cognitive biases that adversely affect the detection of these extraspinal findings.[2] Once radiologists get into the effective habit of reviewing the extraspinal region adequately for incidental findings, they will then have to characterize any discovered abnormalities, determine what they represent, and decide how best to report and manage the incidental findings.[18] In contrast, recognizing and characterizing clinically irrelevant extraspinal findings is important in the context of avoiding further unnecessary imaging or potentially risky interventions.[18] Although many incidentalomas are of no clinical consequence, recommendations for the further evaluation and management of indeterminate or clinically significant findings are available.[19-22] Nevertheless, identifying and documenting these incidental extraspinal findings is an important step in contributing to the subsequent care and management of the patients.

CLINICS CARE POINTS

- While scout and localizer images are obtained for examination planning, they possess information not included in the rest of the examination and must, therefore, be independently reviewed for pathology.

- Though many incidental extraspinal findings are of little clinical significance, there are enough with clinical import that warrant the radiologist consciously seeking them out.

- To minimize susceptibility to cognitive biases, the radiologist should make use of a dedicated extraspinal search pattern when reviewing cross-sectional imaging of the spine.

DISCLOSURE

The authors have nothing to disclose.

REFERENCES

1. Kızılgöz V, Aydın H, Sivrioğlu AK, et al. Incidences and reporting rates of incidental findings on lumbar, thoracic, and cervical spinal magnetic resonance images and extra-neuronal findings on brain magnetic resonance images. Eur Res J 2019;5(3):449–60.
2. Lee CS, Nagy PG, Weaver SJ, et al. Cognitive and system factors contributing to errors in radiology. AJR Am J Roentgenol 2013;201:611–7.
3. Sener RN, Ripeckyj GT, Otto PM, et al. Recognition of abnormalities on computed scout images in CT examinations of the head and spine. Neuroradiology 1993;35(3):229–31.
4. ACR–ASNR–ASSR–SPR Practice parameter for the performance of computed tomography (CT) of the spine. 2016. Available at: https://www.acr.org/-/media/ACR/Files/Practice-Parameters/CT-Spine.pdf. Accessed October 14, 2010.
5. ACR–ASNR–SCBT-MR–SSR Practice parameter for the performance of magnetic resonance imaging (MRI) of the adult spine. 2018. Available at: https://www.acr.org/-/media/ACR/Files/Practice-Parameters/MR-Adult-Spine.pdf. Accessed October 14, 2010.
6. Barboza R, Fox JH, Shaffer LE, et al. Incidental findings in the cervical spine at CT for trauma evaluation. AJR Am J Roentgenol 2009;192(3):725–9.
7. Ergun T, Lakadamyali H. The prevalence and clinical importance of incidental soft-tissue findings in cervical CT scans of trauma population. Dentomaxillofac Radiol 2013;42(10):20130216.
8. Applewhite BP, Buch K, Yoon BC, et al. Lung apical findings in coronavirus disease (COVID-19) infection on neck and cervical spine CT. Emerg Radiol 2020. https://doi.org/10.1007/s10140-020-01822-0.
9. Barajas RF Jr, Rufener G, Starkey J, et al. Asymptomatic COVID-19: what the neuroradiologist needs to know about pulmonary manifestations. AJNR Am J Neuroradiol 2020;41(6):966–8.
10. Dilli A, Ayaz UY, Turanlı S, et al. Incidental extraspinal findings on magnetic resonance imaging of intervertebral discs. Arch Med Sci 2014;10(4):757–63.
11. Beheshtian E, Sahraian S, Yousem DM, et al. Incidental findings on cervical spine computed tomography scans: overlooked and unimportant? Neuroradiology 2018;60(11):1175–80.
12. Zidan MMA, Hassan IA, Elnour AM, et al. Incidental extraspinal findings in the thoracic spine during magnetic resonance imaging of intervertebral discs. J Clin Imaging Sci 2019;9:37.
13. Kamath S, Jain N, Goyal N, et al. Incidental findings on MRI of the spine. Clin Radiol 2009;64(4):353–61.

14. Lee SY, Landis MS, Ross IG, et al. Extraspinal findings at lumbar spine CT examinations: prevalence and clinical importance. Radiology 2012;263(2):502–9.

15. Quattrocchi CC, Giona A, Di Martino AC, et al. Extraspinal incidental findings at lumbar spine MRI in the general population: a large cohort study. Insights Imaging 2013;4(3):301–8.

16. Tuncel SA, Çaglı B, Tekataş A, et al. Extraspinal incidental findings on routine MRI of lumbar spine: prevalence and reporting rates in 1278 Patients. Korean J Radiol 2015;16(4):866–73.

17. Semaan HB, Bieszczad JE, Obri T, et al. Incidental extraspinal findings at lumbar spine magnetic resonance imaging: a retrospective study. Spine 2015; 40(18):1436–43.

18. Raghavan P, Record J, Vidal L. Beyond the spinal canal. Radiol Clin North Am 2019;57(2):453–67.

19. Hoang JK, Langer JE, Middleton WD, et al. Managing incidental thyroid nodules detected on imaging: white paper of the ACR Incidental Thyroid Findings Committee. J Am Coll Radiol 2015;12(2):143–50.

20. Mayo-Smith WW, Song JH, Boland GL, et al. Management of incidental adrenal masses: a white paper of the ACR Incidental Findings Committee. J Am Coll Radiol 2017;14(8):1038–44.

21. Herts BR, Silverman SG, Hindman NM, et al. Management of the incidental renal mass on CT: a white paper of the ACR Incidental Findings Committee. J Am Coll Radiol 2018;15(2):264–73.

22. Gore RM, Pickhardt PJ, Mortele KJ, et al. Management of incidental liver lesions on CT: a white paper of the ACR Incidental Findings Committee. J Am Coll Radiol 2017;14(11):1429–37.

Incidental Thyroid Nodules on Imaging
Relevance and Management

Kedar G. Sharbidre, MD[a],*, Mark E. Lockhart, MD, MPH[b], Franklin N. Tessler, MD, CM[c]

KEYWORDS

- Incidental • Thyroid • Ultrasound • CT • Computed tomography • MR imaging • Diagnosis
- Biopsy

KEY POINTS

- Incidental thyroid nodules are extremely common findings on extrathyroidal imaging examinations of the chest and neck.
- Most of the incidental thyroid nodules are benign and do not require further workup.
- Incidental nodules with increased metabolic activity on PET/computed tomography have a higher risk of malignancy and should be further evaluated by sonography and biopsy.
- Guidelines published by the American College of Radiology are helpful to guide management of incidental thyroid nodules.

INTRODUCTION

Thyroid nodules, defined by the American Thyroid Association (ATA) as discrete focal abnormalities within the thyroid, which are radiologically distinct from the surrounding thyroid parenchyma, are found in up to 68% of adults scanned with high-spatial resolution sonography.[1] Therefore, it is not surprising that they are frequently found on computed tomography (CT), MR imaging, PET, or ultrasound (US) (as well as PET-CT and PET-MR imaging) examinations performed for indications other than evaluation of a known or suspected thyroid nodule. Such findings are termed incidental thyroid nodules (ITNs) and are typically nonpalpable. Notably, some nodules demonstrated on a dedicated thyroid US may also be considered ITNs. For example, if a sonogram is performed to evaluate a palpable nodule in the right lobe, and a nodule is detected on the left side, the latter would be considered incidental. Similarly, thyroid nodules discovered on a carotid sonogram are ITNs.

The reported incidence of ITNs on imaging examinations varies considerably. Extrathyroidal US remains the most common modality that depicts ITNs, accounting for 20% to 67%, followed by CT and MR imaging (9%–25%) and PET/CT (1%–4.3%).[2–7] ITNs are more common in women, and their incidence increases with age.

IMAGING OF INCIDENTAL THYROID NODULES
Extrathyroidal Ultrasound

US examinations performed for indications other than thyroid nodule assessment account for most of the reported ITNs.[8] These include sonograms of the carotid arteries, parathyroids, cervical lymph nodes, internal jugular veins, and other structures in the neck. High-frequency transducers are used in all of these examinations. A dedicated thyroid US usually should be

[a] Department of Radiology, University of Alabama at Birmingham, 619 19th Street South, JT N357, Birmingham, AL 35249, USA; [b] Department of Radiology, University of Alabama at Birmingham, 619 19th Street South, JT N344, Birmingham, AL 35249, USA; [c] Department of Radiology, University of Alabama at Birmingham, 619 19th Street South, GSB 409, Birmingham, AL 35249, USA
* Corresponding author.
E-mail address: ksharbidre@uabmc.edu

Radiol Clin N Am 59 (2021) 525–533
https://doi.org/10.1016/j.rcl.2021.03.004

recommended for complete evaluation, except in situations where no further investigation is warranted because of the ITN's morphology and/or size based on a risk-stratification system or clinical circumstances.

Computed Tomography and MR Imaging

Any imaging examination that includes the lower neck may depict thyroid nodules. Most commonly, they are seen on CT of the chest, neck, or cervical spine; MR imaging of the neck soft tissues or cervical spine; or CT or MR angiography of the neck. The thyroid is also occasionally seen on the axial T2-weighted images of a breast MR imaging. Drake and colleagues[4] reported ITNs in 3.45% of MR imagings, 5.84% of chest CT scans performed with intravenous contrast, and 5.14% of noncontrast chest CT scans, in a population of 98,054 imaging examinations. The rate of malignancy in ITNs detected on CT and MR imaging scans varies from 0% to 11%.[9–11]

Normal thyroid tissue demonstrates intrinsic high attenuation on CT and enhances homogenously following intravenous iodinated contrast administration.[2] Typically, a solid or cystic nodule on CT will seem hypoattenuating compared with the adjacent thyroid tissue. However, neither CT nor MR imaging can be used to accurately characterize thyroid nodules, because they cannot depict the fine architectural features that enable identification of thyroid cancer. Both imaging modalities underestimate thyroid nodule size and number and are not as reliable as US for their characterization.[12]

On CT, an ITN may seem cystic or solid, with or without calcifications. Microcalcifications are strongly associated with papillary thyroid carcinomas (PTCs) but are usually not identified on CT (**Fig. 1**). Che-wei and colleagues found that multiple punctate calcifications were associated with a higher risk of malignancy compared with solitary small calcifications, whereas coarse and peripheral calcifications carried a lesser likelihood of cancer.[13] Another study found that 12% of ITNs were calcified on CT but were not correlated with malignancy.[12] As a result, some experts recommend that calcified nodules on CT should not be managed differently than noncalcified nodules.[14]

Thyroid cysts may be simple or complex, with septations and/or solid components. Simple cysts are less attenuating than cysts that contain hemorrhage or colloid and that may be isodense to muscle.[15] However, CT density measurements do not reliably distinguish cysts from solid nodules due to volume averaging and small size. Importantly, papillary carcinomas may seem cystic on CT. Assessment may also be hampered by beam hardening artifacts, particularly on chest CT, and nodules may not be well seen on nonenhanced CT. Larger thyroid malignancies that exhibit gross extrathyroidal extension or are accompanied by adenopathy should be readily visible, but these are often identified clinically before imaging. Abnormal lymph nodes with cystic components, calcifications, and/or increased enhancement are suspicious for malignancy.

On MR imaging, the normal thyroid is T1 hyperintense and T2 isointense to hypointense on

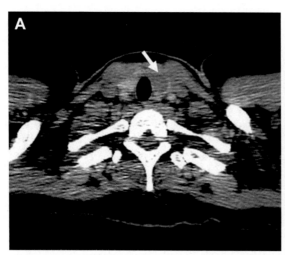
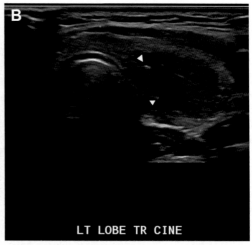

LT LOBE TR CINE

Fig. 1. A 28-year-old woman with an incidental nodule in left thyroid lobe on chest CT. (*A*) The CT shows a well-marginated hypodense nodule measuring 2.1 cm (*white arrow*). (*B*) Dedicated US was recommended, which showed a solid, hypoechoic 1.8 cm nodule with microcalcifications (*white arrowheads*), categorized as ACR TI-RADS-5. Fine-needle aspiration (FNA) biopsy of this nodule showed papillary thyroid cancer.

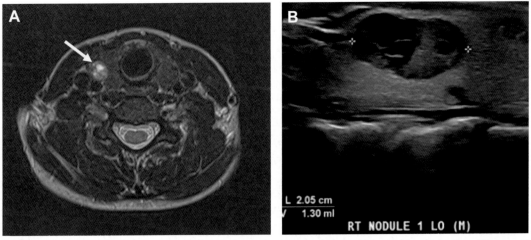

Fig. 2. A 37-year-old woman presented with neck pain and underwent MR imaging cervical spine. (A) On a T2-weighted axial MR image of the cervical spine, there is an incidental 1.8 cm hyperintense nodule (arrow) in the right thyroid lobe. (B) Dedicated ultrasound was recommended, which showed a solid-cystic right thyroid nodule (calipers), which was classified as ACR TI-RADS 3, which is considered as intermediate risk, and follow-up was recommended.

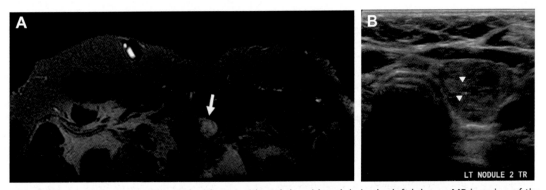

Fig. 3. A 65-year-old woman presented with an incidental thyroid nodule in the left lobe on MR imaging of the breasts. (A) T2-weighted axial images of the breasts that included lower neck show a focal hyperintense nodule (arrow). (B) Ultrasound demonstrated a hypoechoic solid nodule with punctate echogenic foci (white arrowheads) and was classified as ACR TI-RADS 5. FNA biopsy was recommended, which showed follicular neoplasm. Left hemithyroidectomy was subsequently performed, which showed nodular thyroid hyperplasia.

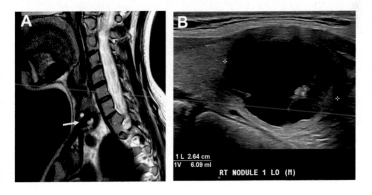

Fig. 4. A 36-year-old woman with an incidental solid-cystic right thyroid nodule on the cervical spine MR imaging performed for neck pain. (A) Sagittal T2-weighted MR image shows a 2.4 cm mixed high and low signal intensity right thyroid nodule (arrow). (B) Dedicated ultrasound was recommended, which showed a predominantly cystic nodule (calipers), classified as ACR TI-RADS 2 (considered benign), without any follow-up or biopsy recommended.

noncontrast images and enhances homogeneously after gadolinium administration. Both malignant and benign thyroid nodules may be isointense on T1-weighted sequences and hyperintense on T2-weighted sequences[16] (**Figs. 2–4**). Some studies have demonstrated that papillary carcinomas may have significantly lower T2 signal intensity than benign thyroid nodules.[17] Diffusion-weighted images, which are often obtained on MR imaging examinations performed for evaluation of the neck soft tissues or cervical spine, may help characterize some ITNs. A significant difference in the apparent diffusion coefficient (ADC) value was found between benign and malignant thyroid nodules, with ADC values in malignant nodules being lower than in benign nodules. Thus, T2 hypointensity and reduced ADC signal in an ITN may indicate malignancy. However, the ADC value in a benign thyroid nodule may be reduced by its contents, including colloid, necrosis and cystic change, hemorrhage, fibrosis, and calcium.[18]

Molecular Imaging Techniques

ITNs may be seen on some molecular imaging examinations, most commonly PET with fluorodeoxyglucose F 18 (^{18}F-FDG PET)/CT. The thyroid usually demonstrates mild homogeneous ^{18}F-FDG avidity. Diffusely increased uptake on ^{18}F-FDG PET-CT may be seen with inflammatory processes, that is, thyroiditis. However, focal increased uptake is a cause for concern (**Fig. 5**). Although the incidence of PET-detected ITNs is low, ranging from 1.2% to 4.3%,[2,5,6] the risk of malignancy can be as high as 30%.[5–7] In a recent study, Guevara and colleagues evaluated 5100 whole-body ^{18}F-FDG-PET/CT examinations and found nodular thyroid uptake in 2.3%, approximately 48% of them were biopsied, of which 50% were malignant on fine-needle aspiration (FNA) or surgery. This study showed that benign nodules showed significantly lower ^{18}F-FDG uptake, with a maximum standardized uptake value of 5.0 as the best threshold value to distinguish between benign and malignant nodules.[19]

Mallick and colleagues reviewed 2413 SPECT-CT examinations and evaluated them for incidental nonparathyroid abnormalities. They found that 27% patients had nonparathyroid findings; the most common were thyroid nodules (49%). Of these nodules, 6.9% were found to be malignant, and papillary microcarcinomas were the most common diagnosis.[20] Papillary thyroid microcarcinoma (PTMC) is a papillary cancer that is 1.0 cm or less in diameter.

ITNs are uncommonly seen on nuclear medicine examinations such as technetium-99m methoxyisobutylisonitrile (MIBI) and indium-111 octreotide scans. Both adenomas and thyroid cancers can show uptake on MIBI and octreotide scans. Two small series of selected patients with incidental MIBI-avid thyroid nodules showed that the rate of malignancy varied from 22% to 66%.[21,22] More recently, whole-body gallium-68 prostate-specific membrane antigen (PSMA)-based PET/CT or MR imaging has been used for whole-body primary staging of

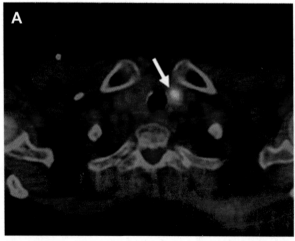
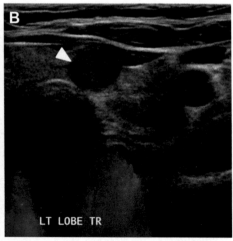

Fig. 5. A 68-year-old woman with an incidental left thyroid nodule on staging PET-CT for lung cancer. (*A*) The fused PET image shows hypermetabolic activity of the left thyroid nodule (*arrow*) in the axial plane. (*B*) The nodule was evaluated with dedicated ultrasound, which showed 1.0 cm round hypoechoic solid nodule (*arrowhead*) in the left thyroid lobe, categorized as ACR TI-RADS 4. Biopsy and thyroidectomy performed subsequently revealed papillary thyroid cancer.

intermediate- or high-risk prostate cancer, and some of these examinations can show thyroid uptake. In a systematic review, Bertagna and colleagues[23] found that 26% of PSMA-detected ITNs were malignant, and these were mostly PTCs.

CLINICAL EVALUATION AND PROBLEMS WITH WORKUP OF INCIDENTAL THYROID NODULES

Before proceeding to further investigations, the referring clinicians should ask the patient about any relevant historical factors associated with thyroid malignancy. These include a prior history of radiation, a personal history of breast cancer, a family history of thyroid cancer, or inherited syndromes associated with thyroid cancer, such as multiple endocrine neoplasia (MEN) type 2, familial non–MEN-associated medullary carcinoma, familial papillary carcinoma, familial polyposis coli, Cowden disease, or Gardner syndrome.

The prevalence of thyroid malignancy increases with age and peaks at a slightly earlier age in women than men. Only a small proportion of ITNs are found in young patients, in part because they undergo fewer imaging examinations than older individuals. However, the ratio of malignant to benign ITNs is likely to be higher in young patients, particularly those younger than 35 years.[2,12] A screening thyroid stimulating hormone (TSH) level should be measured in all patients with ITNs, and a serum calcitonin level should be obtained if there is family history of medullary thyroid cancer or multiple endocrine neoplasia type II. Routine measurement of serum thyroglobulin and serum calcitonin is recommended in patients with ITNs.

Once an ITN is detected, the most important question for the clinician is to whether to do further workup or follow-up. The actual risk of malignancy in ITNs varies from 1.6% to 12%. The highest rate was seen in a study of patients undergoing biopsy.[24,25] This rate of malignancy also depends on the clinical characteristics of the population studied and the percentage of detected ITNs that undergo further workup. Based on available evidence, most small thyroid cancers will have an indolent course without any treatment, and these patients will typically die from causes other than thyroid cancer.[26] The 5-year survival for individuals with most common type, papillary thyroid cancer, was approximately 98.3% (2010–2016).[27]

The last few decades have seen a significant increase in the incidence of thyroid cancer, and this has been attributed to various factors, most important of which is increasing use of highly sensitive imaging modalities along with increasing rates of FNA and thyroid surgery. However, multiple studies have demonstrated that the increased incidence of TC detection has not been associated with a commensurate risk in mortality. This may be due to increasing detection of slow-growing small thyroid cancers and the low potential for recurrence or mortality associated with PTC and PTMC.[28] About 50% to 60% of adults are found to have incidental nodules on autopsy, indicating the benign nature of most such tumors.[29] A 5-year study reported by Ito and colleagues[30] indicated that 70% of nonoperated PTMCs remained stable and/or decreased in size. Thus, overdiagnosis and overtreatment (ie, detection and treatment of disease that would never become clinically relevant or associated with significant mortality or morbidity) is a substantial problem.

Thyroid nodules characterized as suspicious by US are ultimately referred for FNA to obtain tissue for cytologic analysis. Nodules are usually classified by the Bethesda System for Reporting Thyroid Cytopathology, which includes 6 categories: (I) nondiagnostic, (II) benign, (III) atypia of undetermined significance/follicular lesion of undetermined significance, (IV) follicular neoplasm/suspicious for follicular neoplasm, (V) suspicious for malignancy, and (VI) malignant.[31] In the past, Bethesda III and IV nodules, collectively termed indeterminate, were often subjected to a second biopsy. If the repeat biopsy results were still indeterminate, many surgeons preferred resection (diagnostic thyroid lobectomy). However, the introduction of molecular (genomic) testing has offered an additional management option for indeterminate nodules. For example, the 2015 ATA guidelines recommend consideration of molecular testing in lieu of surgery for Bethesda IV nodules after taking into account sonographic and clinical features (see **Fig. 3**). The number of thyroid FNAs performed in the United States doubled between 2006 and 2011, accompanied by a significant increase in thyroidectomy rates.[32] A recent study found high sensitivity (94%) but low specificity rate (54%) for FNA, indicating that some of the patients who undergo surgery will not have cancer on final pathology.[33] However, no studies have evaluated the adverse effects related to treatment of incidental nodules compared with symptomatic nodules, to the authors' knowledge. Although thyroidectomy is generally considered safe, complications such as permanent hypoparathyroidism, hypocalcemia, and recurrent laryngeal nerve palsy are relatively common.[28]

Considering the increasing costs of imaging services and surgery, it is prudent to limit interventions to instances that are likely to meaningfully improve survival and/or quality of life. The annual cost of care for thyroid cancer in the United States is estimated to reach $3.5 billion in 2030, with expenses for imaging, surgery, and adjuvant therapy for newly diagnosed patients constituting the major expenditures.[34] In the United States, the overall costs associated with unnecessary medical care are estimated at around $210 billion annually.[35] Most such treatment is done because of practitioners' fear of being sued for malpractice, a concept that also applies to the thyroid nodule management based on recent surveys.[36,37] These costs will continue to increase due to an enlarging population and increasing thyroid cancer detection. Reducing the rate of overdiagnosis and overtreatment will be critical to limit costs and reduce physical and psychosocial harm to patients. Similar considerations apply in other countries.

GUIDELINES FOR INCIDENTAL THYROID NODULE MANAGEMENT

The first step in ITN management is to decide if a nodule needs further workup, which typically begins with a dedicated thyroid sonogram, followed by application of a sonographic risk stratification system to guide further management. Multiple guidelines published under the auspices of professional societies worldwide are available. They include the American College of Radiology Thyroid Imaging Reporting and Data System (ACRTI-RADS), the ATA guidelines, the European Union EU-TIRADS, and the Korean K-TIRADS. Only a few guidelines provide recommendations on management of ITNs, as summarized here:

A. American College of Radiology white paper[2] (Table 1) by Hoang and colleagues is largely based on the Duke 3-tiered system and provides specific recommendations for evaluation of ITNs on various modalities. Size is the most important imaging feature used for assessment of nodule risk. Thyroid nodule size, although not strongly correlated with risk of malignancy, is associated with prognosis.[38,39]

The ACR ITN white paper recommends no further evaluation be performed in patients for whom the clinician and patient feel that the associated comorbidities or limited life expectancy may increase the risk of morbidity and mortality more than the thyroid cancer treatment itself. At the authors' institution, they follow the ACR ITN recommendations for nodules detected on US, CT, or MR imaging. Occasionally, nonrecommended dedicated thyroid sonograms are still performed at the referring clinician's or patient's request, however.

The thyroid nodule risk stratification system by the ACR TI-RADS committee published in 2017[40]

Table 1
Imaging recommendations for incidental thyroid nodules based on American College of Radiology white paper (2015)[2]

Imaging Modality	Age (y)	Size	Recommendation
CT or MR Imaging	Any	Any	Dedicated US thyroid
• Extrathyroidal invasion, atypical enlarged neck lymph nodes with associated cystic change, calcification, or increased enhancement	<35	≥1 cm	Dedicated US thyroid
	≥35	≥1.5 cm	Dedicated US thyroid
	Any	Any	Dedicated US thyroid
• No above suspicious features: if multiple nodules, recommendation is based on the largest nodule			
• Enlarged heterogenous thyroid without any discrete nodule			
^{18}F-FDG PET avid ITNs:	Any	Any	Dedicated US thyroid and guided FNA
ITNs on MIBI and octreotide scans	Any	Any	Dedicated US thyroid
Extrathyroidal US:	Any	Any	Dedicated US thyroid
• Microcalcifications, marked hypoechogenicity, lobulated or irregular margins, or taller-than-wide shape on transverse view (if any present)	<35	≥1 cm	Dedicated US thyroid
	≥35	>1.5 cm	Dedicated US thyroid
• Without abovementioned features, such nodules should be managed similar to CT/MR detected nodules using size and age criteria			

is now widely used for characterization of ITNs on US. It classifies thyroid nodules into 5 risk levels according to their sonographic features. Management recommendations include no follow-up, US surveillance, and biopsy. This system has been evaluated in multiple comparative studies, which have demonstrated that ACR TI-RADS leads to a significant reduction in biopsy of benign nodules. Although ACR TI-RADS does not recommend sampling of subcentimeter nodules, these may be followed sonographically, lessening the likelihood of missing cancers. In one study, there were fewer recommendations for sonographic workup of findings considered to be insignificant (from 35% to 7%), with estimated cost savings of more than $300,000 for the hospital system.[41]

B. 2015 American Thyroid Association Management guidelines[42]: the ATA guidelines recommend that all ITNs larger than 1 cm in adults be evaluated with a dedicated thyroid sonogram.

Solid hypoechoic nodules 1 cm with or without one or more: irregular margins, microcalcifications, taller than wide shape, rim calcifications with soft tissue extrusion, or extrathyroidal extension.
Solid hypoechoic nodules greater than or equal to 1 cm in greatest dimension with intermediate to high suspicion sonographic pattern (irregular margins, microcalcifications, taller than wide shape, rim calcifications with soft tissue extrusion, or extrathyroidal extension).

C. The British Thyroid Association (BTA) guidelines[43] recommend initial clinical assessment of all ITNs. If no abnormalities are found on clinical evaluation, there is no need for any further assessment. However, suspicious nodules that demonstrate tracheal invasion, extracapsular invasion, or associated abnormal lymph nodes on imaging should undergo further investigation. An important limitation of these guidelines is that the recommended clinical examination is not sensitive for detection of smaller nodules and is subject to interobserver variability. The committee recommends nodules detected by PET-CT with focal FDG activity should be investigated with US and FNA, unless disseminated disease is identified, and the prognosis from an alternative malignancy would preclude further investigation.[43]

D. American Association of Clinical Endocrinologists[44] recommends US evaluation of all ITNs detected by CT or MR imaging before consideration of FNA biopsy, whereas those detected by PET-CT should undergo US evaluation and FNA because of the high risk of malignancy.

E. NCCN (National Comprehensive Cancer Network)[45] recommends all incidental thyroid nodules be evaluated by US thyroid and TSH

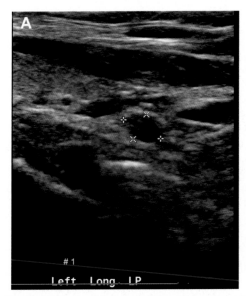 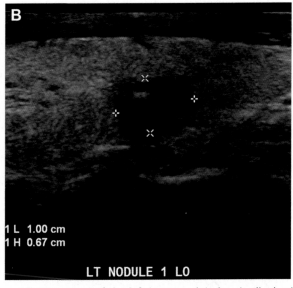

Fig. 6. A 45-year-old man with hyperparathyroidism. (*A*) Ultrasound of the left lower neck in longitudinal axis shows a hypoechoic nodule caudal to the lower pole of left thyroid lobe (calipers). (*B*) An incidental 1.0 cm solid markedly hypoechoic nodule (calipers) with macrocalcification was identified in the left thyroid lobe. This nodule was categorized as TIRADS-5, which was biopsied and subsequently resected in the same setting of parathyroidectomy, which revealed papillary thyroid microcarcinoma, follicular variant. The nodule caudal to the lower pole of left thyroid nodule was a parathyroid adenoma on pathology.

measurement. If TSH levels are normal or elevated, they recommend further assessment based on US characteristics.

F. ITNs on parathyroid US: another scenario involves management of ITNs found during parathyroid US in patients with hyperparathyroidism (**Fig. 6**). A recent study suggested that intermediate- to high-suspicion nodules greater than 1.5 cm may be resected at the same time as parathyroidectomy, potentially eliminating the risk of future reoperation with reduction in surgical complications, operating time and hospital stay, and cost of continued surveillance of such nodules.[46]

It is worth noting that patients are now frequently able to review their radiology reports, facilitating their participation in decision-making. Therefore, radiology reports should be standardized and ITNs should be appropriately addressed in the body and conclusion sections of the report, which should provide specific recommendations.

SUMMARY

The increasing prevalence of thyroid cancer imposes significant clinical and economic burdens on the health care system. Advanced imaging technology has led to an "epidemic" of ITNs, of which fewer than 10% are cancer. Many of these nodules are subjected to further investigations, invasive tests, and sometimes resection, all of which are associated with risks and economic implications. Radiologists should be cautious when recommending further investigations on ITNs. Recommendations should be based on guidelines such as those from the ACR and should be clearly stated. Further workup usually begins with sonography, with subsequent management based on a published risk stratification system in shared decision-making with the referring physician and the patient.

DISCLOSURE

Dr M.E. Lockhart: Deputy Editor, Journal of Ultrasound in Medicine; Chair, ACR Appropriateness Criteria Committee; Book Royalties, Elsevier.

REFERENCES

1. Guth S, Theune U, Aberle J, et al. Very high prevalence of thyroid nodules detected by high frequency (13 MHz) ultrasound examination. Eur J Clin Invest 2009;39(8):699–706.
2. Hoang JK, Langer JE, Middleton WD, et al. Managing incidental thyroid nodules detected on imaging:

white paper of the ACR Incidental Thyroid Findings Committee. J Am Coll Radiol 2015;12:143–50.
3. Starker LF, Prieto PA, Liles JS, et al. Endocrine incidentalomas. Curr Probl Surg 2016;53:219–46.
4. Drake T, Gravely A, Westanmo A, et al. Prevalence of Thyroid Incidentalomas from 1995 to 2016: A Single-Center, Retrospective Cohort Study. J Endocr Soc 2019;4(1):bvz027.
5. Hagenimana N, Dallaire J, Vallée É, et al. Thyroid incidentalomas on 18FDG-PET/CT: a metabolico-pathological correlation. Otolaryngol Head Neck Surg 2017;46(1):22.
6. Kamakshi K, Krishnamurthy A, Karthik V, et al. Positron emission tomography-computed tomography-associated incidental neoplasms of the thyroid gland. World J Nucl Med 2020;19(1):36–40.
7. Nayan S, Ramakrishna J, Gupta MK. The proportion of malignancy in incidental thyroid lesions on 18-FDG PET study: a systematic review and meta-analysis. Otolaryngol Head Neck Surg 2014;151(2):190–200.
8. Steele SR, Martin MJ, Mullenix PS, et al. The significance of incidental thyroid abnormalities identified during carotid duplex ultrasonography. Arch Surg 2005;140:981–5.
9. Nguyen XV, Choudhury KR, Eastwood JD, et al. Incidental thyroid nodules on CT: evaluation of 2 risk-categorization methods for work-up of nodules. AJNR Am J Neuroradiol 2013;34(9):1812–7.
10. Ahmed S, Horton KM, Jeffrey RB Jr, et al. Incidental thyroid nodules on chest CT: review of the literature and management suggestions. AJR Am J Roentgenol 2010;195(5):1066–71.
11. Youserm DM, Huang T, Loevner LA, et al. Clinical and economic impact of incidental thyroid lesions found with CT and MR. AJNR Am J Neuroradiol 1997;18(8):1423–8.
12. Shetty SK, Maher MM, Hahn PF, et al. Significance of incidental thyroid lesions detected on CT: correlation among CT, sonography, and pathology. AJR Am J Roentgenol 2006;187:1349–56.
13. Wu CW, Dionigi G, Lee KW, et al. Calcifications in thyroid nodules identified on preoperative computed tomography: patterns and clinical significance. Surgery 2012;151(3):464–70.
14. Hoang JK. Reply to "Three-tiered system for incidental thyroid nodules: do not forget the calcifications". AJR Am J Roentgenol 2014;203(4):W453.
15. Weber AL, Randolph G, Aksoy FG. The thyroid and parathyroid glands. CT and MR imaging and correlation with pathology and clinical findings. Radiol Clin North Am 2000;38(5):1105–29.
16. Hobbs HA, Bahl M, Nelson RC, et al. Journal Club: incidental thyroid nodules detected at imaging: can diagnostic workup be reduced by use of the Society of Radiologists in US recommendations and the three-tiered system? AJR Am J Roentgenol 2014;202:18–24.

17. Noda Y, Kanematsu M, Goshima S, et al. Thyroid for differential diagnosis of benign thyroid nodules and papillary carcinomas. Am J Roentgenol 2015;3: W332–5.

18. Wu Y, Yue X, Shen W, et al. Diagnostic value of diffusion-weighted MR imaging in thyroid disease: application in differentiating benign from malignant disease. BMC Med Imaging 2013;13:23.

19. Ladrón de Guevara H, David MM, Claudia GS, et al. Frequency of malignancy in thyroid incidentalomas detected by whole body 18F-FDG PET/CT. Rev Med Chil 2020;148(1):10–6.

20. Mallick R, Malik J, Yip L, et al. McCoy, Novel Findings on SPECT-CT Tc-99 sestamibi imaging for primary hyperparathyroidism. J Surg Res 2020;252:216–21.

21. Kresnik E, Gallowitsch HJ, Mikosch P, et al. Technetium-99m-MIBI scintigraphy of thyroid nodules in an endemic goiter area. J Nucl Med 1997;38:62–5.

22. Kostoglou-Athanassiou I, Pappas A, Gogou L, et al. Scintigraphy with [111In]octreotide and 201Tl in a Hurthle cell thyroid carcinoma without detectable radio-iodine uptake. Report of a case and review of the literature. Horm Res 2003;60:205–8.

23. Bertagna F, Albano D, Giovanella L, et al. 68Ga-PSMA PET thyroid incidentalomas. Hormones (Athens) 2019;18(2):145–9.

24. Smith-Bindman R, Lebda P, Feldstein VA, et al. Risk of thyroid cancer based on thyroid US imaging characteristics: results of a population-based study. JAMA Intern Med 2013;173:1788–96.

25. Nam-Goong IS, Kim HY, Gong G, et al. Ultrasonography-guided fine-needle aspiration of thyroid incidentaloma: correlation with pathological findings. Clin Endocrinol 2004;60:21–8.

26. Hoang JK, Nguyen XV. Understanding the risks and harms of management of incidental thyroid nodules: a review. JAMA Otolaryngol Head Neck Surg 2017; 143(7):718–24.

27. SEER cancer Stat Facts: thyroid cancer. National Cancer Institute. Bethesda, MD, Available at: https://seer.cancer.gov/statfacts/html/thyro.html. Accessed August 29, 2020.

28. Lin JS, Bowles EJA, Williams SB, et al. Screening for thyroid cancer: updated evidence report and systematic review for the US preventive services task force. JAMA 2017;317(18):1888–903.

29. Mortensen JD, Woolner LB, Bennett WA. Gross and microscopic findings in clinically normal thyroid glands. J Clin Endocrinol Metab 1955;15:1270–80.

30. Ito Y, Uruno T, Nakano K, et al. An observation trial without surgical treatment in patients with papillary microcarcinoma of the thyroid. Thyroid 2003;13:381–7.

31. Cibas ES, Ali SZ. The 2017 Bethesda system for reporting thyroid cytopathology. Thyroid 2017;27: 1341-1346.

32. Sosa JA, Hanna JW, Robinson KA, et al. Increases in thyroid nodule fine-needle aspirations, operations, and diagnoses of thyroid cancer in the United States. Surgery 2013;154:1420–6.

33. Ronen O, Cohen H, Sela E, et al. Differences in cytopathologist thyroid nodule malignancy rate. Cytopathology 2020;31:315–20.

34. Lubitz CC, Kong CY, McMahon PM, et al. Annual financial impact of well-differentiated thyroid cancer care in the United States. Cancer 2014;120:1345–52.

35. Carroll AE. The high costs of unnecessary care. JAMA 2017;318:1748–9.

36. Kakudo K, Bychkov A, Abelardo A, et al. Malpractice climate is a key difference in thyroid pathology practice between North America and the rest of the world. Arch Pathol Lab Med 2019;143:1171.

37. Labarge B, Walter V, Lengerich EJ, et al. Evidence of a positive association between malpractice climate and thyroid cancer incidence in the United States. PLoS One 2018;13:e0199862.

38. Frates MC, Benson CB, Charboneau JW, et al. Management of thyroid nodules detected at US: Society of Radiologists in US consensus conference statement. Radiology 2005;237:794–800.

39. Cooper DS, Doherty GM, Haugen BR, et al. Revised American Thyroid Association management guidelines for patients with thyroid nodules and differentiated thyroid cancer. Thyroid 2009;19:1167–214.

40. Tessler FN, Middleton WD, Grant EG, et al. ACR thyroid imaging, reporting and data system (TI-RADS): white paper of the ACR TI-RADS committee. J Am Coll Radiol 2017;14:587–95.

41. Martino A. Imaging 3.0 case study: reducing variability. Available at: https://www.acr.org/Practice-Management-Quality-Informatics/Imaging-3/Case-Studies/Quality-and-Safety/Reducing-Variability. Accessed Sept 8, 2020.

42. Haugen BR, Alexander EK, Bible KC, et al. 2015 American Thyroid Association Management Guidelines for Adult Patients with Thyroid Nodules and Differentiated Thyroid Cancer: The American Thyroid Association Guidelines Task Force on Thyroid Nodules and Differentiated Thyroid Cancer. Thyroid 2016;26(1):1–133.

43. Perros P, Colley S, Boelaert K, et al. Guidelines for the management of thyroid cancer. Clin Endocrinol (Oxf) 2014;81:1–122.

44. Patel K, Yip L, Lubitz C, et al. The American Association of endocrine surgeons guidelines for the definitive surgical management of thyroid disease in adults. Ann Surg March 2020;271(3):e21–93.

45. Haddad RI, Bischoff L, Bernet V, et al. NCCN clinical practice guidelines in oncology (NCCN guidelines): thyroid carcinoma. Version 2. 2020.

46. Kyriacou A, Vogiazanos E. A Critical Reflection of British Thyroid Association (BTA) guidelines for the management of thyroid nodules and cancer. J Thyroid Disord Ther 2016;5. https://doi.org/10.4172/2167-7948.

Incidental Lung Nodules on Cross-sectional Imaging
Current Reporting and Management

Lea Azour, MD*, Jane P. Ko, MD, Sophie L. Washer, MD, Amelia Lanier, MD, Geraldine Brusca-Augello, DO, Jeffrey B. Alpert, MD, William H. Moore, MD

KEYWORDS

- Pulmonary nodule • Solid • Subsolid • Lung cancer • Fleischner

KEY POINTS

- Pulmonary nodules are the most common incidental finding in the chest, particularly on computed tomography (CT) examinations that include some or all of the chest.
- Several nodule features may suggest benignity and obviate dedicated chest CT follow-up imaging, whereas others require follow-up.
- Accurate reporting of pulmonary nodules is necessary for characterization in terms of size, attenuation, and morphology.
- Solid and subsolid pulmonary nodules confer differing risks for malignancy. Societal guidelines exist for managing incidental nodules and distinguish the 2 nodule types when recommending management strategy.

INTRODUCTION

Computed tomography (CT) increasingly is utilized, with abdominal and chest CT accounting for approximately two-thirds of all CT examinations.[1] Similarly, the detection rate of pulmonary nodules, defined as a solid, semisolid, or ground-glass focus measuring less than 3 cm, has increased, from 3.9 to 6.6 per 1000 person-years between 2006 and 2012.[2] Many CT-detected pulmonary nodules may be incidental or found on examinations performed for other indications, which can include part (eg, neck CT or abdominal CT) or all of the chest (either alone or including other parts of the body, such as in the setting of trauma).

In a review of 1708 CT pulmonary angiograms, pulmonary nodules represented the most common incidental finding (83 of 223 patients; 37.2%), with further imaging recommended for the majority (86%) of the incidental nodules.[3] An earlier review similarly showed further recommendations were specified for 96% of patients with new incidental nodules, based on existing guidelines at that time.[4] Incidental nodules are frequently identified on CT scans focused on extrapulmonary anatomy, for example, in 12%[5] to 18%[6] of cardiac CTs, with a majority of patients then undergoing further imaging or investigation (33/61[5] and 74/81 patients,[6] respectively) and potentially further management if proving to be lung cancer.[5]

Given their frequency and potential clinical significance, reporting and management guidelines have been established to address the incidentally detected pulmonary nodule. An understanding of available guidelines and the rationale behind the recommendations is critical to all radiologists, both generalists and body and thoracic imagers, when interpreting chest CT. This article reviews the technical considerations in evaluating and reporting both solid and subsolid pulmonary nodules, and the application of currently available guidelines for nodule management.

Department of Radiology, NYU Grossman School of Medicine, NYU Langone Health, Center for Biomedical Imaging, 660 First Avenue, New York, NY 10016, USA
* Corresponding author.
E-mail address: Lea.Azour@nyulangone.org

Radiol Clin N Am 59 (2021) 535–549
https://doi.org/10.1016/j.rcl.2021.03.005
0033-8389/21/© 2021 Elsevier Inc. All rights reserved.

TECHNICAL AND REPORTING CONSIDERATIONS IN NODULE EVALUATION

Pulmonary nodules are characterized in terms of attenuation, size, and interval change. Accurate, consistent characterization and description of nodules[7] and attention to CT technique are essential. Pulmonary nodules are best evaluated on CT scans acquired at full inspiration, with reconstructions in contiguous thin sections of 1.5 mm or smaller thickness. Pulmonary nodules should be evaluated on the high-frequency, sharp reconstruction algorithm in lung windows.[7] The soft tissue low-frequency reconstruction algorithm is helpful for assessing pulmonary nodule features, such as calcification, because images are less noisy than high-frequency algorithm reconstructions.[8]

When measuring pulmonary nodules, all ground-glass or cystic components should be included in total nodule size.[7] For subcentimeter nodules, the average of long-axis and short-axis dimensions should be reported, whereas bidirectional measures are provided for nodules greater than 1 cm in maximum dimension.[7] Any solid component of subsolid nodules (SSNs) is reported as the longest dimension of the largest area[7] (Fig. 1). All nodules should be reported to the nearest millimeter.[7] Nodules less than 3 mm are considered micronodules, for which measurement is not necessary.

Imagers still may encounter pitfalls in characterizing lung nodules, even with current CT technology. For example, thick-section images may cause a solid nodule to appear subsolid due to volume averaging, as may motion. Review of multiplanar sagittal and/or coronal reformatted images may prevent additional interpretive pitfalls. In the axial plane, small fissural or bandlike foci may appear subsolid, while actually triangular or linear in other planes. Areas of paraspinal or apical opacity may similarly appear nodular in 1 plane, and evaluating multiplanar reformatted images may help distinguish true nodularity from fibrosis (Fig. 2). Perifissural nodules (PFNs) can be morphologically assessed in 3-dimensions as well.

MANAGEMENT GUIDELINES: GENERAL CONCEPTS

Incidental nodule management and decision making are pursued on a case-by-case basis, guided by imaging features, patient risk, and patient preference. Existing guidelines for incidentally detected pulmonary nodules include those from the Fleischner Society[9] (Fig. 3), the British Thoracic Society (BTS),[10] and the American College of Chest Physicians (ACCP).[11] The data used to make these guidelines are informed by lung cancer screening trials, including the National Lung Screening Trial (NLST), the Nederlands-Leuvens Longkanker Screenings Onderzoek (NELSON) trial, and the International Early Lung Cancer Action Program (I-ELCAP). Although these trials were conducted for lung cancer screening, they also give substantial insight into the natural history of solid and subsolid pulmonary nodules.

Attention to the patient population addressed by nodule management guidelines is crucial. Although the Fleischner guidelines are restricted to adults ages 35 years or older, the BTS and ACCP guidelines are applicable to incidental nodules in adults of any age. The Fleischner guidelines should be used only in nonimmunocompromised individuals with no known malignancy, because those factors affect the likelihood of infection or malignancy.[9]

Solid nodules and SSNs are managed differently, because their etiologies and clinical

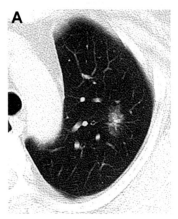
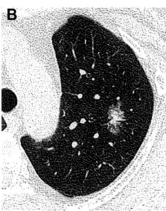

Fig. 1. Technique may influence nodule characterization. (A) A 73-year-old woman presenting for evaluation of lung nodule. On 5-mm, thick-section axial CT image, the borders and nodule solid components are blurred due to partial volume averaging. Thicker-section images can cause solid aspects to appear lower, or ground-glass, in attenuation. (B) Corresponding thin-section, axial 1-mm image better demonstrates the lobulated margins and internal component morphology. Greater soft tissue attenuation is identified on the 1-mm section compared with the thicker image.

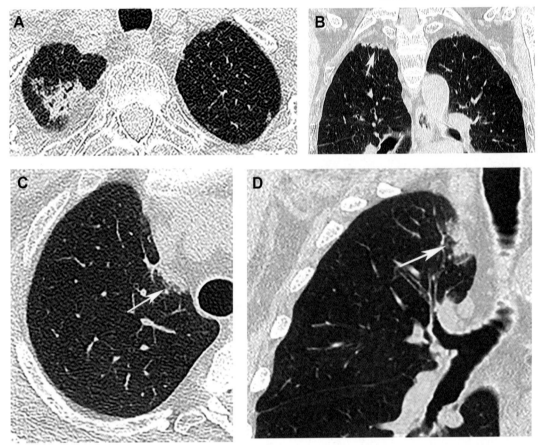

Fig. 2. Multiplanar reformatted images aid in characterizing focal lung abnormalities. (*A, B*) An 84-year-old woman presenting for evaluation of lung nodule. (*A*) Right apical abnormality appears masslike in the axial plane on CT; (*B*) however, on coronal reformatted images, the finding is confined to the immediate subpleural region without dominant convexities (*arrow*). This was confirmed as a benign apical cap upon right lower lobe resection for a different, slowly enlarging dominant part-solid right upper lobe nodule (not shown). (*C, D*) A 69-year-old man presenting for pulmonary nodule follow-up. (*C*) Right upper lobe paramediastinal subpleural focal, predominately soft tissue attenuation finding on CT (*arrow*) appears oblong in the axial plane, initially potentially considered to be an area of focal scarring. (*D*) Coronal reformatted image, however, reveals a nodular shape and that this finding is larger in the craniocaudal dimension (*arrow*). This was micropapillary-predominant adenocarcinoma on resection.

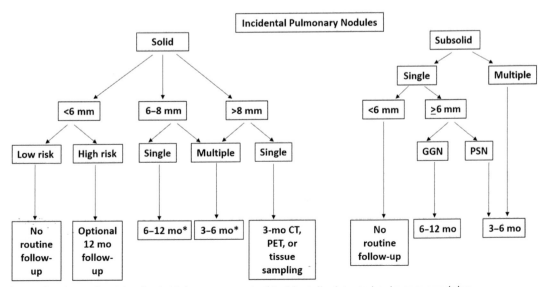

Fig. 3. Fleischner algorithm for initial management of incidentally detected pulmonary nodules.

behavior differ. For example, lung cancers appearing as solid nodules and those as SSNs have different growth rates, thus influencing the time interval for subsequent follow-up CT. For this reason, the most recent Fleischner guidelines[12] address solid nodule[13] and SSN[14] management independently.

Nodule management algorithms from the Fleischner Society, BTS, and ACCP all address patient risk of malignancy. In the ACCP guidelines, the pretest probability of malignancy for solid nodules can be assessed either by clinician judgment or through quantitative, validated risk prediction models to categorize patients into high-risk (>65%), intermediate-risk (5%–65%), and low-risk (<5%) categories.[11] The Fleischner guidelines also support patient risk assessment, and have high-risk and low-risk categories for solid nodules (see Fig. 3); they consider the ACCP high-risk and intermediate-risk groups as the high-risk category.[9] Determining malignancy probability is based on clinical factors, including age, smoking history, and cancer history, and nodule features, such as nodule size, margin, and lobar location. Fluorodeoxyglucose (FDG)-PET and histopathology also are incorporated into the ACCP malignancy risk assessment.[11]

Risk calculators have been validated to assess the likelihood of nodule malignancy, and primarily address solid nodules. Risk calculators incorporate malignancy predictors. For example, in the Brock model, which is based on data from the Pan-Canadian Early Detection of Lung Cancer Study, patient risk factors for malignancy include older age, female sex, family history, and emphysema; and nodule risk factors include larger size, spiculation, upper lobe location, and subsolid attenuation.[15] Risk calculators have optimal performance when applied to populations similar to those on which the model was based.[11,16]

INCIDENTAL SOLID PULMONARY NODULE MANAGEMENT

Incidental solid pulmonary nodules may be consigned to benignity if certain CT features are present, including long-term stability, characteristic benign calcium patterns, or macroscopic fat. Primary considerations for solid nodules include granulomatous disease, lung cancer, solitary pulmonary metastases, hamartoma, and carcinoid tumors (Table 1). The possibility of vascular AVMs and aneurysms may be clarified on intravenous contrast–enhanced examinations. In the absence of prior imaging or characteristic morphology, incidental solid nodules may be indeterminate.

Nodules with Calcification or Fat

Nodules may demonstrate several calcification patterns on CT (Figs. 4 and 5). Diffuse or completely calcified nodules most often represent benign calcified granulomas. Calcified granulomas are the sequela of prior infection, such as tuberculosis or histoplasmosis, and are a common incidental finding, in 57% of an 872-person agrarian cohort, for example.[17] Uncommonly, certain cancer metastases, however, may present as calcified or ossified nodules, including those from sarcomas, thyroid, or mucinous adenocarcinomas.

Typically, benign calcification patterns also include central calcification, lamellated calcification, or popcorn calcification; the BTS guidelines recommend no follow-up for nodules demonstrating these calcification patterns.[10] Central and laminated calcification may be seen in granulomatous nodules. Popcorn calcifications, round or with rings and arcs,[18] are characteristic of hamartoma and also may be seen in pulmonary amyloid or chondroid nodules or masses. It may be difficult to characterize this from dystrophic calcification on CT, and surveillance CT or PET may be pursued. In a series of 47 hamartomas, 26% were reported to have calcification.[19]

Punctate or amorphous calcifications are indeterminate and have been reported in carcinoid tumors and lung neoplasms.[20] [68]Gallium-dotatate PET (somatostatin-receptor functional imaging) may help differentiate carcinoid from hamartoma, although granulomas also may have somatostatin receptors.[21]

Macroscopic fat within a pulmonary nodule on CT usually is considered pathognomonic for benign hamartoma (Fig. 6). Siegelman and colleagues[19] found 38% of hamartomas in their series of 47 cases to show fat. Other rare causes of fat-containing pulmonary nodules include pulmonary lipoma[22] and metastases from fat-containing primaries, such as liposarcoma or renal cell carcinoma. Lipoid pneumonia also may result in opacities with fat attenuation. The BTS guidelines recommend no follow-up for nodules with macroscopic fat.[10]

Perifissural and Subpleural Nodules

PFNs have been defined as triangular, oval, or polygonal-shaped nodules, with smooth, circumscribed borders, contacting or within 5 mm to 10 mm of a fissure[23] (Fig. 7). PFNs are encountered commonly, comprising approximately one-fifth to one-fourth of all noncalcified pulmonary nodules on CT.[23–25]

Initial data regarding the behavior of PFNs were derived from lung cancer screening cohorts.[23,24]

Table 1
Differential considerations for the incidental pulmonary nodule by attenuation

Nodule Attenuation	Benign	Neoplastic/Malignant
Solid	• Noncalcified granuloma • Intrapulmonary lymph node • Infection • Hamartoma • Rheumatoid nodule • Amyloid • Vasculitis (ie, granulomatosis with polyangiitis) • Alveolar sarcoid • Lymphocytic interstitial pneumonia	• Primary lung malignancy • Metastasis • Carcinoid • Lymphoproliferative disorder
Solid with calcifications	• Granulomatous processes (endemic fungal infections, tuberculosis, varicella) • Hamartoma • Amyloid • Rheumatoid nodule • Metabolic (metastatic calcification) • Alveolar microlithiasis	• Metastases • Sarcoma (osteosarcoma, chondrosarcoma) • Mucinous neoplasms (ovarian, pancreatic, gastrointestinal) • Thyroid cancer • Carcinoid • Primary lung malignancy
Subsolid	• Infectious (fungal, viral) • Transient inflammation • Focal interstitial fibrosis • Organizing pneumonia • Eosinophilic pneumonia • Drug reaction • Alveolar sarcoid • Vasculitis • Thoracic endometriosis	• Primary lung adenocarcinoma spectrum (AAH, AIS, MIA, invasive adenocarcinoma) • Mucinous lung adenocarcinoma • Lymphoma (mucosa-associated lymphoid tissue) and lymphoproliferative disorders • Metastases (melanoma, renal, breast, gastrointestinal/pancreatic adenocarcinomas)
Cystic/cavitary	• Fungal • Septic emboli • Amyloid • Granulomatosis with polyangiitis • Necrobiotic nodules (rheumatoid arthritis, inflammatory bowel disease) • Pulmonary Langerhans cell histiocytosis	• Primary lung malignancy • Metastases • Lymphoproliferative disorder

In screening cohorts, Ahn and colleagues[23] found 28% (234 of 837) of noncalcified nodules to be PFNs, and de Hoop and colleagues[24] found PFNs in 19.7% (794 of 4026). A majority of PFNs are triangular (102%; 44%) or ovoid/lentiform (98; 42%) in shape, and located below the level of the carina.[23,25,26] In a nonscreening cohort, 21% of noncalcified nodules on CT were PFNs. In both screening and nonscreening examinations, PFNs may be large and demonstrate growth.[24,25] Long-term follow-up of 7.5 years in Ahn and colleagues'[23] 146-subject cohort and 5.5-year follow-up in de Hoop and colleagues'[24] 1729-subject cohort demonstrated no lung cancers to arise

from nodules qualifying as PFNs. PFNs in oncologic patients with a median follow-up of more than 5 years demonstrated the majority to remain stable or decrease in size, also reassuring for benignity.[27]

Histopathologically, typical-appearing PFNs or subpleural nodules have been found to represent intrapulmonary lymph nodes.[24,26,28,29] Due to the low probability of malignancy associated with typical PFNs and subpleural nodules, the BTS guidelines recommend no follow-up for subcentimeter, smoothly marginated, triangular or lentiform nodules within 1 cm of the pleura or a fissure.[10] The Fleischner guidelines similarly

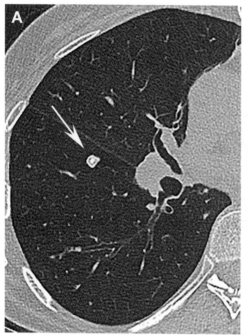
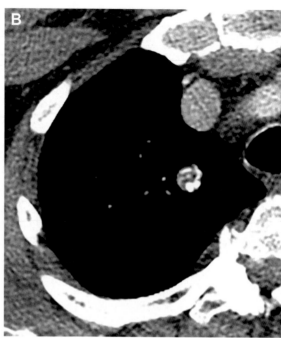

Fig. 4. Benign calcification patterns. (*A*) A 60-year-old woman with bronchiectasis and nontuberculous mycobacterial infection. Nodule (*arrow*) on image from axial CT chest demonstrates a central target calcification compatible with a benign calcified granuloma. (*B*) A 56-year-old man presenting for pulmonary nodule evaluation. Axial CT chest image, mediastinal windows, shows a nodule with coarse popcorn calcifications, consistent with pathology-proved hamartoma; the patient had elected surgical resection.

recommend no CT follow-up for juxtapleural nodules or PFNs with morphology compatible with that of an intrapulmonary lymph node.

Interobserver variation may affect PFN classification, with only moderate agreement reported for thoracic radiologists, particularly when PFNs do not abut a fissure on CT. Also, all nodules abutting fissures are not typical PFNs, and atypical PFNs have a higher rate of malignancy.[30] Atypical

PFN features include irregular shape, convexity of and displacement of the fissure, spiculated margins, or heterogeneity.[24] de Hoop and colleagues[24] found a malignancy rate of 1.7% for atypical PFNs in their screening cohort. For this reason, follow-up is recommended for atypical PFNs, with the Fleischner Society recommending 6 to 12 month follow-up CT. There is limited data regarding large PFNs, to the authors' knowledge,

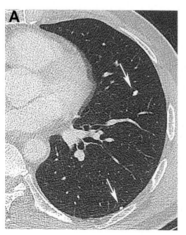
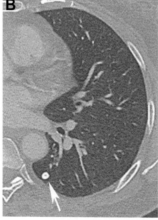

Fig. 5. Indeterminate pulmonary nodules with calcification. (*A*) A 47-year-old man with history of osteosarcoma. Image from axial CT chest demonstrates small calcified nodules abutting the left fissure and subpleural left lower lobe (*arrows*), which initially were indeterminate in this patient with history of osteosarcoma. The nodules subsequently demonstrated progressive growth and were compatible with metastases on continued imaging surveillance (not shown). (*B*) A 61-year-old woman with history of gastric mass. Indeterminate peripheral calcification pattern in small left lower lobe nodule (*arrow*) on axial CT chest, determined to be a metastasis from gastric adenocarcinoma on surveillance.

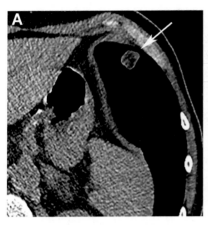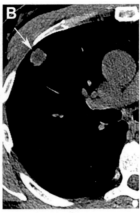

Fig. 6. Nodule attenuation may guide differential considerations. (*A*) A 72-year-old man with emphysema and pulmonary nodules. On axial 2-mm section reconstruction using low-frequency kernel, macroscopic fat within a left lower lobe nodule (*arrow*) in conjunction with smooth margins is compatible with hamartoma. The Hounsfield unit measurement corresponding to the low attenuation region was −81. (*B*) A 48-year-old man with history of Kaposi sarcoma. Low attenuation within a nodule also may be due to necrosis, with fluid attenuation Hounsfield unit measurement in this right upper lobe nodule (*arrow*) on axial CT chest. Pathology from percutaneous lung biopsy revealed abundant necrosis with fungal elements, and no malignancy was identified.

and 10 mm and larger PFNs also can be followed.[10]

Solid Nodule Follow-up and Management

For solid nodules on CT, nodule size is the predominant determinant for management; larger nodules have a higher likelihood of malignancy.[31] Additional features that increase risk are upper lobe location and spiculation.[15] Therefore, even small nodules with suspicious morphology may be surveilled at 12 months, with small size making clinical progression in the interim unlikely.[9] The

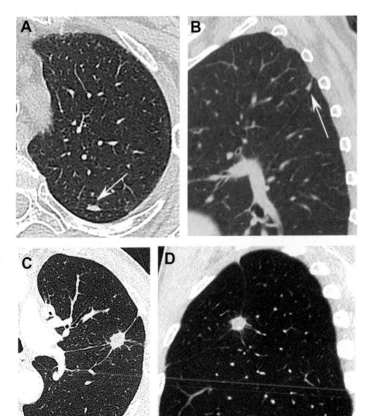

Fig. 7. Typical and atypical PFNs. (*A, B*) A 54-year-old woman with dyspnea and history of smoking. (*A*) Axial chest CT image demonstrates an ovoid left upper lobe nodule abutting the fissure (*arrow*), shorter in anteroposterior than transverse dimension. (*B*) Sagittal reformatted image demonstrates the PFN's triangular shape (*arrow*) to better advantage. On histopathology, this was an intrapulmonary lymph node. (*C, D*) A 61-year-old man with history of previously resected lung cancer. Axial and sagittal images demonstrate an atypical PFN, which is large and spiculated. Morphology is not consistent with a typical PFN representing an intraparenchymal lymph node and warranted further evaluation. Resection was performed, confirming necrotizing granulomatous inflammation.

volume doubling time associated with neoplastic solid nodules often is shorter than that for SSNs, less than 400 days, implying that any prior imaging proving 2-year stability should in most cases suggest solid nodule benignity.[9]

Determining Solid Nodule Follow-up Interval

For solid pulmonary nodules for which benignity cannot be established (**Fig. 8**), the Fleischner Society's initial follow-up recommendations are based on nodule size and patient risk factors (see **Fig. 3**). The 2017 Fleischner guidelines delineate 3 size cutoffs: less than 6 mm (<100 mm^3), 6 mm to 8 mm (100–250 mm^3), and greater than 8 mm (>250 mm^3), and high-risk and low-risk patient categories.[9] Nodules typically are measured in the axial plane, unless maximal dimension is in coronal or sagittal, in which case this measurement plane should be specified.[7]

According to these guidelines, the recommended follow-up for patients with solitary or multiple solid nodules smaller than 6 mm is the same. A solid solitary nodule under 6 mm in a low-risk patient does not require follow-up imaging, because the malignancy risk for small, less than 6 mm nodules is less than 1%.[9,15] A high-risk patient may have a single optional follow-up low dose CT at 1 year.

Solitary solid nodules 6 mm to 8 mm require closer follow-up, regardless of risk factors. Nodules greater than 8 mm (>250 mm^3) require close follow-up or additional work-up regardless of patient risk. For nodules of this size, at least a low-dose chest CT at 3 months is recommended. Additional management options, however, include PET/CT, primarily for staging, or correlation with tissue histology if more suspicious nodule features are present.

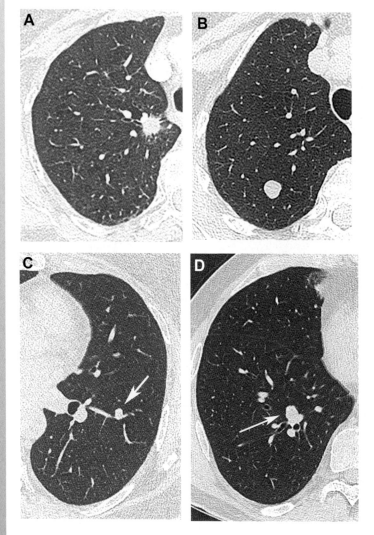

Fig. 8. Benign and malignant solid lung nodules can share similar margin features, and management is directed by a combination of factors, including nodule size, nodule number, and patient risk. (*A*) A 78-year-old woman presenting for lung nodule incidentally detected on chest MRI. Spiculated right upper lobe solid nodule on axial CT chest raises suspicion for cancer, particularly given the large nodule size. Finding confirmed to be primary lung adenocarcinoma on resection. (*B*) An 87-year-old man presenting for evaluation of nodule detected on radiography. Axial CT shows the round, well-circumscribed smoothly marginated right upper lobe nodule, which can be seen with both benign and malignant etiologies. In this patient with renal carcinoma and numerous bilateral pulmonary nodules, this large nodule proved to be a metastasis. (*C*) A 63-year-old woman with history of breast cancer. Indeterminate perivascular left lower lobe nodule (*arrow*) on axial CT chest also had smooth margins. Given size and growth, this was resected and confirmed to be carcinoid, which can demonstrate low or no metabolic uptake on FDG-PET. (*D*) A 64-year-old man presenting with chest pain. Another smoothly marginated indeterminate and incidentally detected right lower lobe nodule (*arrow*). This well-circumscribed nodule was non-FDG avid, and percutaneous tissue sampling confirmed a benign diagnosis of hamartoma.

When multiple solid nodules greater than 6 mm are encountered, the largest nodule or nodule with the most suspicious features determines follow-up management. For multiple nodules greater than 6 mm, the follow-up interval is shorter than that of solitary nodules, with follow-up recommended in 3 months to 6 months.

INCIDENTAL SUBSOLID PULMONARY NODULES

SSNs include both pure ground-glass nodules (GGNs) and part-solid nodules (PSNs) on CT.[32] GGNs are synonymous with nonsolid nodules. PSNs, synonymous with semisolid nodules, have both ground-glass and soft-tissue attenuation components.[32] Due to their subsolid attenuation, underlying structures, such as airways and vessels, can be visualized within these nodules on CT. SSNs may be due to several benign and neoplastic etiologies (see **Table 1**; **Fig. 9**); however, when persistent, they have a high likelihood of representing a neoplasm on the lung adenocarcinoma spectrum.

Subsolid Nodule Follow-up and Management

Management algorithms recommend the initial determination of SSN persistence on CT. This is based on the fact that up to 70% of incidentally detected SSNs may be transient.[33] In screening populations, which are at higher risk for lung cancer, a substantial proportion of SSNs regressed. In the I-ELCAP cohort, 26% (628 of 2392) of nonsolid nodules[34] and approximately 20% (567 of 2892) of PSNs[35] identified on baseline examination either decreased in size or resolved. Similarly, in 622 SSNs selected from the NLST cohort, and 264 SSNs from the NELSON cohort, 28%[36] and 63%[37] of SSNs resolved on follow-up, respectively. An even higher proportion of newly arising SSNs evident on follow-up CT examinations, approximately 70% in the I-ELCAP cohort, decreased in size or resolved.[34,35]

Several factors have been described in association with SSN transience, including younger patient age, male sex, and eosinophilia.[38–40] Imaging features associated with SSN transience include multiplicity,[38,39] ill-defined or nonspiculated margins,[38–40]

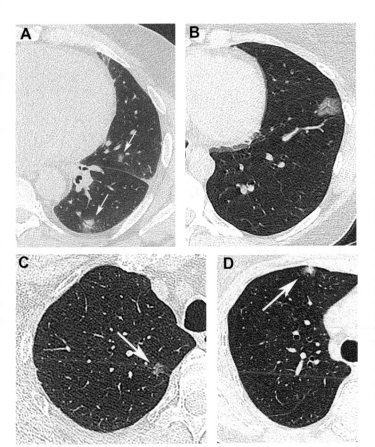

Fig. 9. Persistent SSNs representing benign and neoplastic entities may mimic one another. (*A*) A 56-year-old man with reported history of pneumonia. Subsolid, predominantly soft tissue and with mild ground-glass attenuation left lower lobe nodule (*posterior arrow*), was organizing pneumonia on histopathology. Another SSNs is present in the lingula (*anterior arrow*). (*B*) A 51-year-old woman with cough and elevated antinuclear antibodies. Subsolid ground-glass attenuation left lower lobe nodule, which was mucosa-associated lymphoid tissue lymphoma on histopathology. (*C*) A 77-year-old man with history of pulmonary nodules and intermittent cough. Ground-glass attenuation right upper lobe nodule is shown (*arrow*) with punctate solid components, which proved to be MIA on pathology. (*D*) A 67-year-old woman with pulmonary nodules. Subsolid, predominantly soft tissue with mild ground-glass attenuation right upper lobe nodule with a 7-mm solid component (*arrow*), which was invasive adenocarcinoma on resection.

polygonal shape,[41] mixed attenuation,[41] large solid nodule component,[39] and large overall size.[41] In contradistinction, features including pleural retraction and bubble lucencies may indicate a long-standing or persistent nodule, because such architectural distortion would be expected to develop over time.[38]

Persistent SSNs have a higher rate of malignancy than solid nodules.[42] Neoplastic SSNs most commonly represent tumors on the lung adenocarcinoma spectrum. These often are indolent when purely ground-glass in attenuation, which correlates on histopathology with lepidic tumor growth.[43,44] Lepidic growth is characterized by tumor cell propagation along the surface of intact alveolar walls, without stromal or vascular invasion. Solid component size on CT correlates with invasive components.[45,46]

Lung adenocarcinoma spectrum neoplasms are classified pathologically by the International Association for the Study of Lung Cancer system, which includes preinvasive atypical adenomatous hyperplasia (AAH) (size ≤5 mm) and adenocarcinoma in situ (AIS) (size <3 cm), composed of only lepidic growth, which typically are ground-glass in attenuation. Minimally invasive adenocarcinoma (MIA) (solid component size ≤5 mm) with otherwise lepidic tumor, typically is predominately ground-glass with small solid aspect(s) on CT but can have variable appearances.[47] Invasive adenocarcinomas may be classified further by their predominant subtype, including lepidic, acinar, papillary, micropapillary, and solid. These subtypes confer prognostic information, because lepidic-predominant adenocarcinomas have an excellent 5-year disease-free survival, whereas micropapillary patterns are associated with a poor prognosis.[48,49] This radiology-pathology correlation and associated prognostic implications[50] have shaped management guidelines and nodule follow-up intervals.

Determining Subsolid Nodule Follow-up Interval

Determining initial follow-up interval for SSNs identified on CT is based first on whether there are one or multiple SSNs (see **Fig. 3**). For both GGNs and PSNs, multiplicity warrants a shorter initial follow-up interval of 3 months to 6 months to assess for persistence. Assessing for persistence precludes potentially premature aggressive management. Multiple nodules often may be infectious or inflammatory, although multifocal synchronous indolent primary tumors are a consideration if persistent.

For a solitary SSN 6 mm or larger, the follow-up interval depends on nodule attenuation. For a GGN 6 mm or larger, 6-month to 12-month follow-up is advised to assess for persistence. For a PSN of this size, a more conservative 3-month to 6-month follow-up is advised, because a potentially persistent solid component may correlate with degree of invasiveness. Even pure GGNs, however, may be invasive on histopathology, typically when larger.[51–54] Lee and colleagues[54] found pure ground-glass lesion size 10 mm or greater a specific feature in distinguishing invasive from preinvasive tumors, and Lim and colleagues[52] size 16 mm or greater to be associated with lesion invasiveness.

Cystic Foci

Primary lung malignancy may also present as a cystic focus on CT (**Fig. 10**), which is distinct from a neoplasm that becomes cavitary secondary to necrosis. Based on the I-ELCAP cohort, 3.7% (26/706) of lung cancers were in association with a cystic airspace and were significantly more likely to be identified on follow-up annual screening.[55] In this cohort, 23 of the 26 lung cancers were lung adenocarcinomas, and the others were squamous cell carcinoma, non–small cell carcinoma, and atypical carcinoid tumor.[55] In Tan and colleagues'[56] review of 106 solitary cystic lung cancers, with 93 confirmed by postoperative pathology, 87% (81 of 93) were lung adenocarcinomas, 7.5% (7 of 93) were squamous cell carcinoma, 4.3% (4 of 93) were adenosquamous carcinoma, and 1.1% lymphoma (1 of 93).

Large cystic areas potentially can develop because of tumor. Tumors may have a bronchus in communication with the cystic airspace, and in Tan and colleagues'[56] series, tumor cells directly invaded and occluded the bronchial wall in 34 of 93 (36.6%) of cases. This has been postulated to create a unidirectional check valve that leads to cyst expansion with initial airway narrowing, and subsequent decrease in size with complete airway occlusion.[56,57] In this series, more than 90% of the cystic lung cancers had nonuniform cyst walls, with additional common CT features including septations (58.5%), wall nodularity (54.7%), and surrounding ground-glass (50%).[56] Two-thirds were located in the lung periphery.[56]

Neoplasms originating as cystic foci may become completely solid over time, which may contribute to delayed or missed diagnosis.[58] In the I-ELCAP cohort, the cystic airspace on CT was evident in 25/26 of neoplasms at baseline; nodularity or thickening of the wall became evident at 12 months to 118 months, progressing from a median thickness of 1 mm to 8 mm.[55] In the NELSON cohort, missed lung cancers represented

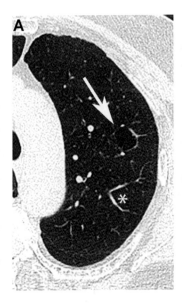
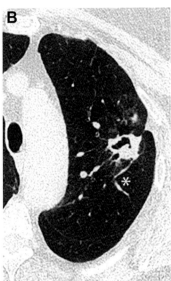

Fig. 10. Cystic cancers. (A) A 75-year-old woman with history of smoking. A 19-mm cystic nodule in the left upper lobe (arrow), with minimal wall thickening, in a patient with emphysema. Mild thickening around a cyst wall can be an early manifestation of neoplastic growth. (B) The patient presented again, now 78 years of age, for a medical clearance radiograph (not shown), which demonstrated a left upper lobe abnormality. The nodule's wall thickening progressed into extensive nodular thickening around the periphery, with increase in overall nodule size and decrease in cystic area over the course of 3 years; note the vessels now pulled anteriorly toward the mass (*). This was adenocarcinoma on histopathology.

0.3% of the screening participants and 8.9% of the cancers; 22.7% of missed lung cancers (5 of 22 tumors) originally manifested as thickening of a bulla wall.[59] Thus, cystic foci with areas of wall thickening should be surveilled, given their potential to develop into lung neoplasms.

NODULES DETECTED ON NONTHORACIC IMAGING

Pulmonary nodules may be incidental on cross-sectional imaging, in particular CT, including examinations that image only portions of the chest/lungs, as discussed previously, such as CT and magnetic resonance imaging (MRI) examinations focusing on the neck, shoulder, abdomen/pelvis, spine, heart, or breasts (Fig. 11). In a review of 395 coronary CTA examinations, noncalcified pulmonary nodules were the most common incidental finding, detected in 23.8% of patients.[60] For nodules detected on nonthoracic imaging, nodule size and level of suspicion guide recommendations and aid in distinguishing those that may be clinically relevant.

The clinical relevance of incidentally detected lung nodules on abdominal CT depends on patient characteristics, mainly history of prior malignancy. Alpert and colleagues[61] found 7.1% (3/42) of nodules incidentally detected on abdominal CT represented metastases, all in patients with a history of malignancy. Another study of 413 patients with incidental pulmonary nodules on abdominal CT found that 11% (46/413) were malignant, and an additional 33% were indeterminate due to limited follow-up.[62] Of the malignant nodules representing metastases (30/43), most patients had known or suspected malignancy.[62] In Wu and colleagues'[62] cohort of 413 patients, only 9% were found to have nodules larger than the original incidentally detected nodule on follow-up CT. Underreporting, however, may be a limitation in determining the clinical implications of incidentally detected pulmonary nodules—Rinaldi and colleagues[63] found incidentally detected nodules on abdominal CT were reported in only 8.4% (8/95) of patients.

For patients without a history of malignancy, the Fleischner Society recommends dedicated chest CT follow-up for 6-mm to 8-mm solid nodules at an interval of 3 months to 12 months, based on risk and multiplicity, and for SSNs an interval of 3 months to 12 months, depending on attenuation and multiplicity.[9] Large or suspicious nodules from incomplete or limited thoracic imaging should be assessed by dedicated CT chest.[9]

Application of the 2017 Fleischner guidelines to nodules incidentally detected on nonthoracic CT may reduce additional imaging follow-up examinations, a source of both radiation exposure and increased medical costs, for nodules with low likelihood of malignancy. For example, application of the 2017 Fleischner guidelines to incidental nodules on coronary CTA examinations was found to reduce the number of recommended follow-up examinations by 64%, from 12.8% of patients to 4.5% of patients.[64]

INFORMATICS APPROACHES FOR STANDARDIZED NODULE FOLLOW-UP AND NOTIFICATION

Once a nodule has been characterized and follow-up recommendations structured, findings must be

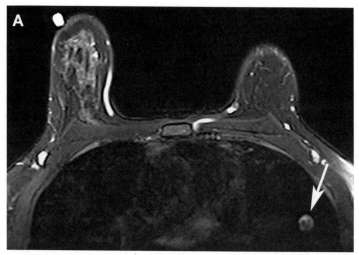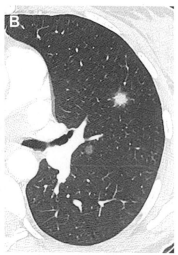

Fig. 11. Nodules are detected incidentally on nonthoracic imaging and can prove clinically significant. (*A*) Breast MRI in a patient with ductal carcinoma in situ revealed a T2 hyperintense and heterogeneously enhancing 1-cm left upper lobe nodule (*arrow*). (*B*) Based on large nodule size, a short-interval, dedicated chest CT was performed, which showed multiple SSNs. The most suspicious and predominately solid left upper lobe nodule was a primary lung adenocarcinoma on percutaneous biopsy.

conveyed successfully to the requesting clinician. The American College of Radiology encourages clear and concise reporting for radiological examinations,[65] and communication of incidental nodule findings can be challenging given various decision nodes in the guidelines and their relative frequency. Gaps in communication and follow-up of incidental nodule findings likely contribute at least partially to the elevated medical malpractice rates in thoracic imaging.[66] Thus, at the local and institutional levels, the need for consensus is essential. The use of consensus guidelines has been shown to improve compliance with pulmonary nodule follow-up guidelines.[67]

Even with the use of structured text reporting, there continues to be low compliance with recommended imaging follow-up guidelines, with up to 55% of patients (151/276) not receiving recommended imaging follow-up in 1 study.[67] Importantly, in this study, 53% (26/49) of patients who had incidentally detected lung nodules greater than 6 mm did not undergo recommended imaging. Information technology can be leveraged to improve compliance with follow-up recommendations. Kang and colleagues[68] created a next-generation informatics system wherein voice dictation result fields were filed within the electronic medical record. This allowed for the creation of worklists composed of patients due for follow-up imaging, potentially facilitating patient outreach. Additionally, portals enabling direct patient communication may further improve compliance with guideline recommendations.[69]

SUMMARY

The general radiologist and body imager, and in addition to the thoracic radiologist, commonly encounter incidental pulmonary nodules, particularly on CT, and guidelines exist addressing nodule management. An awareness of benign nodule features and management recommendations for nodules which are indeterminate in nature is critical when encountering incidental nodules on CT. Additional investigations in screening and non-screening populations will update knowledge of risk assessment and nodule behavior, and thus shape future recommendations.

CLINICS CARE POINTS

- Incidental pulmonary nodule features such as attenuation, number, size and location may guide differential considerations.
- Solid and subsolid nodules confer differing risk of malignancy.
- Individual guidelines exist for the follow-up of incidentally-detected solid and subsolid pulmonary nodules.

DISCLOSURES OF CONFLICTS OF INTEREST

The authors disclose no relevant relationships.

REFERENCES

1. Hess EP, Haas LR, Shah ND, et al. Trends in computed tomography utilization rates. J Patient Saf 2014;10(1):52–8.

2. Gould MK, Tang T, Liu IL, et al. Recent trends in the identification of incidental pulmonary nodules. Am J Respir Crit Care Med 2015;192(10):1208–14.

3. Anjum O, Bleeker H, Ohle R. Computed tomography for suspected pulmonary embolism results in a large number of non-significant incidental findings and follow-up investigations. Emerg Radiol 2019;26(1):29–35.

4. Hall WB, Truitt SG, Scheunemann LP, et al. The prevalence of clinically relevant incidental findings on chest computed tomographic angiograms ordered to diagnose pulmonary embolism. Arch Intern Med 2009;169(21):1961–5.

5. Onuma Y, Tanabe K, Nakazawa G, et al. Noncardiac Findings in Cardiac Imaging With Multidetector Computed Tomography. J Am Coll Cardiol 2006; 48(2):402–6.

6. Iribarren C, Hlatky MA, Chandra M, et al. Incidental Pulmonary Nodules on Cardiac Computed Tomography: Prognosis and Use. Am J Med 2008;121(11):989–96.

7. Bankier AA, MacMahon H, Goo JM, et al. Recommendations for measuring pulmonary nodules at CT: A statement from the Fleischner society. Radiology 2017;285(2):584–600.

8. Ko JP, Azour L. Management of Incidental Lung Nodules. Semin Ultrasound CT MRI 2018;39(3):249–59.

9. MacMahon H, Naidich DP, Goo JM, et al. Guidelines for Management of Incidental Pulmonary Nodules Detected on CT Images: From the Fleischner Society 2017. Radiology 2017;284(1):228–43.

10. Callister MEJ, Baldwin DR, Akram AR, et al. British thoracic society guidelines for the investigation and management of pulmonary nodules. Thorax 2015;70(Suppl 2):ii1–54.

11. Gould MK, Donington J, Lynch WR, et al. Evaluation of Individuals With Pulmonary Nodules: When Is It Lung Cancer? Chest 2013;143(5):e93S–120S.

12. Macmahon H, Naidich DP, Goo JM, et al. Guidelines for Management of Incidental Pulmonary Nodules MacMahon et al. Radiol N Radiol 2017;000(284):228–43.

13. MacMahon H, Austin JHM, Gamsu G, et al. Guidelines for management of small pulmonary nodules detected on CT scans: A statement from the Fleischner Society. Radiology 2005;237(2):395–400.

14. Naidich DP, Bankier AA, MacMahon H, et al. Recommendations for the Management of Subsolid Pulmonary Nodules Detected at CT: A Statement from the Fleischner Society. Radiology 2013;266(1):304–17.

15. McWilliams A, Tammemagi MC, Mayo JR, et al. Probability of Cancer in Pulmonary Nodules Detected on First Screening CT. N Engl J Med 2013;369(10):910–9.

16. Choi HK, Ghobrial M, Mazzone PJ. Models to estimate the probability of malignancy in patients with pulmonary nodules. Ann Am Thorac Soc 2018; 1117–26.

17. Reed RM, Amoroso A, Hashmi S, et al. Calcified Granulomatous Disease: Occupational Associations and Lack of Familial Aggregation. Lung 2014; 192(6):841–7.

18. Hochhegger B, Nin CS, Alves GRT, et al. Multidetector computed tomography findings in pulmonary hamartomas a new fat detection threshold. J Thorac Imaging 2016;31(1):11–4.

19. Siegelman SS, Khouri NF, Scott WW, et al. Pulmonary hamartoma: CT findings. Radiology 1986; 160(2):313–7.

20. Mahoney MC, Shipley RT, Corcoran HL, et al. CT demonstration of calcification in carcinoma of the lung. Am J Roentgenol 1990;154(2):255–8.

21. Balon HR, Brown TLY, Goldsmith SJ, et al. The SNM practice guideline for somatostatin receptor scintigraphy 2.0. J Nucl Med Technol 2011;39(4):317–24.

22. Doulias T, Gosney J, Elsayed H. An intraparenchymal pulmonary lipoma with a high activity on positron emission tomography scan. Interact Cardiovasc Thorac Surg 2011;12(5):843–4.

23. Ahn MI, Gleeson TG, Chan IH, et al. Perifissural nodules seen at CT screening for lung cancer. Radiology 2010;254(3):949–56.

24. de Hoop B, van Ginneken B, Gietema H, et al. Pulmonary Perifissural Nodules on CT Scans: Rapid Growth Is Not a Predictor of Malignancy. Radiology 2012;265(2):611–6.

25. Mets OM, Chung K, Scholten ET, et al. Incidental perifissural nodules on routine chest computed tomography: lung cancer or not? Eur Radiol 2018; 28(3):1095–101.

26. Shaham D, Vazquez M, Bogot NR, et al. CT features of intrapulmonary lymph nodes confirmed by cytology. Clin Imaging 2010;34(3):185–90.

27. Golia Pernicka JS, Hayes SA, Schor-Bardach R, et al. Clinical significance of perifissural nodules in the oncologic population. Clin Imaging 2019;57:110–4.

28. Matsuki M, Noma S, Kuroda Y, et al. Thin-section CT features of intrapulmonary lymph nodes. J Comput Assist Tomogr 2001;25(5):753–6.

29. Miyake H, Yamada Y, Kawagoe T, et al. Intrapulmonary lymph nodes: CT and pathological features. Clin Radiol 1999;54(10):640–3.

30. Schreuder A, Van Ginneken B, Scholten ET, et al. Classification of CT pulmonary opacities as perifissural nodules: Reader variability. Radiology 2018; 288(3):867–75.

31. Horeweg N, van Rosmalen J, Heuvelmans MA, et al. Lung cancer probability in patients with CT-detected

pulmonary nodules: A prespecified analysis of data from the NELSON trial of low-dose CT screening. Lancet Oncol 2014;15(12):1332–41.

32. Hansell DM, Bankier AA, MacMahon H, et al. Fleischner Society: Glossary of Terms for Thoracic Imaging. Radiology 2008;246(3):697–722.

33. Godoy MCB, Sabloff B, Naidich DP. Subsolid pulmonary nodules. Curr Opin Pulm Med 2012;18(4):304–12.

34. Yankelevitz DF, Yip R, Smith JP, et al. CT screening for lung cancer: Nonsolid nodules in baseline and annual repeat rounds. Radiology 2015;277(2):555–64.

35. Henschke CI, Yip R, Smith JP, et al. CT Screening for Lung Cancer: Part-Solid Nodules in Baseline and Annual Repeat Rounds. Am J Roentgenol 2016;207(6):1176–84.

36. Hammer MM, Palazzo LL, Kong CY, et al. Cancer Risk in Subsolid Nodules in the National Lung Screening Trial. Radiology 2019;293(2):441–8.

37. Scholten ET, de Jong PA, de Hoop B, et al. Towards a close computed tomography monitoring approach for screen detected subsolid pulmonary nodules? Eur Respir J 2015;45(3):765–73.

38. Choi WS, Park CM, Song YS, et al. Transient subsolid nodules in patients with extrapulmonary malignancies: their frequency and differential features. Acta Radiol 2015;56(4):428–37.

39. Lee SM, Park CM, Goo JM, et al. Transient part-solid nodules detected at screening thin-section ct for lung cancer: Comparison with persistent part-solid nodules. Radiology 2010;255(1):242–51.

40. Oh JY, Kwon SY, Yoon H II, et al. Clinical significance of a solitary ground-glass opacity (GGO) lesion of the lung detected by chest CT. Lung Cancer 2007;55(1):67–73.

41. Felix L, Serra-Tosio G, Lantuejoul S, et al. CT characteristics of resolving ground-glass opacities in a lung cancer screening programme. Eur J Radiol 2011;77(3):410–6.

42. Henschke CI, Yankelevitz DF, Mirtcheva R, et al. CT Screening for Lung Cancer. Am J Roentgenol 2002;178(5):1053–7.

43. Travis WD, Brambilla E, Noguchi M, et al. International Association for the Study of Lung Cancer/American Thoracic Society/European Respiratory Society International Multidisciplinary Classification of Lung Adenocarcinoma. J Thorac Oncol 2011;6(2):244–85.

44. Lee HY, Choi Y-L, Lee KS, et al. Pure Ground-Glass Opacity Neoplastic Lung Nodules: Histopathology, Imaging, and Management. Am J Roentgenol 2014;202(3):W224–33.

45. Cohen JG, Reymond E, Lederlin M, et al. Differentiating pre- and minimally invasive from invasive adenocarcinoma using CT-features in persistent pulmonary part-solid nodules in Caucasian patients. Eur J Radiol 2015;84(4):738–44.

46. Lee KH, Goo JM, Park SJ, et al. Correlation between the Size of the Solid Component on Thin-Section CT and the Invasive Component on Pathology in Small Lung Adenocarcinomas Manifesting as Ground-Glass Nodules. J Thorac Oncol 2014;9(1):74–82.

47. Travis WD, Asamura H, Bankier AA, et al. The IASLC Lung Cancer Staging Project: Proposals for Coding T Categories for Subsolid Nodules and Assessment of Tumor Size in Part-Solid Tumors in the Forthcoming Eighth Edition of the TNM Classification of Lung Cancer. J Thorac Oncol 2016;11(8):1204–23.

48. Yeh YC, Wu YC, Chen CY, et al. Stromal invasion and micropapillary pattern in 212 consecutive surgically resected stage I lung adenocarcinomas: Histopathological categories for prognosis prediction. J Clin Pathol 2012;65(10):910–8.

49. Miyoshi T, Satoh Y, Okumura S, et al. Early-stage lung adenocarcinomas with a micropapillary pattern, a distinct pathologic marker for a significantly poor prognosis. Am J Surg Pathol 2003;27(1):101–9.

50. Yoshizawa A, Motoi N, Riely GJ, et al. Impact of proposed IASLC/ATS/ERS classification of lung adenocarcinoma: Prognostic subgroups and implications for further revision of staging based on analysis of 514 stage i cases. Mod Pathol 2011;24(5):653–64.

51. Liu Y, Sun H, Zhou F, et al. Imaging features of TSCT predict the classification of pulmonary preinvasive lesion, minimally and invasive adenocarcinoma presented as ground glass nodules. Lung Cancer 2017;108:192–7.

52. Lim H, Ahn S, Lee KS, et al. Persistent Pure Ground-Glass Opacity Lung Nodules ≥ 10 mm in Diameter at CT Scan. Chest 2013;144(4):1291–9.

53. Jin X, Zhao S, Gao J, et al. CT characteristics and pathological implications of early stage (T1N0M0) lung adenocarcinoma with pure ground-glass opacity. Eur Radiol 2015;25(9):2532–40.

54. Lee SM, Park CM, Goo JM, et al. Invasive pulmonary adenocarcinomas versus preinvasive lesions appearing as ground-glass nodules: Differentiation by using CT features. Radiology 2013;268(1):265–73.

55. Farooqi AO, Cham M, Zhang L, et al. Lung Cancer Associated With Cystic Airspaces. Am J Roentgenol 2012;199(4):781–6.

56. Tan Y, Gao J, Wu C, et al. CT Characteristics and Pathologic Basis of Solitary Cystic Lung Cancer. Radiology 2019;291(2):495–501.

57. Xue XY, Wang PL, Xue QL, et al. Comparative study of solitary thin-walled cavity lung cancer with computed tomography and pathological findings. Lung Cancer 2012;78(1):45–50.

58. Mets OM, Schaefer-Prokop CM, de Jong PA. Cyst-related primary lung malignancies: An important and relatively unknown imaging appearance of (early) lung cancer. Eur Respir Rev 2018. https://doi.org/10.1183/16000617.0079-2018.

59. Scholten ET, Horeweg N, de Koning HJ, et al. Computed tomographic characteristics of interval and post screen carcinomas in lung cancer screening. Eur Radiol 2015;25(1):81–8.

60. Lehman SJ, Abbara S, Cury RC, et al. Significance of Cardiac Computed Tomography Incidental Findings in Acute Chest Pain. Am J Med 2009;122(6):543–9.

61. Alpert JB, Fantauzzi JP, Melamud K, et al. Clinical significance of lung nodules reported on abdominal CT. Am J Roentgenol 2012;198(4):793–9.

62. Wu CC, Cronin CG, Chu JT, et al. Incidental pulmonary nodules detected on abdominal computed tomography. J Comput Assist Tomogr 2012;36(6):641–5.

63. Rinaldi MF, Bartalena T, Giannelli G, et al. Incidental lung nodules on CT examinations of the abdomen: Prevalence and reporting rates in the PACS era. Eur J Radiol 2010;74(3). https://doi.org/10.1016/j.ejrad.2009.04.019.

64. Scholtz JE, Lu MT, Hedgire S, et al. Incidental pulmonary nodules in emergent coronary CT angiography for suspected acute coronary syndrome: Impact of revised 2017 Fleischner Society Guidelines. J Cardiovasc Comput Tomogr 2018;12(1):28–33.

65. ACR Practice Parameter for Communication of Diagnostic Imaging Findings. ACR Practice Parameter for Communication of Diagnostic Imaging Findings. Available at: https://Www.Acr.Org/-/Media/ACR/Files/Practice-Parameters/Communication Diag.Pdf.

66. Baker SR, Patel RH, Yang L, et al. Malpractice suits in chest radiology: An evaluation of the histories of 8265 radiologists. J Thorac Imaging 2013. https://doi.org/10.1097/RTI.0b013e3182a21be2.

67. McDonald JS, Koo CW, White D, et al. Addition of the Fleischner Society Guidelines to Chest CT Examination Interpretive Reports Improves Adherence to Recommended Follow-up Care for Incidental Pulmonary Nodules. Acad Radiol 2017. https://doi.org/10.1016/j.acra.2016.08.026.

68. Kang SK, Doshi AM, Recht MP, et al. Process Improvement for Communication and Follow-up of Incidental Lung Nodules. J Am Coll Radiol 2020;17(2):224–30.

69. Amber I, Fiester A. Communicating findings: a justification and framework for direct radiologic disclosure to patients. AJR Am J Roentgenol 2013;200:586.

Incidental Breast Findings on Computed Tomography and MR Imaging

Daniella Asch, MD*, Grace DeWitt, MD, Regina Hooley, MD

KEYWORDS

• Incidental • Breast mass • Breast CT • Breast MR imaging

KEY POINTS

- Examination of the breasts, if included entirely or partially on cross-sectional imaging performed for unrelated reasons, is essential and can result in a substantial number of incidentally detected breast cancers.
- When an incidental breast abnormality is identified, one should evaluate its characteristics, as well as the clinical history and prior imaging examinations, to determine the need for further workup.
- In the absence of long-term stability or previous characterization, most breast masses detected at computed tomography (CT) and magnetic resonance (MR) imaging will require further workup, generally with mammography and targeted ultrasound. Breast imaging evaluation of women younger than the age of 40 should include ultrasound, and mammography can be performed at the discretion of the radiologist/breast imager.
- "Routine" cross-sectional imaging is not sensitive for the detection of breast cancer, and large cancers may be present in the breast but not identified on CT or on non-breast-dedicated MR imaging.
- Evaluation of axillary lymphadenopathy should be based on clinical context and imaging appearance. Biopsy is appropriate for suspected breast cancer metastases and for lymphadenopathy of unknown cause.

INTRODUCTION

A wide range of incidental breast findings may be identified on computed tomography (CT) and magnetic resonance (MR) imaging of the chest/abdomen. It is important to be familiar with the CT and MR imaging appearance of the spectrum of breast abnormalities, which can then be correlated with mammography and ultrasound if necessary. Some findings may be attributable to benign causes on the basis of CT/MR imaging and clinical history alone, whereas others will require evaluation with dedicated breast imaging and possibly biopsy. This article serves to review the gamut of incidental breast findings to help guide management.

NORMAL ANATOMY AND STANDARD IMAGING TECHNIQUE

Normal breast tissue consists of fibroglandular elements and fat. Lactiferous ducts extend from the nipple and branch into excretory, interlobular, and terminal ducts that branch into multiple rounded acini forming the functional unit for milk production. Each lactiferous duct is drained by approximately 15 to 20 lobes in a fanlike distribution. The highest density of glandular tissue is typically present in the upper outer quadrant of the breast. Cooper ligaments are thin, fibrous structures that attach to the skin fascia and pectoralis muscle, surrounding the glandular elements and fat. Between the

Department of Radiology and Biomedical Imaging, Yale School of Medicine, 333 Cedar Street, PO Box 208042, New Haven, CT 06520, USA
* Corresponding author.
E-mail address: daniella.asch@yale.edu

Radiol Clin N Am 59 (2021) 551–567
https://doi.org/10.1016/j.rcl.2021.03.006
0033-8389/21/© 2021 Elsevier Inc. All rights reserved.

glandular elements and the pectoralis muscle is retroglandular fat.[1]

Breast density, the density of glandular tissue compared with fat, varies between patients because of multiple factors and may decrease with age as glandular tissue undergoes fatty involution. The American College of Radiology (ACR) publishes a Breast Imaging Reporting and Data System (BI-RADS) lexicon, which classifies breast density into 4 categories: extremely dense, heterogeneously dense, scattered areas of fibroglandular density, and almost entirely fatty.[1,2]

Lymph nodes are most commonly seen in the axilla and in the upper outer quadrant of the breast along blood vessels but can be found anywhere in the breast (intramammary nodes; **Fig. 1**). Normal lymph nodes classically demonstrate a well-circumscribed, reniform shape with fatty hilum[1] and can vary in size.

Mammography is the foundation of breast imaging and is used for both screening and diagnostic purposes. Breast ultrasound is commonly used for further evaluation of findings on mammography, but also as a screening tool in patients with dense breasts. MR imaging is typically not used as first-line breast imaging, although women with dense breasts as well as high-risk patients may elect supplemental screening breast MR imaging. Other indications for breast MR imaging include breast cancer staging, response evaluation to chemotherapy, and implant evaluation. At a minimum, a standard breast MR imaging examination comprises a T2-weighted/bright fluid sequence, a T1-weighted fat-suppressed precontrast sequence, and T1-weighted fat-suppressed postcontrast sequences. The postcontrast subtraction sequences allow for analysis of dynamic kinetic curves.[3]

PREVALENCE AND CLINICAL RELEVANCE
Epidemiology

Breast cancer is the second most common malignancy in women (after skin cancer), and approximately 1 in 8 women in the United States will develop breast cancer during her lifetime.[4] The World Health Organization estimates 2,261,419 new cases of breast cancer worldwide in 2020, with 684,996 deaths.[5]

Prevalence of Incidental Breast Findings and Frequency of Malignancy

Numerous studies have investigated incidental breast findings on cross-sectional imaging performed for unrelated reasons, most of which are retrospective. Overall, the prevalence of incidental breast findings on CT is reported to be approximately 0.10% to 7.63%,[6–8] noting that these numbers reflect findings explicitly dictated in the radiology report and may underestimate the true prevalence.

The reported malignancy rates regarding incidental breast findings on CT vary widely, ranging from 9% to 70%.[7–16] Overall, the incidental cancer detection rates in women are approximately 0.004% to 0.30%.[2,17] Because of the high frequency of malignancy, the workup of incidental breast findings identified on cross-sectional imaging reflects a very low economic burden compared with primary breast screening.[12] Furthermore, an even higher rate of malignancy (~50%) can be seen when examining only those breast findings for which further workup is explicitly recommended by the interpreting radiologist.[14] Unsurprisingly, a significantly increased rate of malignancy has been shown in older patients.[6]

Data on incidental breast findings on MR imaging are even more limited compared with data on

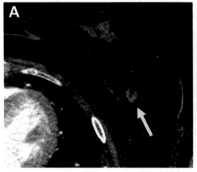
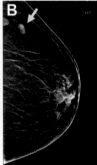
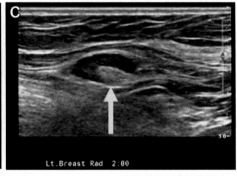

Fig. 1. 68-year-old woman with a normal intramammary lymph node. Axial CT image (*A*) demonstrates a mass (*arrow*) in the left breast with central low density, corresponding to fatty hilum within a lymph node. Mammogram (*B*) and ultrasound (*C*) show the typical appearance of a benign intramammary lymph node (*arrow*).

CT. The reported rate of abnormality detection on MR imaging is less than on CT, at 0.1% to 3%.[6,18] In a study of incidental breast findings on abdominal MR imaging, 3% (292/11,462) of examinations reported a breast abnormality, and dedicated breast imaging was recommended in 66%. The frequency of incidental breast cancer was 11% of patients who underwent follow-up imaging at their institution, 3% of all patients with reported abnormalities, and 0.99% of patients who underwent abdominal MR imaging.[18] Other studies have reported cancer rates of 8% to 14%.[6,19]

APPROACH
Diagnostic Criteria (Imaging Findings Predictive of Malignancy)

When an incidental breast mass is identified, the initial question is raised: is it malignant? The assessment begins by characterization of features, such as shape, margins, density, pattern of enhancement, and associated findings.[20] Ideally, differentiation of benign and malignant breast findings on CT and MR imaging would be straightforward. However, imaging features of benign and malignant disorders are variable and not specific, with most studies evaluating breast findings on CT showing conflicting results. Some investigators report that ill-defined, spiculated, irregular, or lobular shapes/margins are predictive of malignancy when identified on CT.[11,15,21,22] However, others have found no significant difference in shape and margin characteristics between benign and malignant processes, and 1 study even found that what proved to ultimately be benign findings were more often lobular with spiculated margins.[9,10]

A significant difference in enhancement between benign and malignant breast abnormalities has been shown.[10,21] However, most CT scans are performed as single-phase examinations, and, even in multiphasic examinations, quantitative enhancement analysis is not routinely performed. Nonetheless, contrast-enhanced examinations can reveal nonmass enhancement,[21] and breast findings with fibroglandular background may be obscured on nonenhanced CT.[16] It has even been shown that some abnormalities that could not be detected on mammography or sonography were identified on CT.[22] Abnormalities can be better seen on CT than mammography particularly in the setting of dense breasts or location adjacent to the chest wall.[23] However, it is important to note that CT is not sensitive and can lead to missing large, biopsy-proven breast cancers (**Fig. 2**).

CT and MR imaging can also show local invasion of a malignant breast tumor into the pectoralis muscle or other structures.[24] Although prior work has shown potential utility of CT for assessing the local spread of breast cancer,[25] dedicated breast MR imaging is now used for this purpose.

Finally, axillary lymphadenopathy may be associated with malignant breast tumors. However, this is infrequently seen[9,15] and may be due to non–breast conditions, including lymphoma, arthritis/connective tissue disorders, sarcoid, and infectious disease.

Prior Studies

Although many incidentally discovered breast findings on cross-sectional imaging will require dedicated breast imaging, it is important to review the patient's chart for any prior examinations that may be useful in the diagnosis or prevent the need for further imaging. It may also be prudent to review prior relevant examinations with a breast imaging colleague to correlate with findings seen on CT or MR imaging with the patient's prior mammogram. Review may potentially obviate further workup, as demonstrated in a study on breast incidental findings on abdominal and chest MR imaging, where 92% (240/261) of documented abnormalities corresponded to known benign breast findings.[19]

Guidelines/Imaging Workup

No published guidelines exist for the evaluation of incidentally detected breast findings, to the authors' knowledge. The ACR does address workup of palpable breast abnormalities in the ACR Appropriateness Criteria, which could potentially be used as a framework. The criteria recommend initial evaluation with mammography for patients older than age 40 and initial evaluation with ultrasound for patients younger than age 30. Equal rating is given to mammography and ultrasound for patients between 30 and 39 years of age. It should also be noted that ultrasound is often performed after mammography to work up an indeterminate finding, unless the mammogram is clearly benign (BI-RADS 2).[26]

Although there are no established guidelines, it is generally suggested that radiologists recommend diagnostic mammogram and targeted ultrasound for evaluation of incidental breast abnormalities[2,19] for women older than the age of 40. Ultrasound should be recommended for women younger than age 40, and mammography can be performed at the discretion of the breast imager. In addition, a study found that radiologist recommendation for a specific imaging examination (rather than "per clinician") was associated with a 40% increase in compliance for subsequent diagnostic imaging.[19]

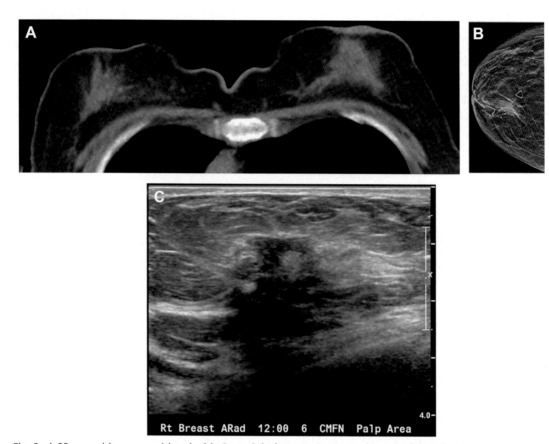

Fig. 2. A 93-year-old woman with palpable 2-cm right breast cancer, occult on CT. (*A*) Right breast mass appears occult on staging CT. Corresponding to the palpable abnormality, there is a spiculated mass seen on right cranio-caudal (CC) mammogram (*B*), with hypoechoic, shadowing appearance on ultrasound (*C*).

IMAGING FINDINGS OF BREAST ABNORMALITIES
Malignant Breast Tumors

Primary breast cancer
Invasive ductal carcinoma Invasive ductal carcinoma (IDC) is the most common subtype, accounting for up to 90% of all invasive breast cancers. If visible on CT/MR imaging, typical findings include a spiculated mass with early and/or peripheral enhancement, although imaging appearance can vary, and a circumscribed process does not exclude malignancy (**Fig. 3**). The microcalcifications and architectural distortion of associated breast cancer detected on mammography are generally not appreciated on CT.[20,27]

Invasive lobular carcinoma Approximately 10% to 15% of invasive breast cancers are invasive lobular carcinomas. This malignancy is more likely to be bilateral and multifocal compared with IDC. As the tumor diffusely infiltrates the breast parenchyma, a discrete mass is often absent. Subtle architectural distortion on mammography is

unlikely to be appreciated on CT. CT and MR imaging may show asymmetric soft tissue and non-mass enhancement (**Fig. 4**).[20,28]

Inflammatory breast carcinoma Inflammatory breast carcinoma is an aggressive malignancy with poor prognosis. It produces the classic "peau d'orange" appearance of the breast on physical examination owing to dermal lymphatic invasion. The breast demonstrates erythema, warmth, induration, and possibly nipple retraction. Clinically, inflammatory carcinoma may resemble mastitis/abscess, but unlike infection, will not completely respond to antibiotic therapy. On imaging, findings of breast edema may be seen, including skin and trabecular thickening, as well as diffusely increased density. Skin thickening is often the most obvious CT finding (**Fig. 5**), and a discrete mass may or may not be visualized. Axillary lymphadenopathy is common[20,23,27] and may be identified on CT.

Mucinous carcinoma Mucinous (colloid) carcinoma is a rare type of well-differentiated

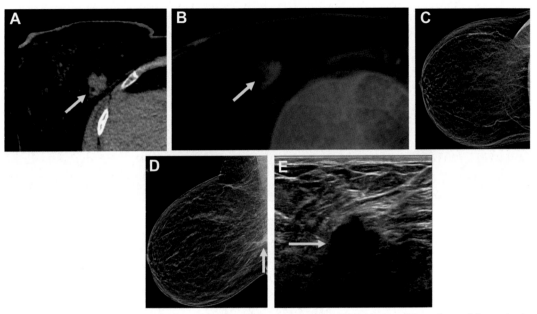

Fig. 3. 70-year-old woman with incidentally detected breast cancer. Axial CT image (A) performed for restaging of a gynecologic malignancy, and subsequent MRI (B), performed for evaluation of a liver mass, demonstrate an irregular, enhancing mass in the right breast (arrow). Note that the mass (arrow) is poorly seen on mammography (C, D) due to its location near the chest wall and is partially visualized on the mediolateral oblique (MLO) (D) view only. Ultrasound (E) demonstrates an irregular, hypoechoic mass (arrow). Biopsy yielded invasive ductal carcinoma.

adenocarcinoma, representing less than 2% of all invasive breast carcinomas, and usually has a good prognosis. Because of the large extracellular mucin composition, these tumors demonstrate hyperintensity on T2-weighted MR images (**Fig. 6**) and may mimic a simple cyst or benign fibroadenoma because classic features of mucinous carcinoma also include a well-circumscribed margin and oval shape. Most mucinous tumors show gradual and progressive enhancement. The imaging features of mucinous carcinoma make it difficult to distinguish from benign processes, particularly on a noncontrast CT or MR image.[29] When seen incidentally, caution must be taken not to dismiss these as inconsequential.

Papillary carcinoma Papillary carcinoma is a rare cause of primary breast cancer, accounting for 1% to 2% of breast carcinomas. They are typically

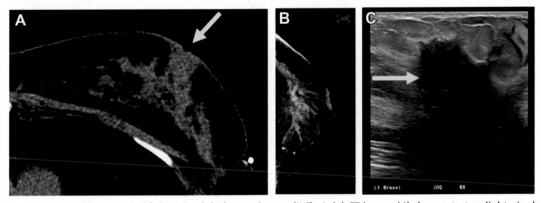

Fig. 4. 60-year-old woman with invasive lobular carcinoma (ILC). Axial CT image (A) demonstrates slight nipple retraction in the left breast (arrow). No discrete mass is appreciated. CC view mammogram (B) shows subtle architectural distortion and nipple retraction ("shrinking breast"), and ultrasound (C) demonstrates a poorly defined, shadowing mass (arrow).

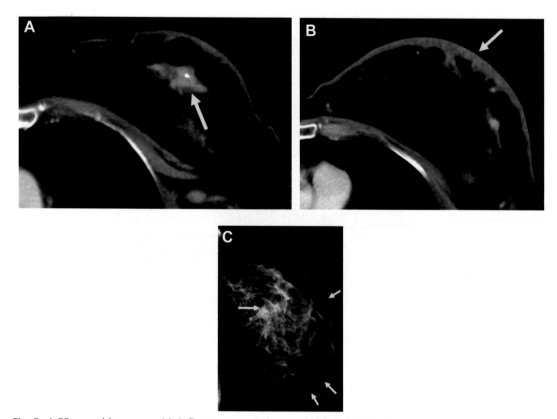

Fig. 5. A 55-year-old woman with inflammatory carcinoma. Axial CT images demonstrate an irregular mass (*arrow* in *A*) with associated biopsy clip (*A*) as well as skin thickening (*arrow* in *B*) (*A, B*). Left CC view mammogram before biopsy (*C*) shows architectural distortion with microcalcifications and skin thickening.

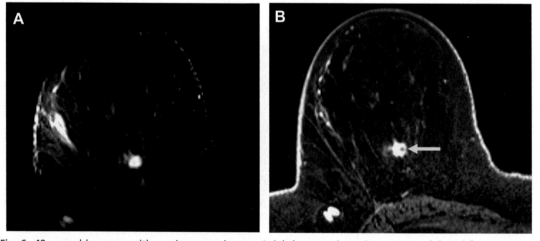

Fig. 6. 49-year-old woman with mucinous carcinoma. Axial short tau inversion recovery (*A*) and fat-suppressed T1-weighted post-contrast (*B*) MR images demonstrate a right breast mass (*arrow*) with high signal intensity on T2-weighted images (*A*) and enhancement (*B*). Artifact from biopsy clip is seen along the medial margin of the mass in (*B*).

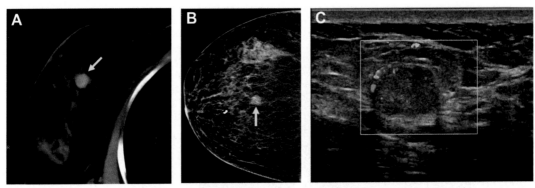

Fig. 7. 59-year-old woman with incidentally detected papillary carcinoma. Axial CT image (*A*) shows a hyper-dense/enhancing, circumscribed right breast mass (*arrow*). Mammogram (*B*) again demonstrates a round mass (*arrow*) and ultrasound (*C*) demonstrates increased vascularity.

circumscribed masses with round, oval, or lobulated shape (**Fig. 7**). Spiculation is rare. These tumors can be entirely solid or have cystic components.[23] Almost half of papillary carcinomas arise in the retroareolar region and are usually found in postmenopausal women.[30]

Paget disease Paget disease is characterized by skin changes of the nipple-areolar complex owing to neoplasia and is most often associated with ductal carcinoma in situ. Paget disease may be occult on imaging and typically is not associated with a discrete mass, but intravenous contrast-enhanced CT or MR imaging may show abnormal enhancement and thickening of the nipple-areolar complex.[31]

Lymphoma

Lymphoma of the breast can be primary or secondary, with secondary more common. Lymphadenopathy is the most common finding, with enlarged, rounded nodes demonstrating loss of fatty hila. Lymphoma can also manifest as diffuse parenchymal thickening, one or more discrete nodules, or as an ill-defined mass that appears similar to primary breast cancer (**Fig. 8**).[20,24] However, when a new breast mass is seen in a patient with lymphoma, although it may reflect secondary lymphomatous involvement of the breast, primary breast cancer should be the top differential diagnosis.[20]

Metastases

Metastatic disease to the breast from a nonmammary primary malignancy is rare, representing approximately 2% of breast cancers. Some common cancers to metastasize to the breast are lymphoma, melanoma, lung, and carcinoid/neuroendocrine tumor. Other sites of metastatic disease are typically present in addition to the breast. Although it may not be possible to distinguish a metastasis from a primary breast cancer on CT/MR imaging, metastases are more frequently

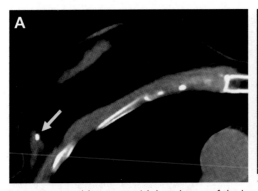
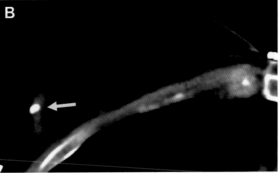

Fig. 8. 62-year-old woman with lymphoma of the breast. Axial CT images (*A, B*) demonstrate multiple right breast masses (*arrows*) with associated biopsy clips. Patient initially presented with a palpable mass and dedicated breast imaging prompted biopsy. The appearance on CT is non-specific, and the masses may not have been detected prospectively. Pathology confirmed low-grade B cell lymphoma. PET scan showed no other lymphadenopathy/masses.

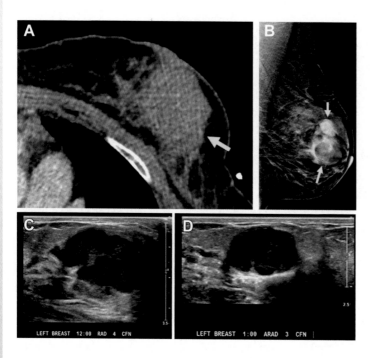

Fig. 9. A 52-year-old woman with melanoma. Axial CT (*A*) demonstrates left breast mass. Mammogram (*B*) and ultrasound (*C*, *D*) show multiple adjacent left breast masses. Biopsy-diagnosed melanoma. No other definite site of disease was identified.

multiple, bilateral, and superficially located (**Fig. 9**).[24,27] Most breast metastases are reported to be round or oval, with homogeneous enhancement and circumscribed margins.[10] They typically do not show the spiculation, microcalcifications, and architectural distortion associated with IDCs.[27]

Benign Breast Abnormalities

Benign masses

Fibroadenoma The most common benign breast tumor, a fibroadenoma, reflects proliferation of connective tissue within a breast lobule. They are usually seen in women of reproductive age. Approximately 20% of patients have multiple and bilateral fibroadenomas. They appear as circumscribed, enhancing masses, which are round or oval (**Fig. 10**). On CT, they may demonstrate the pathognomonic popcorn-shaped calcifications (**Fig. 11**), particularly in postmenopausal patients, although they are often not calcified.[20,24,27] On MR imaging, they can demonstrate nonenhancing fibrous septations, which are considered relatively specific features for fibroadenomas. Hyperintensity on T2-weighted is typically seen in younger patients, whereas hypointensity on T2-weighted images is more common in older patients.[20,28] In the absence of popcorn calcifications on CT or the specific MR imaging features above, confirmation with dedicated breast imaging is needed.

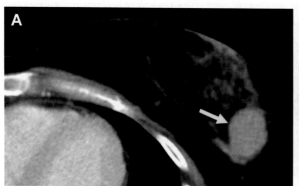
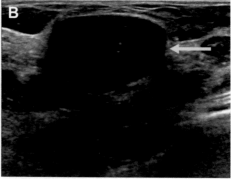

Fig. 10. 35-year-old woman with an incidental breast mass, a presumed fibroadenoma. Axial CT image (*A*) demonstrates a large, mildly lobulated, oval mass (*arrow*) in the left breast. Subsequent ultrasound (*B*) shows an oval, hypoechoic mass (*arrow*). At 9 years of follow-up (not shown), the mass had mildly decreased in size. Findings are compatible with a fibroadenoma.

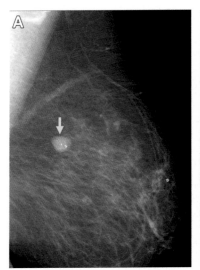
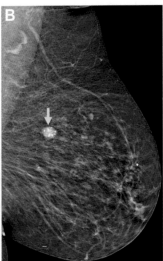
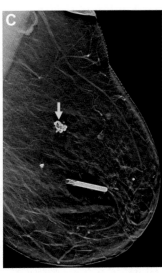

Fig. 11. Mammograms depicting evolution of calcifications in degenerating fibroadenoma. Initial mammogram at age 67 years (*A*) shows a left breast mass with a few small, coarse calcifications. Subsequent mammograms at ages 73 years (*B*) and 79 years (*C*) show increase in associated calcifications over time. A cardiac loop recorder is also present in panel (*C*).

Hamartoma A breast hamartoma, also known as a fibroadenolipoma, is a mass that contains fat and glandular tissue ("breast within a breast"). On CT or MR imaging, they appear as heterogenous, circumscribed masses with macroscopic fat.[20] Hamartomas with this classic appearance can be diagnosed as such without further evaluation with mammography/ultrasound.

Intraductal papilloma Papillomas are benign intraductal masses that may present with nipple discharge. Solitary papillomas are typically central/retroareolar in location (**Fig. 12**), whereas multiple papillomas are usually peripherally located, as they arise from the terminal ductal lobular units. Multiple papillomas are more commonly associated with atypia or malignancy; however, solitary intraductal papilloma also confers an increased

risk of breast malignancy. Smaller papillomas can be difficult to detect, as they may be obscured by retroareolar breast tissue. When visualized, they typically appear round or oval, with circumscribed margins. Mammography may show associated calcifications. Ultrasound, galactography, or MR imaging may better depict the intraductal location of the mass.[30] Most papillomas present as small masses (<1 cm) and may not be detected on cross-sectional imaging.

Fat necrosis Fat necrosis is a common finding seen after surgery or breast trauma, but sometimes no corresponding history is present. It is a sterile inflammation owing to compromised blood supply.[32] On CT, a mass with variable enhancement, rim calcification, and central fat can be seen (**Fig. 13**).[2,32] MR imaging will also demonstrate the

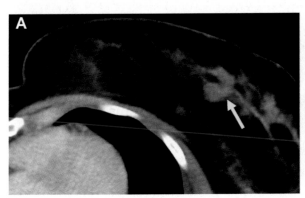
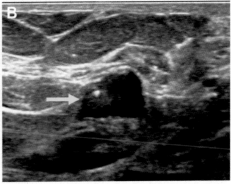

Fig. 12. 48-year-old woman with papilloma. Axial CT image (*A*) shows a non-specific, lobulated mass (*arrow*) in the central left breast. Ultrasound (*B*) shows a complex cystic mass (*arrow*). Pathology yielded papilloma.

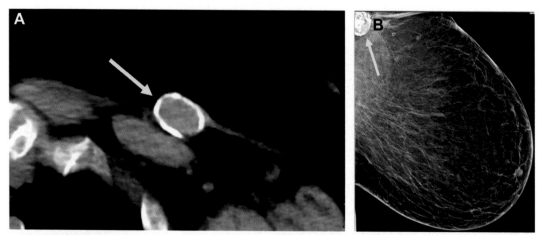

Fig. 13. A 68-year-old woman with fat necrosis. Axial CT image (*A*) and MLO mammogram (*B*) show a peripherally calcified mass in the axillary tail of the left breast. Note that the central fat with rim calcification on CT is diagnostic for fat necrosis in this case.

fat component, although the signal intensity will otherwise be variable if hemosiderin is present. Enhancement is also variable and may be rim or non-mass-like. The presence of central fat, as well as clinical history, will aid in differentiating fat necrosis from tumor recurrence. Nonetheless, the appearance of fat necrosis can mimic malignancy, and further workup with mammography, ultrasound, and even biopsy may be necessary.[32]

Asymmetric/accessory breast tissue Otherwise normal breast tissue typically does not appear symmetric bilaterally (**Fig. 14**). Patients may also have additional glandular tissue in the posterior upper outer quadrant and axilla, separate from the main gland, referred to as accessory breast tissue. Accessory breast tissue can also occur anywhere along the "milk line," which spans from the axilla to the groin. On imaging, accessory breast tissue demonstrates the same characteristics as normal glandular tissue. It should be noted that malignancy can also occur in the accessory tissue, so this should be scrutinized similar to the remainder of the breast.[24]

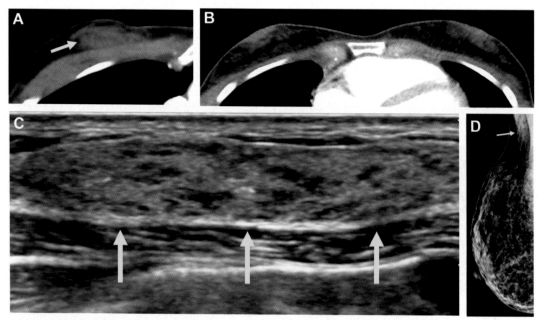

Fig. 14. 43-year-old woman with asymmetric breast tissue. Axial CT (*A*) shows mass-like tissue (*arrow*) in the upper inner quadrant of the right breast, separate from the central breast tissue (*B*). Mammogram (*C*) and targeted ultrasound (*D*) demonstrate normal-appearing, dense, fibroglandular tissue (*arrows* in *C, D*).

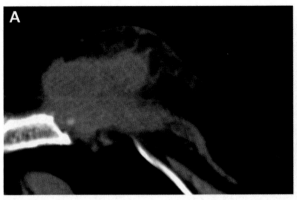
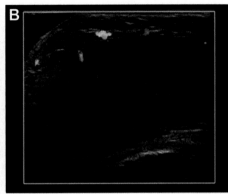

Fig. 15. A 97-year-old woman with left breast abscess. Axial CT image (*A*) demonstrates a multiloculated left breast abscess extending to the chest wall. Ultrasound (*B*) shows an avascular, complex cystic mass with surrounding edema.

Abscess Breast abscesses occur in the setting of infectious mastitis, typically from bacterial infection from skin contamination. Abscesses can develop in women who are breastfeeding (puerperal) or outside of the breastfeeding period. Clinical symptoms include pain, erythema, warmth, and sometimes a palpable mass. The presence of an abscess complicating mastitis may not be clinically apparent. If an abscess is suspected, evaluation with ultrasound is the most appropriate imaging examination. However, CT and MR imaging can show the collection (**Fig. 15**). Clinical history should aid in distinguishing an abscess from other collections, such as a hematoma or seroma, although overlap exists, particularly in the postoperative setting. Treatment consists of antibiotics and ultrasound-guided drainage.[33]

Calcifications

Breast calcifications are common incidental findings on CT but are poorly seen on MR imaging. However, although calcifications are often seen in association with malignancy on mammography, almost all calcifications visualized at CT are benign, owing to limited spatial resolution. If possible, morphology and distribution should be described, noting that some calcifications are associated with an underlying mass, such as a degenerating fibroadenoma. The patterns of calcifications classically associated with benignity include lucent-centered, eggshell or rim, coarse or popcorn, large rodlike, and round. The fine pleomorphic calcifications often associated with malignancy are generally not visualized on CT.[20]

Nipple inversion

Nipple retraction and inversion can be unilateral or bilateral, congenital, or acquired. Although nipple retraction is usually benign, development over a short time is suspicious for malignancy. Benign causes include fibrosis and duct ectasia-periductal mastitis complex.[27] If nipple inversion or retraction is identified incidentally on CT/MR imaging (**Fig. 16**) and prior examinations demonstrating long-term stability are not available, further evaluation with dedicated breast imaging should be performed.[31]

Lactation

During pregnancy and breastfeeding, the breasts become engorged, with increase in milk volume, lymphatic and vascular congestion, and edema. CT and MR imaging will demonstrate cordlike and masslike tissue (**Fig. 17**). The findings can appear asymmetric and mimic pathologic condition, necessitating investigation of clinical history or further imaging. Differential diagnosis may include entities such as lymphoma, inflammatory breast carcinoma, and inflammation.[34] As discussed previously, abscesses are frequently seen in the setting of breastfeeding (puerperal abscess). In addition, cancer does occur during pregnancy and the postpartum period, so it remains important to scrutinize the lactating breast for concomitant pathologic conditions.

Gynecomastia

Gynecomastia is characterized by breast enlargement caused by proliferation of ductal and stromal tissue. It is the most common abnormality of the male breast with numerous causes, including hormonal imbalance, cirrhosis, renal disease, and drug use, among others. Clinically, patients may present with breast enlargement, a palpable lump, or breast pain.[24] There are 3 patterns of gynecomastia seen on imaging: nodular, dendritic, and diffuse glandular.[35] Findings can be symmetric or asymmetric, but the tissue seen in

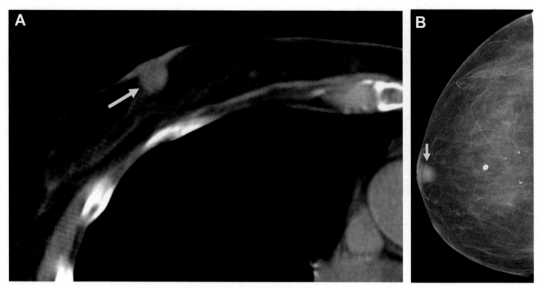

Fig. 16. 93-year-old woman with inverted nipple. Axial CT image (*A*) shows a rounded subareolar mass (*arrow*) in the right breast, compatible with an inverted nipple. Mammogram (*B*) from years prior demonstrates long-term stability of nipple inversion (*arrow*), illustrating importance of correlating with prior imaging to avoid unnecessary workup.

gynecomastia is always retroareolar (**Fig. 18**).[35] Tissue that is eccentric to the nipple and does not demonstrate the classic flame shape of gynecomastia is suspicious for male breast cancer.[27] About 0.7% of breast cancers are diagnosed in men, with risk factors including Klinefelter syndrome, BRCA1 or BRCA2, family history, hyperestrogenism, advanced age, a history of chest radiation, and exogenous estrogen treatment.[35] Note that there is overlap in risk factors for gynecomastia and male breast cancer. Delay in diagnosis often results in men presenting at a more advanced stage than women with breast cancer.[35] Mammography has a high sensitivity (92%) and specificity (90%) for the differentiation between benign and malignant male breast disease[36] and should be recommended for indeterminate findings on CT/MR imaging.

Postoperative findings

Hematoma/seroma Fluid collections are common findings in the postoperative breast, usually reflecting hematoma or seroma (**Fig. 19**). Hematomas are typically high attenuation on CT and hyperintense on T1-weighted MR images, although appearance varies based on age of blood products. Hematomas can be circumscribed or ill-defined and may exhibit spiculated margins owing to fibrosis from healing. Therefore, hematomas can sometimes mimic malignancy, making clinical history crucial. A hematoma or seroma will also decrease in size over time.[20,23,24]

Scar Fibrous scars may develop at biopsy or excision sites. Immediately after the procedure, air and fluid will be present at the site. Subsequent healing will form a scar with architectural distortion or a spiculated mass with central density (**Fig. 20**). Consequently, these findings can also mimic malignancy, and clinical history with location of prior intervention is necessary. If a patient develops increased tissue at the site of a prior scar, recurrent malignancy should be suspected,[20] and a diagnostic mammogram should be performed.

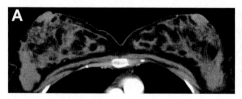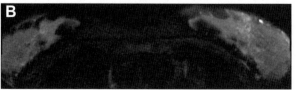

Fig. 17. Lactating breasts. Axial CT (*A*) in a postpartum patient demonstrates dense breasts with cordlike and masslike tissue. Axial T2-weighted fat-suppressed MR image (*B*) in a different postpartum patient demonstrates engorgement of the bilateral breasts.

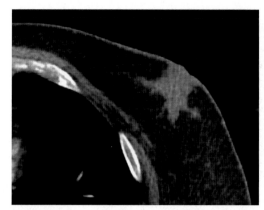

Fig. 18. 66-year-old man with unilateral gynecomastia. Axial CT image shows subareolar dendritic tissue in the left breast, which is highly consistent with gynecomastia.

Autologous tissue flap Myocutaneous and muscle-sparing free flap autologous tissue transfers are popular options for breast reconstruction following mastectomy. Free flaps, specifically the deep inferior epigastric perforator flap, has gained favor because of reduction in donor site morbidity. On CT and MR imaging, the breast will be homogeneous fat tissue (**Fig. 21**). Compromise of vascular supply can lead to flap necrosis, which is a clinical, not imaging, diagnosis.[32]

Implant complications Multiple breast implant findings can be seen on imaging. Capsular contracture or fibrosis manifests as thickened tissue surrounding the implant with development of calcification and possible change in shape of the implant.[2,37] The breast may become inflamed and painful. Contracture is most frequently observed in the first few months after implant placement.[37]

Although rupture of a saline implant results in decompression of the breast and is clinically apparent, rupture of a silicone implant may be clinically occult.[2,37] Symptoms of implant rupture may include contour deformity, displacement, palpable mass, pain, and inflammation.[38] Intracapsular rupture is more common than extracapsular, and the risk increases with age of the implant. With intracapsular rupture, the fibrous capsule remains intact, preventing translation of silicone into the surrounding breast tissue (**Fig. 22**). There are multiple radiologic signs describing intracapsular rupture, the classic being the "linguine sign," typically visualized on MR imaging but sometimes seen on CT.[2,37] The linguine sign reflects collapsed layer of the implant shell floating in silicone. MR imaging has high sensitivity and specificity for implant rupture.[39]

Intracapsular rupture is typically not visible on mammography. With extracapsular rupture, free silicone is seen outside of the fibrous capsule, in the breast parenchyma, or in axillary lymph nodes.[37]

Breast implant-associated anaplastic large-cell lymphoma (BIA-ALCL) is a rare peripheral T-cell lymphoma associated with textured implants (textured surface developed to diminish risk of tight scar capsule) but is increasing in incidence. Patients typically present with an enlarging breast because of a malignant fluid collection surrounding the implant, although some cases may be

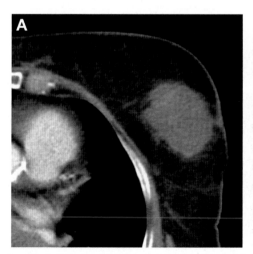
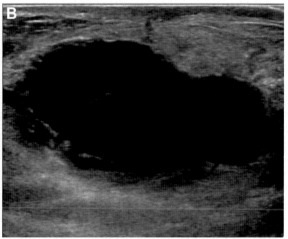

Fig. 19. A 78-year-old woman with seroma. Axial CT image (*A*) shows a mildly lobulated, left breast mass with density of 20 HU. Ultrasound (*B*) demonstrates an anechoic, circumscribed mass consistent with a seroma. Patient had a left breast lumpectomy 4 months before CT.

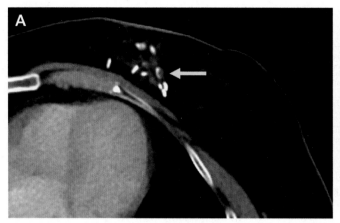
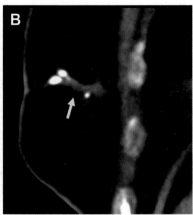

Fig. 20. 70-year-old woman with history of left breast lumpectomy. Axial (*A*) and sagittal (*B*) CT images show clips and calcifications associated with left breast linear scar (*arrows*).

associated with a mass.[40] Ultrasound is the first-line imaging modality of choice in symptomatic patients. However, because patients may not always be attentive to the changes in the breast, it is important to include BIA-ALCL in the differential diagnosis of a unilateral peri-implant effusion, which may be detected on CT or MRI.

Interstitial mammoplasty/injection granulomas
Interstitial mammoplasty is an augmentation technique consisting of direct injection of silicone or paraffin into the breast. These procedures are no longer legally performed in the United States but can be seen in other countries. Injection can result in development of granulomas and calcifications. When silicone has been injected, the typical appearance is well-defined, round, dense, or peripherally calcified nodules (**Fig. 23**). Paraffin injections are more ill-defined, with associated distortion and dense, streaky opacities that may have ring calcifications.[24,25,37]

AXILLARY LYMPHADENOPATHY

There are numerous causes of axillary lymphadenopathy, the most common being nonspecific reactive hyperplasia and breast cancer metastases. Vaccination in the ipsilateral arm is a common cause of reactive hyperplasia. Other malignancies that frequently involve axillary nodes include lymphoma and leukemia as well as melanoma and ovarian cancer. Infection (tuberculosis, cat-scratch disease, human immunodeficiency virus, and mononucleosis), connective tissue diseases (rheumatoid arthritis, systemic lupus erythematosus, psoriatic arthritis, dermatomyositis-polymyositis, and scleroderma), and granulomatous diseases

(sarcoidosis, granulomatosis with polyangiitis) can also cause axillary lymphadenopathy.[41] Given the myriad causes of lymphadenopathy, obtaining a detailed history can be invaluable.

Radiologically, it can be difficult to distinguish benign from pathologic lymph nodes. Some imaging findings suggestive of pathologic condition include increased size, rounded or irregular shape, asymmetric cortical thickening, loss of fatty hilum, and poorly circumscribed margins. A single abnormal-appearing node is suspicious for malignancy, whereas multiple, bilateral abnormal-appearing nodes are often seen in reactive, nonneoplastic processes.[41]

Evaluation of axillary lymphadenopathy should incorporate radiologic appearance and clinical context. Biopsy is appropriate for suspected

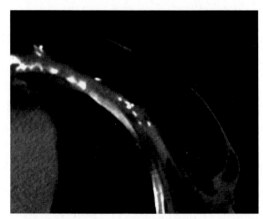

Fig. 21. A 79-year-old woman with left breast free flap reconstruction. Axial CT image demonstrates entirely fatty appearance of the left breast flap with surgical clips along the chest wall.

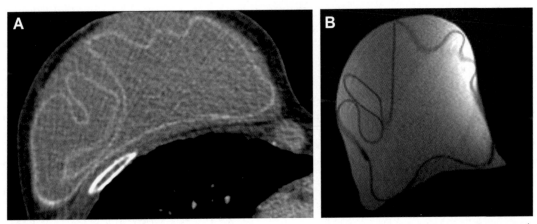

Fig. 22. A 56-year-old woman with ruptured implant. Axial CT (*A*) and MR imaging (*B*) demonstrate intracapsular rupture of right breast silicone implant.

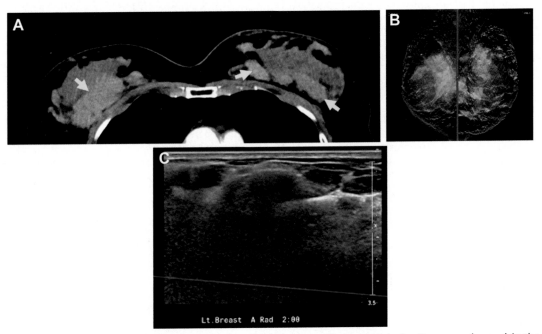

Fig. 23. 60-year-old woman with injected silicone. Axial CT image (*A*) shows high-density masses (*arrows*) in the breasts bilaterally. Bilateral mammogram (*B*) demonstrates extremely dense breasts with numerous silicone granulomas. Ultrasound (*C*) shows "dirty" acoustic shadowing posterior to the silicone.

breast cancer metastases and for lymphadenopathy of uncertain cause.[41]

SUMMARY

Although routine cross-sectional imaging is not sensitive for the detection of breast cancer, incidental breast findings are common, and evaluation of the breasts is essential. It is important for radiologists to recognize the CT and MR imaging appearance of these entities in order to appropriately guide management.

CLINICS CARE POINTS

- Examination of the breasts on cross-sectional imaging is essential and can result in significant numbers of incidentally detected breast cancers.

- When an incidental breast finding is identified, one should evaluate its characteristics as well as the clinical history and prior imaging examinations to determine need for further workup.

- In the absence of long-term stability or previous characterization, most breast masses detected at computed tomography and MR imaging will require further workup, generally with mammography and targeted ultrasound. Breast imaging evaluation of women younger than the age of 40 should include ultrasound, and mammography can be performed at the discretion of the radiologist/breast imager.

- Routine cross-sectional imaging is not sensitive for detection of breast cancer, and large cancers may be present in the breast but not identified on computed tomography or non-breast-dedicated MR imaging.

- Evaluation of axillary lymphadenopathy should be based on clinical context and imaging appearance. Biopsy is appropriate for suspected breast cancer metastases and for lymphadenopathy of unknown cause.

DISCLOSURE

Dr R. Hooley is a consultant for Hologic. The other authors have nothing to disclose.

REFERENCES

1. Ikeda D, Miyake KK. Mammogram analysis and interpretation. In: Thrall JH, editor. Breast imaging: the requisites. 3rd edition. St Louis (MO): Elsevier; 2016. p. 30–74.
2. Gossner J. Intramammary findings on CT of the chest- a review of normal anatomy and possible findings. Pol J Radiol 2016;81:415–21.
3. Miyake KK, Ikeda DM, Daniel BL. Magnetic resonance imaging of breast cancer and magnetic resonance imaging-guided breast biopsy. In: Thrall JH, editor. Breast imaging: the requisites. St Louis (MO): Elsevier; 2016. p. 259–320.
4. How common is breast cancer?. 2020. Available at: https://www.cancer.org/cancer/breast-cancer/about/how-common-is-breast-cancer.html. Accessed August 25, 2020.
5. Global cancer observatory: Breast. Available at: https://gco.iarc.fr/today/data/factsheets/cancers/20-Breast-fact-sheet.pdf. Accessed March 15, 2021.
6. Falomo E, Strigel RM, Bruce R, et al. Incidence and outcomes of incidental breast lesions detected on cross-sectional imaging examinations. Breast J 2018;24:743–8.
7. Monzawa S, Washio T, Yasuoka R, et al. Incidental detection of clinically unexpected breast lesions by computed tomography. Acta Radiol Diagn 2013; 54:374–9.
8. Hussain A, Gordon Dixon A, Almusawy H, et al. The incidence and outcome of incidental breast lesions detected by computer tomography. Ann R Coll Surg Engl 2010;92:124–6.
9. Bach AG, Abbas J, Jasaabuu C, et al. Comparison between incidental malignant and benign breast lesions detected by computed tomography: a systematic review. J Med Imaging Radiat Oncol 2013;57: 529–33.
10. Surov A, Fiedler E, Wienke A, et al. Intramammary incidental findings on staging computer tomography. Eur J Radiol 2012;81:2174–8.
11. Moyle P, Sonoda L, Britton P, et al. Incidental breast lesions detected on CT: what is their significance? Br J Radiol 2010;83:233–40.
12. Schramm D, Jasaabuu C, Bach AG, et al. Costs associated with evaluation of incidental breast lesions identified on computed tomography. Br J Radiol 2016;89:20140847.
13. Healey TT, Agarwal S, Patel R, et al. Cancer yield of incidental breast lesions detected on chest computed tomography. J Comput Assist Tomogr 2018;42(3):453–6.
14. Parvaiz MA, Isgar B. Letter to the editor- incidental breast lesions detected on diagnostic CT scans: a 4-year prospective study. Breast J 2013;19(4):457–9.
15. Poyraz N, Emlik GD, Keskin S, et al. Incidental breast lesions detected on computed thorax tomography. Eur J Breast Health 2015;11:163–7.
16. Lin W-C, Hsu H-H, Li C-S, et al. Incidentally detected enhancing breast lesions on chest computed tomography. Korean J Radiol 2011;12:44–51.

17. Hiroko Shojaku HS, Iwai H, Kitazawa S, et al. Detection of incidental breast tumors by noncontrast spiral computed tomography of the chest. Jpn J Radiol 2008;26:362–7.

18. Prabhu V, Chhor CM, Ego-Osuala IO, et al. Frequency and outcomes of incidental breast lesions detected on abdominal MRI over a 7-year period. AJR Am J Roentgenol 2017;208:107–13.

19. Larson KE, Rios S, Amin AL, et al. Breast incidental findings on abdominal and chest MRI. Breast J 2020;00:1–3.

20. Harish MG, Konda SD, MacMahon H, et al. Breast lesions incidentally detected with CT: what the general radiologist needs to know. RadioGraphics 2007; 27:S37–51.

21. Lin Y-P, Hsu H-H, Ko K-H, et al. Differentiation of malignant and benign incidental breast lesions detected by chest multidetector-row computed tomography: added value of quantitative enhancement analysis. PLoS One 2016;11(4):e0154569.

22. Inoue M, Sano T, Watai R, et al. Dynamic multidetector of breast tumors: diagnostic features and comparison with conventional techniques. AJR Am J Roentgenol 2003;181:679–86.

23. Kin SM, Park JM. Computed tomography of the breast- abnormal findings with mammographic and sonographic correlation. J Comput Assist Tomogr 2003;27:761–70.

24. Son JH, Jung HK, Song JW, et al. Incidentally detected breast lesions on chest CT with US correlation: a pictorial essay. Diagn Interv Radiol 2016;22: 514–8.

25. Nishino M, Hayakawa K, Yamamoto A, et al. Multiple enhancing lesions detected on dynamic helical computed tomography-mammography. J Comput Assist Tomogr 2003;27(5):771–8.

26. Moy L, Heller SL, Bailey L, et al. ACR appropriateness criteria- palpable breast mass. J Am Coll Radiol 2017;14(5):S203–24.

27. Yi JG, Kim SJ, Marom EM, et al. Chest CT of incidental breast lesions. J Thorac Imaging 2008;23: 148–55.

28. Macura KJ, Ouwerkerk R, Jacobs MA, et al. Patterns of enhancement on breast MR images: interpretation and imaging pitfalls. RadioGraphics 2006;26: 1719–34.

29. Bitencourt AGV, Graziano L, Osorio CABT, et al. MRI features of mucinous cancer of the breast: correlation with pathologic findings and other imaging methods. AJR Am J Roentgenol 2016;206:238–46.

30. Eiada R, Chong J, Kulkarni S, et al. Papillary lesions of the breast: MRI, ultrasound, and mammographic appearances. AJR Am J Roentgenol 2012;198: 264–71.

31. Nicholson BT, Harvey JA, Cohen MA. Nipple-areolar complex: normal anatomy and benign and malignant processes. RadioGraphics 2009;29:509–23.

32. Neal CH, Yilmaz ZN, Noroozian M, et al. Imaging of breast cancer-related changes after surgical therapy. AJR Am J Roentgenol 2014;202:262–72.

33. Isabelle Trop M, Alexandre D, David J, et al. Breast abscesses: evidence-based algorithms for diagnosis, management, and follow-up. RadioGraphics 2011;31:1683–99.

34. Brook OR, Guralnik L, Keidar Z, et al. Pitfalls of the lactating breast on computed tomography. J Comput Assist Tomogr 2004;28(5):647–9.

35. Nguyen C, Kettler MD, Swirsky ME, et al. Male breast disease: pictorial review with radiologic-pathologic correlation. RadioGraphics 2013;33: 763–79.

36. Evans GF, Anthony T, Turnage RH, et al. The diagnostic accuracy of mammography in the evaluation of male breast disease. Am J Surg 2001;181(2): 96–100.

37. Yang N, Muradali D. The augmented breast: a pictorial review of the abnormal and unusual. AJR Am J Roentgenol 2011;196:W451–60.

38. Juanpere S, Perez E, Huc O, et al. Imaging of breast implants- a pictorial review. Insights Imaging 2011;2: 653–70.

39. Ikeda DM, Borofsky HB, Herfkens RJ, et al. Silicone breast implant rupture: pitfalls of magnetic resonance imaging and relative efficacies of magnetic resonance, mammography, and ultrasound. Plast Reconstr Surg 1999;104:2054–62.

40. Sharma B, Jurgensen-Rauch A, Pace E, et al. Breast-implant-associated anaplastic large cell lymphoma: review and multiparametric imaging paradigms. RadioGraphics 2020;40(3):609–28.

41. Cao MM, Hoyt AC, Bassett LW. Mammographic signs of systemic disease. RadioGraphics 2011;31: 1085–100.

Incidental Liver Findings on Cross-sectional Imaging

Adam C. Searleman, MD, PhD, Lejla Aganovic, MD, Cynthia S. Santillan, MD*

KEYWORDS

- Incidental finding • Hepatocellular carcinoma • Hepatic cyst • Hepatic adenoma • Hemangioma
- CT • MR imaging • Ultrasound

KEY POINTS

- Hepatic incidental findings often are seen on ultrasound, computed tomography, and MR imaging examinations; however, not all such findings require additional evaluation, which otherwise can be relatively costly and result in patient anxiety.
- A focal hepatic finding is more likely to require further evaluation in high-risk patients, including those patients with underlying liver disease or known malignancy.
- Simple cysts identified on ultrasound are unlikely to require further evaluation due to a high likelihood of benignity.
- Focal hepatic findings less than 1 cm in low-risk patients are unlikely to require further evaluation.

INTRODUCTION

Focal hepatic findings frequently are discovered incidentally on cross-sectional imaging performed for reasons other than for evaluation of the liver. Because these examinations often are not optimized for characterization of such hepatic findings, careful consideration should be given to whether these incidental liver findings (ie, incidentalomas) require further characterization. The role of the radiologist is to recognize and attempt to characterize these findings and, if required, to suggest appropriate follow-up. It is important to identify clinically actionable findings correctly, while making appropriate use of health care resources. The Incidental Findings Committee of the American College of Radiology (ACR) published their recommendations in 2010, with updates in 2017, that provide guidance on the management of liver incidentalomas detected by computed tomography (CT).[1]

In the general population, a vast majority of incidental liver findings are benign entities: most commonly cysts, hemangiomas, and perfusion alterations. More than 5% of patients have liver metastases at the time of diagnosis of an extrahepatic malignancy, most commonly breast and colorectal cancer; therefore, a radiologist's recognition of an incidental possible malignant hepatic nodule or mass may be the first step toward the diagnosis of an extrahepatic malignancy.[2] Primary hepatic malignancies also may be detected incidentally but occur much less commonly than metastases.

The general approach for evaluating an incidental focal hepatic finding is to (1) consider whether technical factors allow for adequate interpretation; (2) determine the presence of features supporting benignity and/or malignancy; (3) compare to any prior imaging, including across modalities; and (4) interpret the risk of malignancy in the context of patient-specific factors, including age, gender, any history of malignancy or concurrent imaging/clinical findings suggesting malignancy, and the presence or absence of chronic liver disease.

Department of Radiology, University of California San Diego, UCSD Medical Center, 200 West Arbor Drive, #8756, San Diego, CA 92103, USA
* Corresponding author.
E-mail address: csantillan@health.ucsd.edu

Radiol Clin N Am 59 (2021) 569–590
https://doi.org/10.1016/j.rcl.2021.03.007
0033-8389/21/© 2021 Elsevier Inc. All rights reserved.

The liver often is included, at least partially, on CT and MR imaging examinations of the abdomen, thorax, thoracolumbar spine, pelvis, and breast as well as on ultrasound examinations, including renal ultrasound. As such, incidental focal liver findings may be detected under circumstances that do not provide sufficient information to make a confident specific diagnosis. For ultrasound examinations, factors that influence the adequacy of the examination for characterization of focal liver findings include the transducer, frequency, focal zone, depth, and gain; in some cases, the finding may be more fully interrogated by the sonographer and in other cases recognized only retrospectively. For CT examinations, the resolution, reconstruction method, and phase of contrast (if any) are important considerations. Slice thickness may limit evaluation of small focal findings. MR examinations have similar considerations as CT examinations; however, the liver may be included only in a few sequences or only localizer sequences, and, for spine MR imaging, the liver may be obscured by the suppression band. Additionally, all imaging modalities have potential artifacts that may obscure all or part of the suspected liver finding, particularly when the focus of the examination was not the liver.

This article describes the multimodality imaging features of various focal liver findings and proposes an algorithmic approach for management of such incidental liver findings on ultrasound, CT, and MR examinations, which are inadequate for complete characterization of the liver. The authors' recommended approach is to evaluate first whether there are any imaging features that are suspicious for malignancy and then to assess for the presence of features that suggest benignity. These imaging features include morphology, location, multiplicity, echogenicity/attenuation/signal, and growth (**Table 1**). Additionally, the liver should be evaluated for secondary findings, including the presence of mass effect, perfusion alterations, biliary obstruction, capsular retraction, or underlying chronic liver disease, in particular, cirrhosis or steatosis.

The imaging features of focal hepatic findings can overlap: atypical manifestations of benign processes can simulate malignancy, and some malignant tumors can resemble benign processes. This is true for dedicated liver imaging, and thus is particularly salient for imaging examinations that were not optimized for liver evaluation. It is crucial to understand patient-specific risk factors when evaluating a focal liver abnormality, because an atypical appearance of a benign process is far more common in patients who are at low risk of malignancy. For instance, focal liver findings less than 1 cm in size almost always are benign in low-risk patients, whereas in patients with known malignancy, approximately 10% demonstrate progressive growth and are presumed to represent metastases.[3] Additionally, patients with most forms of cirrhosis or chronic hepatitis B infections should be evaluated based on the Liver Imaging Reporting and Data System (LI-RADS) criteria due to the markedly increased risk of primary liver malignancy. For simplicity, patients can be stratified into low-risk and high-risk categories, as proposed by the ACR in 2017, and as shown in **Box 1**.[1] In practice, the ordering provider also should consider a patient's wider clinical context when considering the recommendations of the interpreting radiologist.

Table 1	
Key imaging features of incidental focal liver findings	
Morphology	Size
	Shape
	Margin
	Internal architecture
Location	Central vs peripheral
	Segment vs lobe vs diffuse
	Peribiliary vs periportal
Multiplicity	Single
	Multiple
Growth	Stable vs enlarging vs shrinking

Box 1
Patient risk factors
Low-risk patients[a]
No known malignancy
No hepatic dysfunction
No hepatic risk factors[b]
High-risk patients
Known malignancy with a propensity to metastasize to the liver
Cirrhosis
Presence of hepatic risk factors[b]

[a] Within the low-risk patient category, patients greater than 40 years old are considered at higher risk than younger patients. [b] Hepatic risk factors include hepatitis, nonalcoholic steatohepatitis, sclerosing cholangitis, primary biliary cirrhosis, choledochal cysts, hemochromatosis, anabolic, and steroid use.
From Gore RM, et al., Management of incidental liver lesions on CT: a white paper of the ACR Incidental Findings Committee. J Am Coll Radiol, 2017. 14(11): p. 1429-1437; with permission.

CYSTIC INCIDENTAL FINDINGS

When an incidental finding is primarily cystic, attention should be given to the size, distribution, complexity, margins, relationship to the biliary tract, and enhancement patterns, to assess the risk of malignancy. Additional imaging may be needed if these features are not well evaluated or appear atypical, especially in high-risk patients. Both benign and malignant cystic processes can have mass effect, which may manifest as biliary obstruction or perfusion alteration. The most common cystic liver processes are discussed later. Uncommon cystic findings not discussed further here include very unusual findings, such as hepatic lymphangioma and mesenchymal hamartoma; those secondary to trauma, such as seroma/liquefied hematoma; and biloma as well as infectious or inflammatory cysts.[4]

Definitely Benign: Simple Hepatic Cyst

Hepatic cysts are extremely common and can be found in 2% to 18% of the general adult population, with a slight female predilection.[5] True simple cysts are developmental and are composed of a thin wall lined with cuboidal epithelium, which do not communicate with the biliary tract.[6] A vast majority of hepatic cysts are asymptomatic. Hepatic cysts are round or ovoid foci, ranging from several millimeters to multiple centimeters in size, but most are less than 3 cm. All have well-defined margins. Most cysts are unilocular and can have up to 2 thin and nonenhancing septations.[7] Hepatic cysts may be solitary or multiple. On ultrasound, cysts appear as anechoic structures with thin or imperceptible walls and a clearly defined posterior wall. Increased through-transmission should be seen except with small cysts. On CT, cysts are homogeneous, fluid attenuation structures (<20 Hounsfield units [HU] when large enough to measure accurately) with sharp margins and no internal or mural enhancement. On MR imaging, they are homogeneous with sharp margins, very high signal on T2-weighted imaging (T2WI), similar to urine, bile, and cerebrospinal

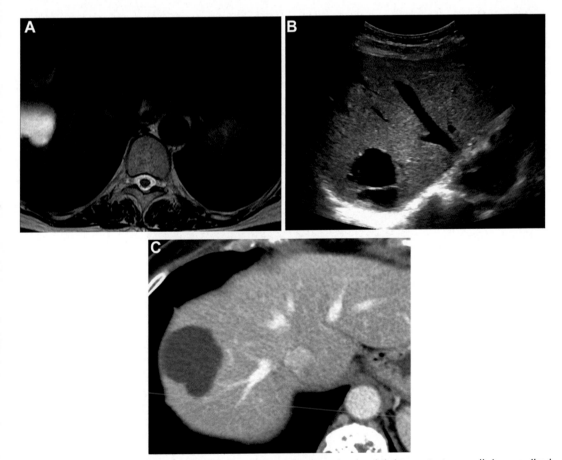

Fig. 1. Hepatic cyst. Axial T2-weighted MR image from a spine examination (*A*) demonstrates a well circumscribed cyst in the liver dome. Transabdominal ultrasound image shows a septated cyst in the posterior right hepatic lobe (*B*). The same cyst is shown as a well circumscribed low attenuation focal process on an IV contrast-enhanced axial CT image (*C*).

fluid, and low signal on T1-weighted imaging (T1WI) **(Fig. 1)**. They exhibit no enhancement and have no restricted diffusion.

Atypical manifestations

True hepatic cysts sometimes can contain hemorrhage or other debris, resulting in mild complexity or layering components, in which cases the cyst no longer is considered simple. Wall calcifications can develop as sequelae of hemorrhage or infection. Hemorrhagic or highly proteinaceous cysts can have increased signal on T1WI and decreased signal on T2WI but should demonstrate no enhancement with CT or MR imaging (or ultrasound) contrast media.

Suspicious features

Wall or septal thickening, nodularity, and enhancement are suspicious features warranting further evaluation.

Definitely Benign: Biliary Hamartomas

Also known as von Meyenburg complexes, biliary hamartomas are benign ductal plate malformations composed of disorganized dilated bile ducts within a fibrous stroma that result from failure of embryonic bile ducts to involute.[6] In most cases, there is no communication with the biliary tract. The prevalence is approximately 3% to 6% at autopsy and 1.5% by imaging.[8] In rare cases, malignant degeneration to cholangiocarcinoma has been described.[9] Biliary hamartomas typically present as numerous small rounded or irregular structures throughout the liver, with well-defined margins and a predilection for the subcapsular region. Biliary hamartomas typically are 0.5 cm to 1.5 cm and relatively uniform in size.[10] Many hamartomas are less than 5 mm in size and, therefore, can be difficult to detect by ultrasound and CT but usually are well seen on MR with T2WI due to the high internal signal intensity **(Fig. 2)**. On ultrasound, visualized foci can appear hypoechoic,

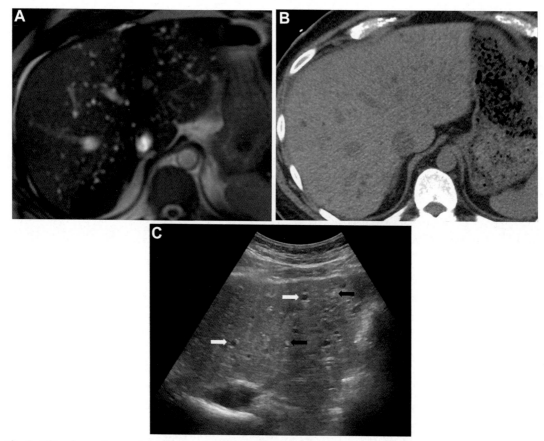

Fig. 2. Biliary hamartomas. Axial steady-state free-precession image from a cardiac MR imaging examination (*A*) demonstrates numerous hyperintense small foci throughout the liver. Axial nonenhanced CT image in the same patient (*B*) shows many low attenuation foci, although fewer than those visible on the MR examination. Overall, the foci are smaller than 1 cm. Transverse ultrasound image of the left hepatic lobe demonstrates several small cysts (*white arrows*); small echogenic foci represent smaller hamartomas (*black arrows*) (*C*).

hyperechoic, or mixed, depending on the size and composition. Foci below ultrasound resolution may appear as a region of heterogeneous parenchymal echotexture. Comet-tail artifact can be seen with hyperechoic foci.[10] On CT, hamartomas typically are seen as homogeneous fluid attenuation (<20 HU) structures with sharp and sometimes irregular margins. On MR imaging, they present as well-defined cysts with high signal on T2WI, low signal on T1WI, and no diffusion restriction. Predominantly solid foci, when present, are isointense to liver parenchyma on T1WI, and have intermediate signal on T2WI.[11] On postcontrast images, larger foci may have a subtly enhancing rim from adjacent compressed hepatic parenchyma.

Atypical manifestations

Most biliary hamartomas are predominantly cystic, although sometimes a nodular area or rim of the solid fibrous component is visible and can show mild enhancement.[12] The sonographic and CT appearance can resemble metastatic disease or hepatic abscesses in some cases.[11] Alternative or concurrent diagnoses should be considered when there is marked variation in size or size greater than 3 cm.

Excluding or suspicious features

Prominent enhancement, interval growth, restricted diffusion, and calcifications warrant consideration of alternative, possibly malignant, diagnoses.

Definitely Benign: Peribiliary Cysts

Peribiliary cysts develop from peribiliary glands, are lined by a single layer of epithelium, and do not communicate with the biliary tract.[13] A recent classification framework has been proposed: type I hepatic peribiliary cysts are numerous and develop in the presence of chronic liver disease; type II extrahepatic cysts have a predilection for women without chronic liver disease or portal hypertension, often are solitary, and often present with biliary obstruction due to mass effect; and type III are mixed hepatic and extrahepatic.[14] Peribiliary cysts typically present as multiple, less than 1 cm cystic structures seen on both sides of the portal vein, often most pronounced at the hepatic hilum and central portal triads, which has been described as a string-of-beads pattern[15] (**Fig. 3**). The typical distribution of noncommunicating cystic structures is key to diagnosis of hepatic peribiliary cysts in the appropriate clinical setting. Involvement may be segmental or diffuse. Increased size or number of hepatic peribiliary cysts is correlated with worsening chronic liver disease.[14] On ultrasound, they appear as small

cysts, which are most pronounced along the central intrahepatic portal veins. On CT, peribiliary cysts present as multiple nonenhancing, well-defined, low-attenuation structures along the sides of portal veins. In cases of confluent cysts, where individual foci are not resolvable, involvement of both sides of the portal vein can help distinguish it from intrahepatic biliary dilation but can resemble periportal edema. On MR imaging, they appear as well-defined cysts with high signal on T2WI, low signal on T1WI, and no diffusion restriction, enhancement, or communication with the biliary system.

Atypical manifestations

Confident diagnosis can be challenging when the number of peribiliary cysts is small and their distribution is unclear or when the number is too high and the bile ducts are obscured.

Excluding or suspicious features

Thickened or nodular walls, septations, or atypical distribution suggest other diagnoses.

Definitely Benign: Polycystic Liver Disease

Polycystic liver disease (PCLD) is an autosomal dominant condition resulting in diffuse hepatic cystic disease. PCLD is present in 75% to 90% of patients with autosomal dominant polycystic kidney disease, and isolated PCLD has a prevalence of less than 0.01%.[16] Two types of cysts can be seen: intrahepatic cysts that likely arise from biliary hamartomas and peribiliary cysts.[17] Cyst formation continues over time, and cysts often start to become large enough to be symptomatic at approximately the fifth decade. Treatment options include cyst aspiration, sclerosis, fenestration, enucleation, and liver transplantation, depending on symptom burden, liver function, and other clinical factors.[16] The sonographic, CT, and MR imaging appearance of individual cysts is similar to simple hepatic cysts and peribiliary cysts, except in the setting of complications, such as hemorrhage or infection.[17] Numerous cysts of varying sizes usually are present, often but not always with diffuse hepatic involvement (**Fig. 4**). The cysts slowly increase in size with age, and at least 10 enlarging cysts must be present for the diagnosis of PCLD.[5] No enhancement of the cyst walls or contents should be present.

Definitely Benign: Choledochal Malformation (Caroli Disease)

Choledochal malformations are a rare spectrum of developmental conditions affecting the biliary ductal plate with an autosomal recessive inheritance. Caroli disease results from abnormal

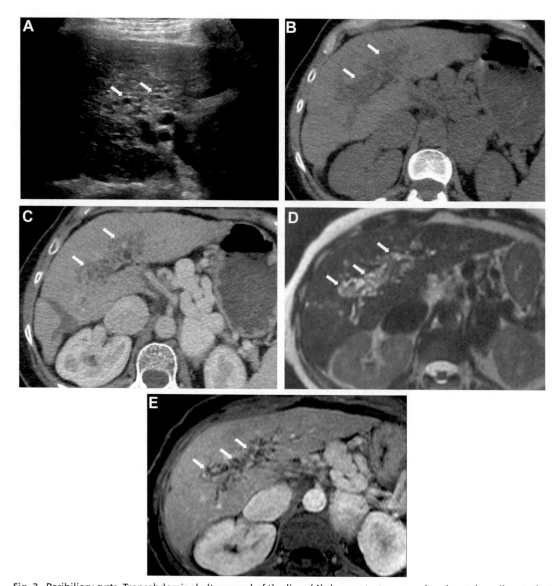

Fig. 3. Peribiliary cysts. Transabdominal ultrasound of the liver (*A*) demonstrates several periportal small cysts that appear to track along the portal vessels (*arrows*). Nonenhanced axial CT image (*B*) shows ill-defined regions of low attenuation in the region of the central portal vessels and bile ducts (*arrows*). Axial portal venous phase CT image (*C*) shows that the low attenuation corresponds to numerous small cysts adjacent to the portal veins (*arrows*). Diffuse surface nodularity of the liver is present, which is highly consistent with cirrhosis. Axial T2-weighted MR image (*D*) demonstrates innumerable small T2 hyperintense round structures lining the portal veins (*arrows*). These structures do not demonstrate enhancement on the axial portal venous phase T1-weighted fat-suppressed axial image (*E* [*arrows*]). Also note the large, tortuous left abdominal varices.

cavernous ectasia of the large bile ducts, whereas Caroli syndrome affects all levels of the biliary tract, including the small ducts which can result in congenital hepatic fibrosis.[18] Patients with this condition are at increased risk of cholangitis, strictures, choledocholithiasis, cirrhosis, and malignancies, including cholangiocarcinoma and papillary adenocarcinomas. There also is an association with multiple cystic conditions of the kidneys. Caroli disease manifests as saccular and fusiform biliary dilation from persistent ectatic embryonic bile ducts within the ductal plate, which communicate with the biliary tract.[18] Segmental intrahepatic involvement is more common than diffuse disease with predilection for the left lobe. Extrahepatic involvement can be present. Periductal fibrosis of the portal triad can manifest as the central dot sign, although this fibrovascular bundle can be eccentrically located or not visualized. The size of the dilated ducts

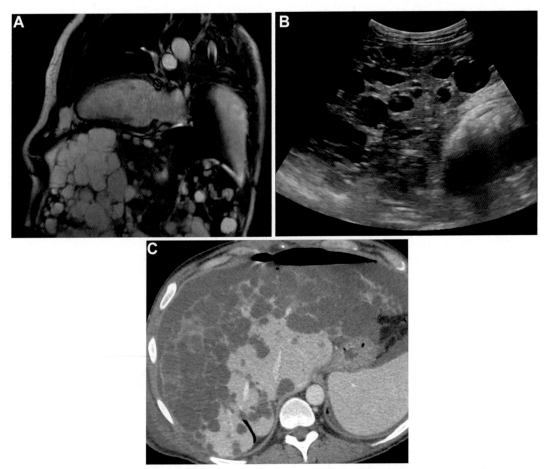

Fig. 4. PCLD. Vertical long-axis bright-blood sequence from a cardiac MR imaging examination demonstrates numerous hyperintense thin-walled structures in the liver (*A*). Transverse transabdominal ultrasound in the same patient shows anechoic cysts of varying sizes throughout the liver (*B*). Axial IV contrast-enhanced CT image shows numerous cysts of varying sizes involving both lobes of the liver (*C*). The cysts do not track along the portal vessels and appear to replace much of the parenchyma. Free intraperitoneal air on this image was due to a recent surgery.

varies but typically is less than 3 cm in diameter.[18] On ultrasound, Caroli disease presents as intrahepatic biliary dilation in a typical distribution. If a central dot sign is visualized, Doppler examination can demonstrate its fibrovascular nature.[19] On CT and MR imaging, homogeneous fluid attenuation/signal saccular or fusiform biliary dilation with sharp margins is present. A central dot sign is characteristic (**Fig. 5**). Communication with the biliary tract often is seen best with MR cholangiopancreatography. No restricted diffusion is present. On postcontrast images, the only enhancing component should be the fibrovascular bundle, which follows the enhancement pattern of the hepatic arteries and portal veins. Hepatobiliary phase contrast can demonstrate communication with the biliary tract, which can be helpful with the diagnosis in uncertain cases.

Atypical manifestations

The presence of saccular intrahepatic biliary dilation is a key distinguishing feature of Caroli disease from alternative diagnoses, such as primary sclerosing cholangitis and recurrent pyogenic cholangitis.[20]

Excluding or suspicious features

Signs of malignancy include presence of solid masses or strictures with shoulders or irregular margins. Because patients with Caroli disease have an increased risk for malignancy, these patients need to have follow-up with liver specialists, even in the absence of imaging findings specific for malignancy.

Indeterminate: Ciliated Hepatic Foregut Duplication Cyst

Ciliated hepatic foregut duplication cyst is a rare congenital cyst composed of ciliated

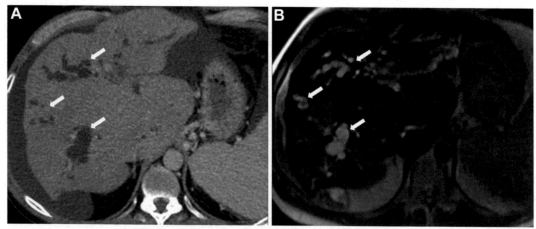

Fig. 5. Caroli disease. Axial IV contrast-enhanced CT image (*A*) demonstrates multiple saccular low attenuation regions, which represent dilated bile ducts (*arrows*). These same areas demonstrate T2 hyperintensity on axial T2-weighted MR imaging (*B* [*arrows*]), where their continuity with the bile ducts is better demonstrated. Caroli disease was confirmed on explant in this patient. Ascites is also present, as well as findings of cirrhosis.

pseudostratified columnar epithelium. Most cases are asymptomatic; however, cases of malignant transformation to squamous cell carcinoma have very uncommonly been described.[21] On imaging, a unilocular cyst typically is seen in an anterior subcapsular location in segment 4, or less commonly segments 5 or 8.[4] There is a predilection for men. On ultrasound, the duplication cysts appear as an anechoic or hypoechoic cystic focus with sharp margins and no internal vascularity. On CT, a nonenhancing low to isoattenuation cyst is present in a typical location with sharp margins. Attenuation may be higher than simple fluid due to mucinous or proteinaceous contents (**Fig. 6**). On MR imaging, this process presents with high signal on T2WI and variable signal on T1WI, depending on the cyst contents.

Resection can be considered when there are atypical features, such as solid components, enlargement, or enhancement, given the risk of malignant transformation.

Indeterminate: Mucinous Cystic Neoplasms and Intraductal Papillary Neoplasm of the Bile Ducts

Mucinous cystic neoplasms of the bile ducts likely arise from either ectopic rests of embryonic bile ducts or peribiliary glands given the presence of endocrine cells in approximately half, which are found in fewer than 5% of all hepatic cysts.[22] The presence of hormonally responsive ovarian-type mesenchymal stroma may explain a strong predilection for women, with a mean age at presentation of 45 years.[22] In 2010, the World Health Organization

terminology of biliary cysts was revised due to striking similarity between neoplasms, formerly known as biliary cystadenomas and mucinous pancreatic neoplasms, and these now are referred to as intraductal papillary neoplasms (IPNs) of the bile ducts.[23] IPNs have a similar incidence between genders and an increased risk of malignant transformation.[22] A majority are intrahepatic, with fewer than 10% arising from the extrahepatic bile ducts.[5] Mucinous cystic neoplasms are slow-growing complex mucinous processes with thick walls that can have thin or thick septations and rarely papillary or nodular components. These often but not always solitary, are at least 1.5 cm in size, and have a predilection for the left hepatic lobe. The walls are densely fibrotic and can have thin calcifications (**Fig. 7**). Whereas mucinous cystic neoplasms rarely communicate with the biliary tract, IPNs must communicate.[23] On ultrasound, these appear as multiloculated masses with internal contents ranging from anechoic to hypoechoic. Hyperechoic wall or septal calcifications also can be present. Doppler imaging may demonstrate flow within the walls or septations. On CT, these appear as multiloculated masses with internal contents ranging from simple fluid attenuation to hyperattenuating to liver parenchyma.[24] On MR imaging, a multiloculated mass is present with internal contents, which vary in signal on T1WI and T2WI, depending on whether the contents are predominantly mucinous, proteinaceous, or hemorrhagic. Fluid-fluid levels can be observed. The solid components often enhance on postcontrast images (**Fig. 8**).

Mucinous cystic neoplasms and IPNs are considered indeterminate for malignancy since they can

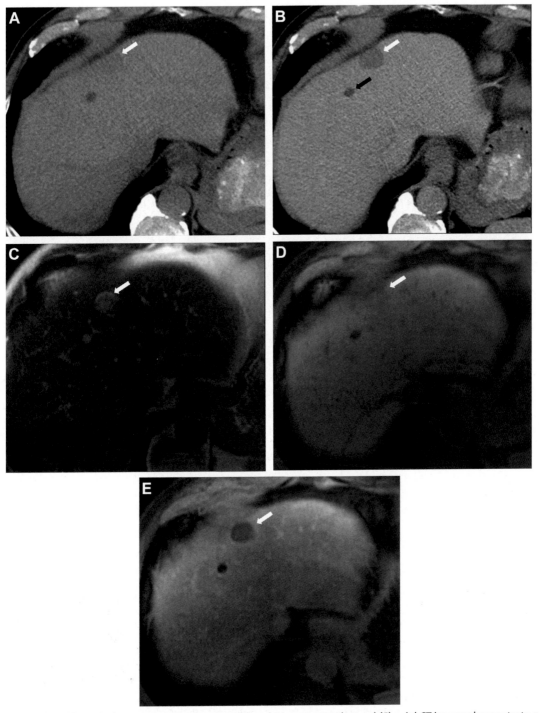

Fig. 6. Ciliated hepatic foregut cyst. Noncontrast (*A*) and IV contrast-enhanced (*B*) axial CT images demonstrate a round structure in the periphery of segment 4 that does not enhance (*white arrows*). This structure is higher in attenuation than a small simple cyst, which also is in segment 4 (*black arrow*). Axial T2-weighted MR image shows the structure has moderately hyperintense dependent material nearly filling the structure, with a crescent of fluid anteriorly (*C* [*arrow*]). Noncontrast (*D*) and IV contrast-enhanced (*E*) axial T1-weighted fat-saturated MR images demonstrate that there is no enhancement within the structure (*white arrows*).

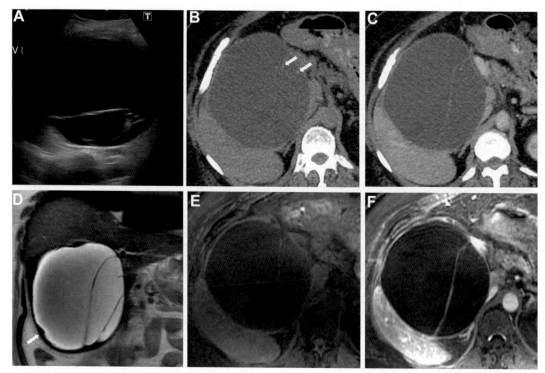

Fig. 7. Mucinous cystic neoplasm. Transabdominal ultrasound image of the liver demonstrates a large cystic mass with multiple septations (*A*). The septations did not demonstrate blood flow on Doppler. Axial precontrast (*B*) and postcontrast (*C*) CT images show a large cystic mass arising from the left hepatic lobe. A few punctate calcifications are present along the septations (*arrows*). The septations enhance following contrast. Coronal T2-weighted MR image shows the mass extending caudally from the left hepatic lobe (*D*). The wall of the cyst is hypointense, consistent with a fibrous nature (*arrow*). Axial precontrast (*E*) and postcontrast (*F*) T1-weighted fat saturated MR images better demonstrate the enhancing septations.

have dysplastic and neoplastic foci, even without definite enhancing soft tissue nodules. Given this uncertainty, these patients should be evaluated by surgeons to assess for possible resection.

Cystic Malignant Entities

A wide variety of malignancies can present primarily as liver cysts. These include metastases, hepatocellular carcinoma (HCC), or rarely undifferentiated embryonal carcinoma in young adults.[4] In patients with a known extrahepatic malignancy evaluated at a tertiary care cancer center and subcentimeter cysts on CT, approximately 11% demonstrated interval growth and were considered metastatic.[3] A predominantly cystic appearance may be due to mucin, hemorrhage, necrosis, or cystic degeneration and has been described for many primary tumors, including but not limited to, colorectal, breast, lung, and ovarian cancers as well as neuroendocrine tumors, gastrointestinal stromal tumors, and multiple sarcomas.

When the imaging features of a hepatic cyst are not definitely benign, then the risk of malignancy

should be considered based on patient risk factors, size, and imaging features, although the imaging features of small cystic foci may be difficult to adequately assess due to volume averaging and other technical factors. Features that are suspicious for malignancy include ill-defined or enhancing margins, peripheral enhancement or T2WI signal abnormalities, restricted diffusion, or prominent solid components, including thick walls, thick septations, or mural nodularity.

SOLID INCIDENTAL FINDINGS
Definitely Benign: Perfusion Alterations

The liver has a dual blood supply with inflow provided by both the portal vein and hepatic artery. Differences in the proportion of hepatic arterial versus portal venous perfusion can manifest as altered enhancement of the affected areas of the liver on intravenous (IV) contrast-enhanced CT and MR imaging.[25] In some cases these abnormalities are associated with an underlying focal process, which may cause adjacent perfusion alterations due to siphoning, arterial bed enlargement, internal

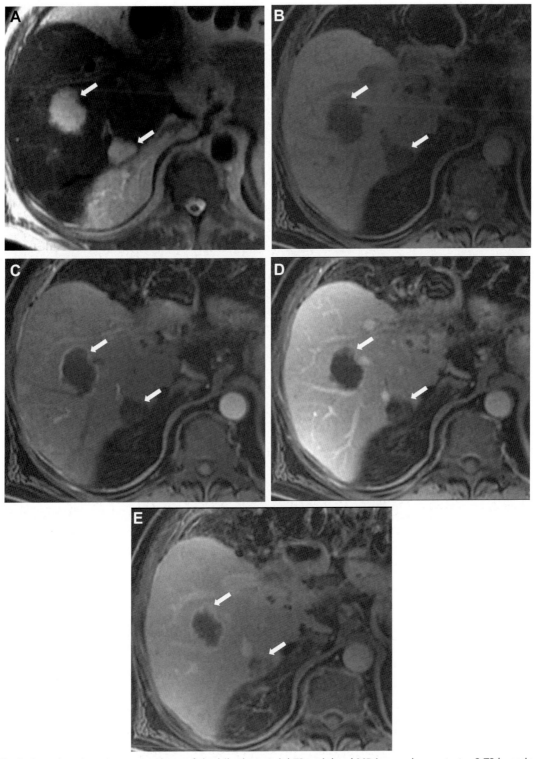

Fig. 8. Intraductal mucinous neoplasm of the bile duct. Axial T2-weighted MR image demonstrates 2 T2 hyperintense foci in the right hepatic lobe, with mildly ill-defined and irregular margins (*A* [*arrows*]). Axial T1-weighted fat-saturated precontrast (*B*) and IV contrast-enhanced arterial (*C*), portal venous (*D*), and delayed phase (*E*) MR images show how both foci have peripheral enhancement and regions of progressive mural based nodular enhancement (*arrows*). This patient had a history of hepatic resection for an intraductal mucinous neoplasm of the bile duct, and these were just 2 of many metastases which developed several years after surgery.

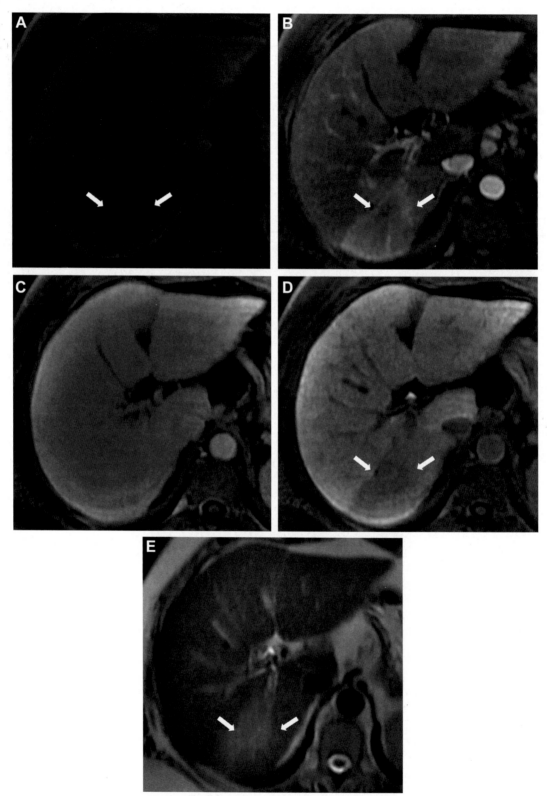

Fig. 9. Perfusion alteration. Axial T1-weighted fat-saturated MR image demonstrates an ill-defined slightly hypo-intense wedge-shaped region in the posterior right hepatic lobe (*A* [*arrows*]). Postcontrast arterial phase image following administration of a hepatobiliary contrast agent shows a wedge-shaped region of hyperenhancement in the same distribution (*B* [*arrows*]). The region is isointense to the background liver during the transitional

arterioportal shunting, or portal vein narrowing or occlusion.[26] In cases without an associated focal abnormality, perfusion alterations can be due to portal hypoperfusion, sinusoidal congestion or obstruction, vascular shunts, extrinsic parenchymal compression, hyperemia from adjacent inflammation, or accessory or anomalous vascular supply, such as in the gallbladder fossa, adjacent to the falciform ligament, or periportal region.[27] Focal fat deposition or sparing in the same distribution suggests chronicity when present. The size and morphology of a perfusion alteration depend on the underlying cause and may be sectorial/wedge-shaped, lobar, polymorphous, peribiliary, or diffuse.[26,27] Perfusion alterations are not seen on noncontrast CT, unless associated with focal fat deposition/sparing. On MR imaging, they sometimes may be associated with focal fat deposition/sparing, mild increased signal on T2WI, or abnormal diffusion. On postcontrast images, the geographic area of arterial hyperenhancement typically partially or completely fades to background parenchymal enhancement in the later contrast phases and often is referred to as transient hepatic attenuation or intensity differences on CT and MR imaging, respectively. Perfusion alterations sometimes can be visible as a region of hypointensity on the hepatobiliary phase of postcontrast MR imaging (**Fig. 9**).

The apex and entire region of the alteration should be examined carefully for an underlying focal abnormality, which can be benign or malignant. Small rounded perfusion abnormalities can mimic an enhancing focus when only a single phase of contrast imaging is available.[27]

Definitely Benign: Focal Fat Deposition or Sparing

Abnormal accumulation of triglycerides in the liver may occur from increased delivery or decreased secretion related to perfusion alterations or altered metabolism, which may be secondary to systemic metabolic abnormalities (eg, insulin resistance and hyperlipidemia), substances including alcohol or steroids, chronic viral hepatitis, or congenital disorders.[28] Some cases of diffuse steatosis are associated with inflammation, cellular injury, and fibrosis, which can progress to chronic liver disease or cirrhosis.

Several patterns of hepatic steatosis have been described, some of which can mimic tumors.[29] Common areas of focal fat deposition or sparing

are similar to those that often have alternate inflow, such as the gallbladder fossa, adjacent to the falciform ligament or ligamentum venosum, and hepatic hilum. These areas of focal fat sparing or deposition should not displace or distort the traversing blood vessels. Uncommonly, multifocal rounded or oval areas of focal fat deposition can be seen in atypical locations and resemble nodular focal masses. In rare cases, perivascular deposition occurs along the portal or hepatic veins. Subcapsular rounded or confluent deposition can be seen when insulin is added to peritoneal dialysate in patients with renal failure and insulin-dependent diabetes mellitus. On ultrasound, hepatic lipid droplets result in increased echogenicity compared with normal kidney, spleen, or spared liver parenchyma (**Fig. 10**). Larger areas of steatosis can result in decreased acoustic penetration and poor delineation of the hepatic vessels, diaphragm, or underlying focal abnormalities. On non-enhanced CT, lipid is hypoattenuating to the liver parenchyma, and the degree of hypoattenuation correlates with lipid content. Common attenuation thresholds for hepatic steatosis include absolute values of 40 HU or at least 10 HU less than spleen. MR imaging is the most sensitive, specific, and accurate method for detection and quantification of hepatic steatosis.[28] Focal fat demonstrates signal drop out between in-phase and out-of-phase T1WI (see **Fig. 10**). Most cases of focal fat deposition enhance similarly to uninvolved liver parenchyma; however, occasionally an underlying perfusion alteration may be detected.

Focal fat deposition or sparing should not cause mass effect or demonstrate peripheral or internal abnormal enhancement. When fat deposition or sparing is suspected in atypical locations, particularly in a high-risk patient, MR imaging is recommended for confirmation.

Definitely Benign: Hepatic Hemangioma

Hepatic hemangiomas are the most common benign tumor of the liver, with a prevalence between 1% to 20% and a predilection for women.[10] Hepatic hemangiomas are a venous malformation composed of expanded endothelialized vascular spaces, with 1 or more nonenlarged or minimally enlarged feeding arteries.[30] Hemangiomas have well-defined rounded or lobulated margins. In most cases, hemangiomas are solitary and less than 3 cm in size. Giant hemangiomas have been

---

phase (*C*). During the hepatobiliary phase, this region is slightly hypointense to the background liver (*D* [*arrows*]), a finding suggestive of hepatocyte dysfunction which can be seen with abnormal perfusion. T2-weighted MR images demonstrated mild hyperintensity in this region, indicating mild edema due to the altered perfusion (*E* [*arrows*]).

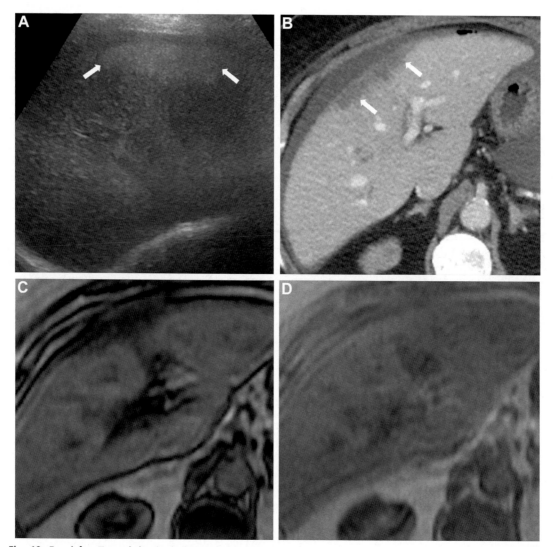

Fig. 10. Focal fat. Transabdominal ultrasound image demonstrates a region increased echogenicity along the anterior liver (*A [arrows]*). IV contrast-enhanced axial CT image shows a corresponding region of hypoattenuation without associated mass effect on the remainder of the liver (*B [arrows]*). The patient was on peritoneal dialysis, which accounts for the free fluid and small amount of free intraperitoneal gas. Axial T1-weighted opposed-phase (*C*) and in-phase (*D*) MR images show loss of signal on the out-phase image, indicative of focal fat.

variously defined in the literature as greater than 4 cm, 6 cm, or larger.[30] Hemangiomas often are stable or slowly growing in size, but in rare cases may grow rapidly, particularly during pregnancy or with exogenous estrogen exposure. Hemangiomas can be seen throughout the liver but tend to be peripheral and even may be pedunculated. On ultrasound, hemangiomas present as a well-circumscribed mass, which typically is hyperechoic. Approximately 10%, however, are isoechoic or hypoechoic with a hyperechoic rim. Hemangiomas may appear hypoechoic if the background liver is abnormally echogenic due to steatosis or fibrosis. Posterior acoustic enhancement should be present for hemangiomas of sufficient size. Low-velocity internal

vascular flow may be seen by Doppler examination. Arterioportal shunting can be demonstrated by color Doppler in some cases.[31] On nonenhanced CT, hemangiomas appear as well-circumscribed homogeneous hypoattenuating masses. On MR imaging, they are well circumscribed and are hypointense on T1WI to liver, very hyperintense on T2WI, and have no restricted diffusion (**Fig. 11**). Classically, hemangiomas demonstrate peripheral discontinuous globular/nodular enhancement on the arterial phase of imaging, with progressive centripetal fill-in during later phases. The enhancing portion follows the arterial blood pool on all phases. Giant hemangiomas may have a nonenhancing central scar. Small hemangiomas, typically less than 2 cm in size, can have a flash-filling enhancement pattern, with homogeneous arterial hyperenhancement that fades on later phases. Rapidly enhancing hemangiomas may have associated arterioportal shunting or other perfusion alteration of the adjacent liver parenchyma. Extreme caution, particularly in high-risk patients, should be used when attempting to diagnose a hemangioma on a single-phase, IV contrast-enhanced CT examination due to the importance of the progressive pattern of enhancement for the diagnosis.

Atypical manifestations

Myriad atypical appearances of hepatic hemangiomas have been described.[30,32] Atypical enhancement patterns likely are secondary to variant internal architecture, with large vascular spaces associated with very slow fill-in.[33] Some cases may not have the characteristic very hyperintense T2WI signal due to the internal architecture. Larger hemangiomas often have an atypical heterogeneous appearance and may demonstrate central areas of hemorrhage, fibrosis, thrombosis, cystic degeneration, necrosis, internal septations, either central or peripheral calcifications, and atypical enhancement patterns. Hyalinized or sclerosed hemangiomas have thrombosed or fibrotic vascular channels, resulting in delayed enhancement, lower T2WI signal than expected, and adjacent capsular retraction. In these cases, comparison with prior imaging demonstrating a typical hemangioma at the same location can be considered diagnostic of a sclerosed hemangioma. Some hemangiomas have fluid-fluid levels, which are thought to represent sedimentation in large vascular spaces and can be seen by CT or MR imaging but not ultrasound.

Features suspicious for malignancy

Some malignant liver tumors also can be very hyperintense on T2WI, such as neuroendocrine tumors and breast or colon cancer metastases.

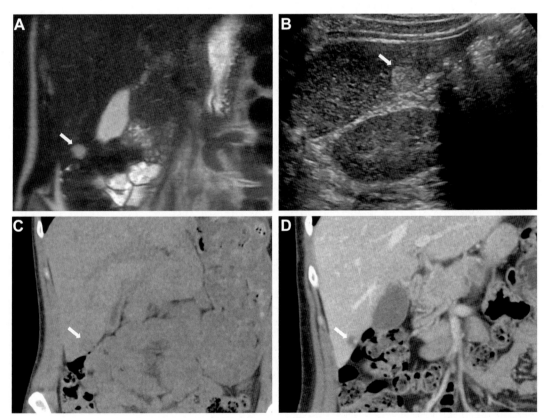

Fig. 11. Hepatic hemangioma. Coronal T2WI from a pelvic MR examination demonstrates a round hyperintense focus in the inferior tip of the liver (*A* [*arrow*]). Note that the focus is slightly lower in signal intensity compared to fluid in the stomach and adjacent bowel. The focus is homogeneously hyperechoic to the surrounding liver parenchyma on transabdominal ultrasound (*B* [*arrow*]). Noncontrast coronal CT image (*C*) demonstrates a slightly hypoattenuating round hepatic focus (*arrow*). Venous phase IV contrast-enhanced examination shows peripheral round areas of contrast enhancement within the process, which is consistent with the peripheral puddling typical of hepatic hemangiomas (*D* [*arrow*]).

Some hypervascular tumors, such as angiosarcoma, can demonstrate globular regions of enhancement with progressive fill-in, although the pattern typically is far more disorganized than what normally is seen with hemangiomas.[33] In contrast to malignant tumors, however, areas of an atypical hemangioma that enhance do not show washout. Atypical hemangiomas may require dedicated multiphasic liver imaging or tissue sampling to confirm the diagnosis.

Definitely Benign: Focal Nodular Hyperplasia

Focal nodular hyperplasia (FNH) is the second most common primary liver tumor, with a prevalence of approximately 1% to 3%.[5] FNH is found most commonly between the third and fifth decades, and there is a strong predilection for women.[34] The precise etiology is unknown to the authors' knowledge but is thought to be a hyperplastic regenerative response to an arteriovenous malformation between the hepatic arteries and veins, with no portal venous supply. The components of normal hepatic parenchyma are present but with malformed vascular structures, cholangiolar proliferation, and nodular architecture with hepatocytes and Kupffer cells.[35,36] Typical FNH is notable for a stellate area of central fibrosis with radiating septa. Nonclassic FNH (telangiectatic FNH, FNH with cytologic atypia, and mixed hyperplastic and adenomatous FNH) lack either the nodular architecture or malformed vessels but still have cholangiolar proliferation.[36] Intralesional steatosis is present in approximately 20% of cases, usually mild and associated with nonclassical FNH.[37] There is no risk of malignant transformation, and a vast majority of individuals with FNH are asymptomatic.

Classic FNH has well-defined lobulated margins with a central scar and radiating fibrous septations, typically less than 5 cm in size.[10] Large classic FNHs may have more than 1 central scar. Nonclassic FNHs without a macroscopic central scar may be more heterogeneous and with less lobulated margins. There is no capsule between the FNH and normal liver parenchyma; however, larger foci can have a pseudocapsule of compressed normal parenchyma, peripheral vessels, and inflammation.[36] Approximately 20% of cases have multiple areas of FNH, which often are nonclassic.[36] Slow interval growth or regression can be observed but is not associated with estrogen levels.[38] On ultrasound, FNH often is isoechoic to normal liver due to similar composition, although it may be hyperechoic or hypoechoic. A central scar may be seen with pulsatile waveforms on Doppler examination. When present, the pseudocapsule typically is hypoechoic. On nonenhanced CT, classic FNH typically is isoattenuating or hypoattenuating due to the variable presence of steatosis. Classic FNH demonstrates homogeneous arterial phase enhancement, which fades on later stages and, therefore, can be indistinguishable from the surrounding liver on portal venous phase or delayed phase imaging. The central scar has delayed enhancement owing to the expanded extracellular volume. When present, there can be delayed enhancement of the pseudocapsule. On MR imaging, the following criteria are required for diagnosis of typical FNH: isointense or hypointense signal on T1WI, isointense or mildly hyperintense signal on T2WI, typical enhancement characteristics, central scar, and lack of a fibrous capsule. A several-millimeter thick T2WI hyperintense pseudocapsule can be present and can be distinguished from a fibrous capsule, which is hypointense on T1WI and T2WI.[36] The central scar typically is hypointense on T1WI and hyperintense on T2WI. FNH typically is hyperintense to liver parenchyma on hepatobiliary phase imaging and rarely can show peripheral ringlike hyperintensity[39] (**Fig. 12**).

Atypical manifestations

Nonclassic FNHs often have atypical imaging features, most commonly an absent or abnormal central artery and scar. Some FNHs may be slightly hypointense on T1WI, usually due to sinusoidal dilation or steatosis of the background liver. For foci that are less than 3 cm with either no central scar or mild hyperintensity on T1WI in a low-risk population, a diagnosis of FNH can be suggested when the other classic MR imaging and enhancement features of FNH are present.[35] Heterogeneity other than the central scar and radiating septations also is atypical and is seen more commonly in nonclassic FNH.

Features suspicious for malignancy

Important differential diagnostic considerations include hepatocellular adenoma, HCC, and hypervascular metastases. Calcifications, cystic areas, fibrous capsule, washout, and hemorrhage should suggest a diagnosis other than FNH. In addition to these features, size greater than 4 cm and multiple foci should increase suspicion for alternative diagnoses. In particular, when the central scar is hypointense or isointense on T2WI, does not demonstrate late enhancement, or has calcifications, fibrolamellar HCC should be considered.[10] FNH rarely should be diagnosed conclusively in high-risk populations.

Indeterminate: Hepatocellular Adenoma

Hepatocellular adenomas (HCAs) are proliferations of benign-appearing hepatocytes that are

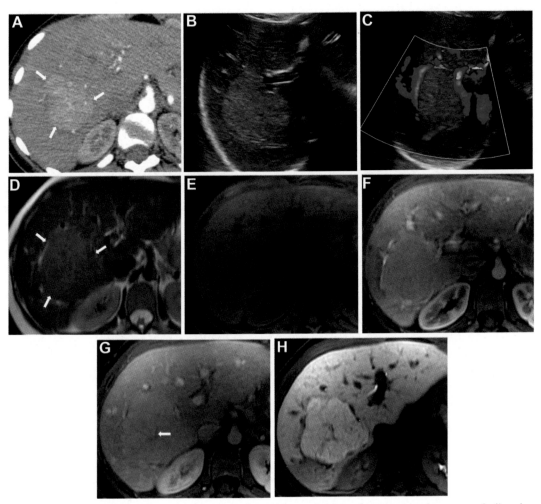

Fig. 12. FNH. Axial image from a CT angiogram performed for evaluation of suspected pulmonary embolism demonstrates an ill-defined region of hyperenhancement in the right hepatic lobe (*A* [*arrows*]). Transabdominal ultrasound shows a corresponding hyperechoic region (*B*), which displaces regional vessels (*C*). The mass is mildly hyperintense to the background liver on axial T2-weighted MR (*D* [*arrows*]). Axial T1-weighted fat-saturated precontrast (*E*) and postcontrast arterial phase (*F*) and portal venous phase (*G*) MR images show hyperenhancement of the mass, with a central linear region of hypoenhancement, which is consistent with a central scar (*arrow*). Hepatobiliary-phase postcontrast T1-weighted fat-saturated axial MR image shows diffuse contrast uptake of the mass resulting in hyperintensity to background parenchyma (*H*). The imaging findings, as well as absence of chronic liver disease or known malignancy, are highly consistent with FNH.

associated with estrogen or other hormonal disturbances, including exogenous hormone supplementation in the form of oral contraceptives or anabolic steroids, pregnancy, and metabolic syndrome. HCAs also are found in patients with underlying type I or type III glycogen storage disease.[40] The prevalence is approximately 0.05%, with a strong predilection for women of child-bearing age.[5] As of 2017, there are 8 subtypes of hepatic adenoma that vary in their clinical behavior, imaging appearance, and risk of malignancy, with the most frequent ones being inflammatory, hepatocyte nuclear factor (HNF)-1α–mutated, and β-catenin–mutated.[41] Inflammatory adenomas account for

30% to 35% of HCAs and are driven by overactivation of the JAK-STAT pathway. These HCAs are prone to bleeding due to abnormal arteries, sinusoidal dilation, and peliotic areas and have a 10% risk of malignancy.[40] The second most common adenoma subtype, at 30% to 35%, is characterized by biallelic inactivation of the HNF-1α tumor suppressor gene and is associated with maturity-onset diabetes of the young.[42] HNF-1α inactivated HCAs often are asymptomatic, contain fat, and have a very low risk of malignancy.[42] Approximately 20% of adenomas are driven by activating mutations of the β-catenin pathway which also is a known driver of HCC.[41] Of these, the most frequent

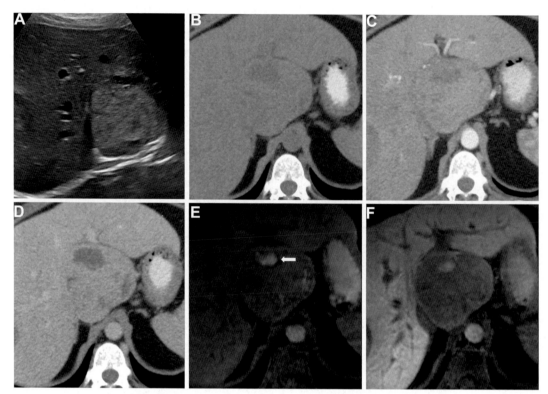

Fig. 13. HCA. Transabdominal ultrasound image (*A*) shows a large heterogeneously hyperechoic mass replacing the caudate lobe. Note homogeneous echogenicity and smooth surface contour of the liver, which is consistent with absence of known chronic liver disease. Precontrast (*B*) and postcontrast arterial phase (*C*) and portal venous phase (*D*) axial CT images demonstrate a heterogeneous enhancing mass in the caudate lobe. T1-weighted fat-suppressed axial MR image demonstrates areas of hyperintensity indicating internal hemorrhage of the mass (*E* [*arrow*]). Hepatobiliary phase axial MR images after the administration of a hepatobiliary contrast agent show absence of contrast retention within the mass, supporting the diagnosis of HCA (*F*).

subtype has a mutation at exon 3, which has the highest risk of malignant transformation to HCC.

HCAs typically are solitary expansile round or ovoid masses, which are 5 cm to 15 cm at diagnosis (**Fig. 13**). The architecture often is heterogeneous with areas of hemorrhage, focal fat, necrosis, and calcifications, and there is no central scar. Diffusely and extensively steatotic adenomas, often in a background of hepatic steatosis, often are of the HNF-1α–mutated subtype. Hepatic adenomatosis is defined as greater than 10 adenomas. HCAs on ultrasound typically are hypoechoic and heterogeneous with areas of hyperechogenicity, which may be due to focal steatosis or blood products. Doppler examination may show internal or peripheral vascularity with blunted waveforms.[5] On nonenhanced CT, HCAs range from isoattenuating to hypoattenuating related to the amount of steatosis, with hyperdense components corresponding to blood products. HCAs on MR imaging typically have a heterogeneous appearance on T1WI depending on the composition. Inflammatory adenomas are

characterized by diffuse hyperintensity on T2WI. The HNF-1α subtype may be hyperintense or isointense to liver on T1WI and T2WI, with prominent diffuse signal loss on opposed-phase T1WI. Inflammatory adenomas tend to have arterial hyperenhancement, which persists on portal venous and delayed imaging. HNF-1α–mutated adenomas are less hyperenhancing on the arterial phase and often completely fade on portal venous and delayed imaging. β-Catenin–mutated adenomas have variable enhancement patterns that may resemble HCC.[42]

Imaging features of inflammatory or β-catenin–mutated subtypes, size greater than 5 cm, male gender, anabolic steroid use, and underlying glycogen storage disease are known risk factors for malignancy.[42] In addition, progressive increased size and vascular invasion are concerning for malignant transformation.[43] In general, HCAs cannot be diagnosed confidently on nondedicated liver imaging, and those that are suspicious for HCA require either further imaging evaluation or comparison with prior dedicated liver imaging.

Solid Malignant Entities

Solid hepatic lesions that do not demonstrate definitely benign features should be further characterized by dedicated imaging or, in some cases, by tissue sampling, to evaluate for possible primary or metastatic malignancy. Metastases tend to be expansile and rounded in morphology with ill-defined margins. Identification of a suspicious incidental hepatic process should prompt careful evaluation for an occult primary tumor.

In patients with cirrhosis or chronic liver disease, the primary consideration for a solid focus is HCC. Major features of HCC include arterial phase hyperenhancement, washout appearance, and capsule appearance.[44,45] The presence of these 3 features in the appropriate clinical context has high specificity for HCC with risk categories defined by the ACR-supported LI-RADS manual.[45] LI-RADS classification should be used only in the correct clinical setting, because a tumor that would be classified as definite HCC (LR-5) often is treated as diagnostic of HCC in high-risk patients but is not as specific for HCC in low-risk patients. Not all HCC develops in the setting of chronic liver disease, and it can be particularly difficult to diagnose accurately in those cases.

The second most common primary liver malignancy is cholangiocarcinoma, which also can present as a solid mass.[46] The mass-forming manifestation of cholangiocarcinoma tends to be homogeneously hypoattenuating, hypointense on T1WI, and mildly hyperintense on T2WI with irregular margins. Encasement of the portal veins is common, because these tumors arise from portal triads, but tumor-in-vein is seen less frequently than with HCC. Obstructive biliary dilation variably is present. A desmoplastic or fibrotic reaction is common and can result in capsular retraction and obliteration of portal veins. The central region tends to be more fibrotic and to a lesser extent necrotic, and the periphery tends to be more cellular. This often manifests as a targetoid appearance, and irregular rim arterial enhancement and centripetal fill-in.[45]

Regardless of patient risk factors, morphologic features suspicious for malignancy include ill-defined margins, heterogeneous or mosaic architecture, a nodule-in-nodule appearance, prominent necrosis or cystic areas, capsular retraction, mass effect out of proportion to size, biliary obstruction, and rapid growth. The sonographic features of malignant entities often overlap with those of benign entities. Doppler examination may or may not demonstrate internal vascularity. Calcifications may be present. On MR imaging, malignant tumoral foci tend to be heterogeneous on both T1WI and T2WI. Most homogeneous very hyperintense T2WI focal findings are benign, although some malignancies can have this appearance when combined with irregular margins. Highly cellular tumors tend to have restricted diffusion. Malignant tumors can have variable enhancement patterns and intensity, including rim hyperenhancement, delayed enhancement, and washout. In some cases, with CT, hypervascular tumors may be detectable only on arterial phase imaging and can mimic small flash-filling processes, including hemangiomas and other benign shunts. Some malignancies can mimic the benign enhancement patterns of typical hemangiomas and classic FNH, but in most cases other features raise concern for an alternative diagnosis.

INCIDENTAL HEPATIC FINDINGS ALGORITHMS

Based on this review of common benign entities and importance of patient risk factors, the authors propose the following algorithms for assessment of incidental hepatic findings first identified on ultrasound, CT, or MR imaging examinations. The algorithms attempt to avoid unnecessary work-up and evaluation of focal processes, which are highly likely to be benign, while recognizing the importance of prompt assessment of focal findings that may be malignant or carry a risk of malignancy that may be detectable on dedicated liver imaging.

The first step in detection of a focal liver finding should be comparison with prior imaging of the liver. If the finding has been adequately characterized on prior imaging, the radiologist can presume that this is unlikely to require further evaluation unless it has definitely changed in morphology or size. The proposed algorithms presume that prior adequate liver imaging is either not available or has not been performed. These algorithms also do not apply if the current imaging of the finding is considered adequate for evaluation of the liver, which includes multiphasic postcontrast imaging for CT and MR and T2WI for MR imaging.

The ultrasound algorithm (Fig. 14) begins by asking the radiologist to distinguish between cystic and solid processes. Because ultrasound provides excellent characterization of cysts, a simple cyst is highly likely to be benign and not require further evaluation. For characterization of complex cysts, MR is considered superior to CT given its sensitivity for enhancing nodules or septations. Ultrasound, however, is not as specific for many benign solid entities as other modalities. In high-risk patients, solid incidental findings should be considered possibly malignant unless they definitely meet all imaging criteria for focal fat sparing or focal fat deposition.[47]

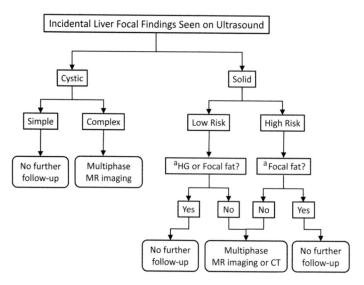

Fig. 14. Algorithm for focal incidental liver findings first seen on ultrasound. Refer to **Box 1** for description of high-risk versus low-risk patients. To be considered a hemangioma or focal fat sparing/deposition, the finding must meet all of the listed criteria. [a]Hemangioma (HG) = round, sharp edges, hyperechoic, no blood flow on Doppler; and focal fat sparing/deposition = typical location, sharp edges, geographic.

The CT and MR imaging algorithm (**Fig. 15**) begins by evaluating size. The proposed binary distinction between less than 1 cm versus greater than or equal to 1 cm is a simplification of prior algorithms and reflects a similar distinction currently used by LI-RADS, version 2018.[45] Because focal findings that are less than 1 cm may not be well characterized on immediate dedicated liver imaging, the authors recommend waiting 3 months to 6 months before providing additional imaging in high-risk patients, because growth may support possible malignancy and allow better evaluation of imaging features. For focal findings greater than or equal to 1 cm, nondedicated CT or MR imaging may be adequate to diagnose a definite benign entity in some circumstances. Due to the importance of multiphasic imaging for their diagnosis, solid hepatic nodules or masses often are not adequately assessed when seen incidentally, so if the finding does not meet all criteria for a definite benign entity, then further dedicated liver imaging should be performed.

SUMMARY

Incidental focal hepatic findings are a common problem on CT, MR imaging, and ultrasound, given the inclusion of this large solid organ within the field of view of many different types of imaging examinations. Further evaluation of ultimately benign liver focal findings can result in increased patient anxiety, health care costs, and risks associated with additional procedures or imaging examinations.

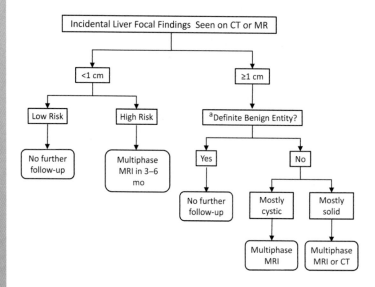

Fig. 15. Algorithm for incidental liver findings first seen on CT or MR. Refer to **Box 1** for description of high-risk versus low-risk patients. [a]To be considered a definite benign entity, the finding must meet all of the criteria for specific entity as follows: cyst = sharp margin, homogeneous, less than 20 HU or marked T2WI hyperintensity; focal fat deposition/sparing = geographic, typical location, sharp edges, no mass effect; perfusion alteration = sharp margin, wedge-shaped, no mass effect; and hemangioma (MR) = sharp margin, homogeneous, moderate to marked T2WI hyperintensity.

The proposed algorithms rely on several key factors, including size and patient risk factors. Radiologists also need to be familiar with the discussed benign entities, so they can make these benign diagnoses even when dedicated liver imaging has not been performed. The authors hope that this review and proposed algorithms can act as a guide for radiologists to more confidently assess the need for further imaging of incidental focal liver findings on cross-sectional imaging examinations and which modality is preferred in each scenario.

CLINICS CARE POINTS

- An incidental liver lesion should be assessed in the context of patient specific risk factors for liver malignancy.
- In a low risk patient, findings on ultrasound typical of hemangioma or focal fat deposition/sparing do not require further work up.
- In a high risk patient, any solid finding on ultrasound except focal fat deposition/sparing requires further imaging with multiphasic CT or MR.
- Incidental liver finding < 1 cm on CT or MR in a low risk patient does not require further work up.
- Incidental liver finding < 1 cm on CT or MR in a high risk patient requires follow up imaging in 3-6 months with multiphase MRI.

ACKNOWLEDGMENTS

A.C. Searleman is supported by NIH grant T32 EB005970.

DISCLOSURE

The authors have nothing to disclose.

REFERENCES

1. Gore RM, Pickhardt PJ, Mortele KJ, et al. Management of incidental liver lesions on CT: a white paper of the ACR incidental findings committee. J Am Coll Radiol 2017;14(11):1429–37.
2. Horn SR, Stoltzfus KC, Lehrer EJ, et al. Epidemiology of liver metastases. Cancer Epidemiol 2020; 67:101760.
3. Schwartz LH, Gandras EJ, Colangelo SM, et al. Prevalence and importance of small hepatic lesions found at CT in patients with cancer. Radiology 1999; 210(1):71–4.
4. Borhani AA, Wiant A, Heller MT. Cystic hepatic lesions: a review and an algorithmic approach. AJR Am J Roentgenol 2014;203(6):1192–204.
5. Tran Cao HS, Marcal LP, Mason MC, et al. Benign hepatic incidentalomas. Curr Probl Surg 2019; 56(9):100642.
6. Vachha B, Sun MR, Siewert B, et al. Cystic lesions of the liver. AJR Am J Roentgenol 2011;196(4): W355–66.
7. Mavilia MG, Pakala T, Molina M, et al. Differentiating cystic liver lesions: a review of imaging modalities, diagnosis and management. J Clin Transl Hepatol 2018;6(2):208–16.
8. Chung EB. Multiple bile-duct hamartomas. Cancer 1970;26(2):287–96.
9. Jain D, Ahrens W, Finkelstein S. Molecular evidence for the neoplastic potential of hepatic Von-Meyenburg complexes. Appl Immunohistochem Mol Morphol 2010;18(2):166–71.
10. Gore RM, Newmark GM, Thakrar KH, et al. Hepatic incidentalomas. Radiol Clin North Am 2011;49(2): 291–322.
11. Horton KM, Bluemke DA, Hruban RH, et al. CT and MR imaging of benign hepatic and biliary tumors. Radiographics 1999;19(2):431–51.
12. Liu S, Zhao B, Ma J, et al. Lesions of biliary hamartoms can be diagnosed by ultrasonography, computed tomography and magnetic resonance imaging. Int J Clin Exp Med 2014;7(10):3370–7.
13. Terayama N, Matsui O, Hoshiba K, et al. Peribiliary cysts in liver cirrhosis: US, CT, and MR findings. J Comput Assist Tomogr 1995;19(3):419–23.
14. Bazerbachi F, Haffar S, Sugihara T, et al. Peribiliary cysts: a systematic review and proposal of a classification framework. BMJ Open Gastroenterol 2018; 5(1):e000204.
15. Baron RL, Campbell WL, Dodd GD 3rd. Peribiliary cysts associated with severe liver disease: imaging-pathologic correlation. AJR Am J Roentgenol 1994;162(3):631–6.
16. Cnossen WR, Drenth JP. Polycystic liver disease: an overview of pathogenesis, clinical manifestations and management. Orphanet J Rare Dis 2014;9:69.
17. Morgan DE, Lockhart ME, Canon CL, et al. Polycystic liver disease: multimodality imaging for complications and transplant evaluation. Radiographics 2006;26(6):1655–68 [quiz: 1655].
18. Levy AD, Rohrmann CA Jr, Murakata LA, et al. Caroli's disease: radiologic spectrum with pathologic correlation. AJR Am J Roentgenol 2002;179(4): 1053–7.
19. Wu KL, Changchien CS, Kuo CM, et al. Caroli's disease - a report of two siblings. Eur J Gastroenterol Hepatol 2002;14(12):1397–9.
20. Mamone G, Carollo V, Cortis K, et al. Magnetic resonance imaging of fibropolycystic liver disease: the

spectrum of ductal plate malformations. Abdom Radiol (NY) 2019;44(6):2156–71.

21. Bishop KC, Perrino CM, Ruzinova MB, et al. Ciliated hepatic foregut cyst: a report of 6 cases and a review of the English literature. Diagn Pathol 2015; 10:81.

22. Soares KC, Arnaoutakis DJ, Kamel I, et al. Cystic neoplasms of the liver: biliary cystadenoma and cystadenocarcinoma. J Am Coll Surg 2014;218(1): 119–28.

23. Park HJ, Kim SY, Kim HJ, et al. Intraductal papillary neoplasm of the bile duct: clinical, imaging, and pathologic features. AJR Am J Roentgenol 2018; 211(1):67–75.

24. Kim JY, Kim SH, Eun HW, et al. Differentiation between biliary cystic neoplasms and simple cysts of the liver: accuracy of CT. AJR Am J Roentgenol 2010;195(5):1142–8.

25. Desser TS. Understanding transient hepatic attenuation differences. Semin Ultrasound CT MR 2009; 30(5):408–17.

26. Colagrande S, Centi N, Galdiero R, et al. Transient hepatic intensity differences: part 1, those associated with focal lesions. AJR Am J Roentgenol 2007;188(1):154–9.

27. Colagrande S, Centi N, Galdiero R, et al. Transient hepatic intensity differences: part 2, those not associated with focal lesions. AJR Am J Roentgenol 2007;188(1):160–6.

28. Zhang YN, Fowler KJ, Hamilton G, et al. Liver fat imaging-a clinical overview of ultrasound, CT, and MR imaging. Br J Radiol 2018;91(1089):20170959.

29. Hamer OW, Aguirre DA, Casola G, et al. Fatty liver: imaging patterns and pitfalls. Radiographics 2006; 26(6):1637–53.

30. Vilgrain V, Boulos L, Vullierme MP, et al. Imaging of atypical hemangiomas of the liver with pathologic correlation. Radiographics 2000;20(2):379–97.

31. Lim KJ, Kim KW, Jeong WK, et al. Colour Doppler sonography of hepatic haemangiomas with arterioportal shunts. Br J Radiol 2012;85(1010):142–6.

32. Mathew RP, Sam M, Raubenheimer M, et al. Hepatic hemangiomas: the various imaging avatars and its mimickers. Radiol Med 2020;125(9):801–15.

33. Jang HJ, Kim TK, Lim HK, et al. Hepatic hemangioma: atypical appearances on CT, MR imaging, and sonography. AJR Am J Roentgenol 2003;180(1): 135–41.

34. Bioulac-Sage P, Balabaud C, Wanless IR. Diagnosis of focal nodular hyperplasia: not so easy. Am J Surg Pathol 2001;25(10):1322–5.

35. Ferlicot S, Kobeiter H, Tran Van Nhieu J, et al. MRI of atypical focal nodular hyperplasia of the liver: radiology-pathology correlation. AJR Am J Roentgenol 2004;182(5):1227–31.

36. Hussain SM, Terkivatan T, Zondervan PE, et al. Focal nodular hyperplasia: findings at state-of-the-art MR imaging, US, CT, and pathologic analysis. Radiographics 2004;24(1):3–17 [discussion: 18–9].

37. Ronot M, Paradis V, Duran R, et al. MR findings of steatotic focal nodular hyperplasia and comparison with other fatty tumours. Eur Radiol 2013;23(4): 914–23.

38. Halankar JA, Kim TK, Jang HJ, et al. Understanding the natural history of focal nodular hyperplasia in the liver with MRI. Indian J Radiol Imaging 2012;22(2): 116–20.

39. Fujiwara H, Sekine S, Onaya H, et al. Ring-like enhancement of focal nodular hyperplasia with hepatobiliary-phase Gd-EOB-DTPA-enhanced magnetic resonance imaging: radiological-pathological correlation. Jpn J Radiol 2011;29(10):739–43.

40. Nault JC, Bioulac-Sage P, Zucman-Rossi J. Hepatocellular benign tumors-from molecular classification to personalized clinical care. Gastroenterology 2013;144(5):888–902.

41. Zulfiqar M, Sirlin CB, Yoneda N, et al. Hepatocellular adenomas: understanding the pathomolecular lexicon, MRI features, terminology, and pitfalls to inform a standardized approach. J Magn Reson Imaging 2020;51(6):1630–40.

42. Katabathina VS, Menias CO, Shanbhogue AK, et al. Genetics and imaging of hepatocellular adenomas: 2011 update. Radiographics 2011;31(6):1529–43.

43. Kwok WY, Hagiwara S, Nishida N, et al. Malignant transformation of hepatocellular adenoma. Oncology 2017;92(Suppl 1):16–28.

44. Kitao A, Zen Y, Matsui O, et al. Hepatocarcinogenesis: multistep changes of drainage vessels at CT during arterial portography and hepatic arteriography–radiologic-pathologic correlation. Radiology 2009;252(2):605–14.

45. American College of Radiology Committee on LI-RADS. CT/MRI LI-RADS v2018. American College of Radiology. Available at: https://www.acr.org/Clinical-Resources/Reporting-and-Data-Systems/LI-RADS. Accessed January 1, 2021.

46. Chung YE, Kim MJ, Park YN, et al. Varying appearances of cholangiocarcinoma: radiologic-pathologic correlation. Radiographics 2009;29(3):683–700.

47. American College of Radiology Committee on LI-RADS. Ultrasound LI-RADS v2017. American College of Radiology. Available at: https://www.acr.org/Clinical-Resources/Reporting-and-Data-Systems/LI-RADS/Ultrasound-LI-RADS-v2017. Accessed January 1, 2021.

Incidental Adrenal Nodules

Daniel I. Glazer, MD[a],*, Michael T. Corwin, MD[b], William W. Mayo-Smith, MD[a]

KEYWORDS

- Adrenal nodule • Incidentaloma • Adrenal CT • Adrenal MR imaging

KEY POINTS

- Incidental adrenal nodules are common and almost all are benign.
- If benign imaging features are present, no further imaging is necessary.
- If additional imaging is indicated, adrenal CT is the preferred diagnostic test.

INTRODUCTION

Adrenal incidentalomas are defined as nodules greater than 1 cm incidentally discovered during imaging performed for nonadrenal disorders. Adrenal nodules are common, occurring in 4.4% of patients undergoing computed tomography (CT), and in 6% of the population in a large autopsy series.[1,2] Because the prevalence of adrenal nodules increases with age, and as cross-sectional imaging use continues to expand, the overall number of incidental adrenal nodules detected is expected to increase.

Most incidentally detected adrenal nodules are benign, most commonly nonfunctioning adenomas.[3,4] Although almost all small adrenal nodules can safely be ignored, a small percentage of incidentally discovered adrenal nodules require further work-up to determine if they represent clinically relevant neoplasms (adrenocortical carcinoma [ACC], metastases, or pheochromocytoma). One of the major challenges in managing incidentally discovered adrenal nodules is that professional guidelines differ between radiology and endocrinology societies.[3,5,6] This article reviews appropriate clinical management of adrenal nodules incidentally detected on CT examinations performed for nonadrenal disorders.

CURRENT EVIDENCE

Although adrenal nodules are common, almost all nodules in patients without a history of malignancy are benign. In a large series of more than 1000 consecutive unilateral adrenal nodules, no malignant tumors were identified.[4] Even in patients with bilateral nodules, the risk of malignancy is negligible.[7] In patients with a history of malignancy, although the chance of metastases is increased, nodules are still more likely benign than malignant (risk of metastases is estimated at between 26% and 36%).[8]

In contrast to the importance of clinical history, morphologic features alone are insufficient to differentiate between benign and malignant adrenal disease.[9] However, there are specific CT features that confer a high likelihood of benignity and therefore obviate further diagnostic imaging or biopsy. Conversely, because large adrenal masses have a greater chance of being malignant, masses greater than 4 cm are typically referred for surgical management. A recent series of more than 2000 patients demonstrated an overall risk of ACC in incidentally detected adrenal nodules of 1.7%.[10] This analysis demonstrated that the risk of ACC was 0.1% for nodules less than 4.0 cm, which increased to 19.5% for masses greater than 6 cm.[10] Although highly insensitive,

[a] Department of Radiology, Brigham and Women's Hospital, Harvard Medical School, 75 Francis Street, Boston, MA 02115, USA; [b] Department of Radiology, University of California, Davis, 4860 Y Street, Suite 3100, Sacramento, CA 95817, USA
* Corresponding author.
E-mail address: dglazer@bwh.harvard.edu

Radiol Clin N Am 59 (2021) 591–601
https://doi.org/10.1016/j.rcl.2021.03.008
0033-8389/21/© 2021 Elsevier Inc. All rights reserved.

CT features including irregular margins, central low density, and enhancing rim suggest malignancy.[9]

Imaging features that imply a benign diagnosis on CT (or MR imaging) are determined by the amount and type of fat within an adrenal nodule.[11] When a nodule contains greater than 50% macroscopic fat, that is diagnostic of a myelolipoma.[12] It is, however, possible for adrenal adenomas to contain macroscopic fat because of areas of myelolipomatous degeneration. In these instances, macroscopic fat makes up a small portion of the total tumor volume.[13,14] When an adrenal nodule volume is encountered that is primarily soft tissue density but with small focal areas of macroscopic fat, adenoma should be in the differential diagnosis. Although myelolipomas and adenomas are benign, the distinction is important because myelolipomas are not hyperfunctioning, whereas adenomas may be. Macroscopic fat has also been rarely reported in ACC; however, the tumors were large (>6 cm) and contained small proportions of fat.[15]

Lipid-rich adenomas are low in attenuation on CT because of the presence of microscopic fat. When an adrenal nodule measures less than or equal to 10 Hounsfield units (HU) in attenuation, the diagnosis of lipid-rich adenoma is made without the need for additional imaging.[5] As with the presence of macroscopic fat, there are rare instances of overlap in attenuation between adrenal adenomas and other malignancies (most commonly clear cell subtype renal cell carcinoma [RCC] and hepatocellular carcinoma [HCC] metastases, and rarely pheochromocytoma).[16–18] Appropriate clinical history can typically help avoid confusion.

If these features (macroscopic or microscopic fat) are present at the time of nodule detection, no further imaging work-up is necessary. Additionally, if precontrast and postcontrast images are available and the nodule is nonenhancing (indicating a cyst), no further investigation is necessary. However, in the absence of benign features, the nodule is considered indeterminate. Strategies for diagnosing incidentally detected adrenal nodules are presented next.

ADDITIONAL TESTS
Adrenal Protocol Computed Tomography

Adrenal protocol CT is the preferred diagnostic test to characterize an indeterminant adrenal nodule, because it is able to differentiate lipid-rich and lipid-poor adenomas from other adrenal processes.[5] CT characterization of adrenal nodules relies on nonenhanced attenuation measurements, and intravenous (IV) contrast washout if necessary. Lipid-rich adenomas are low in attenuation on nonenhanced images because of the presence of intracellular lipid. Using a cutoff of 10 HU, the diagnosis of adenoma is made with 98% specificity.[19] For nodules or masses with a nonenhanced attenuation of greater than 10 HU, then adrenal washout is performed (Fig. 1). This technique allows the differentiation between lipid-poor adenomas (approximately 20% of adenomas) and other adrenal masses, with a sensitivity of 86% and a specificity of 92%.[20] If the absolute washout is greater than or equal to 60% ([enhanced HU – delayed HU]/[enhanced HU – nonenhanced HU]), then a diagnosis of lipid-poor adenoma is made.[20] It should be noted that approximately one-third of pheochromocytomas can washout greater than or equal to 60%, and therefore should remain in the differential diagnosis if there is biochemical evidence of pheochromocytoma (Fig. 2).[18] It is also important to note that hypervascular metastases, including HCC and RCC, can washout greater than 60%.[16,21] In these patients the diagnosis of HCC or RCC is usually known, so characterizing the adrenal mass is less of a conundrum, particularly if there are other sites of metastases on imaging. Clinical context is important when characterizing an incidental adrenal nodule, because patients rarely present with an HCC or RCC diagnosed by the presence of an incidental adrenal mass. If washout is less than 60%, then the nodule remains indeterminate, and further testing or follow-up imaging may be warranted. However, because of the high prevalence of adenomas, an indeterminate adrenal nodule less than 4 cm that does not washout greater than or equal to 60% is still statistically likely to be an adenoma.

Generally, an adrenal protocol CT consists of a nonenhanced acquisition through the abdomen using reduced radiation dose techniques, followed by radiologist review. If the adrenal nodule measures less than or equal to 10 HU, no further imaging is necessary because the nodule is diagnostic of a lipid-rich adenoma. If the nodule measures greater than 10 HU, then IV contrast is administered, and images are obtained at 60 to 70 seconds and at 15 minutes following injection. This allows for the absolute washout calculation described previously. If the nodule being evaluated has suspicious morphologic features (central low density, irregular margins) or greater than 4 cm, performing a washout CT may not be necessary because surgical consultation is recommended.

Adrenal MR Imaging

Similar to adrenal CT, characterization of adrenal nodules with MR imaging relies on the presence

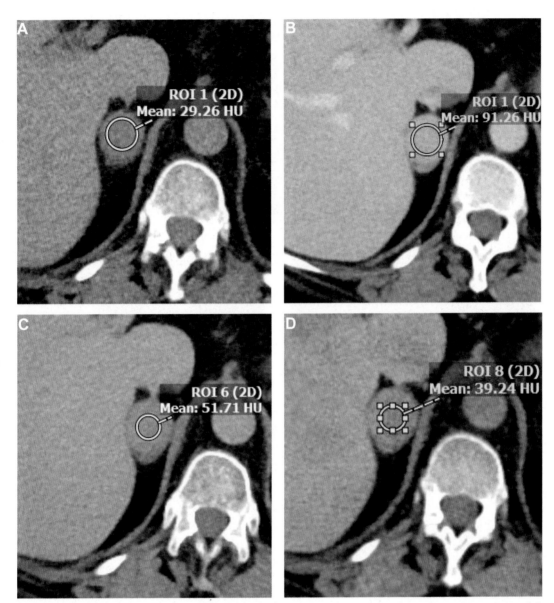

Fig. 1. A 59-year-old woman with a right adrenal nodule incidentally detected on prior imaging obtained for work-up of suspected kidney stones. On this adrenal CT the nodule measures 29 HU in attenuation on nonenhanced images (*A*). Therefore, IV contrast was administered to calculate washout. The nodule measured 91 HU in attenuation at 70 seconds (*B*) and 52 HU in attenuation at 15 minutes (*C*). This resulted in an absolute washout of 62.9%, diagnostic of a lipid-poor adenoma. Interestingly, attenuation measured on virtual noncontrast images (*D*) derived from the postcontrast images was 10 HU higher than the true nonenhanced attenuation in *A*, illustrating a potential pitfall of using dual-energy images to diagnose adenomas.

of microscopic or macroscopic fat within benign processes.[11] Microscopic fat results in diffuse signal loss on out-of-phase compared with in-phase images (chemical shift imaging [CSI]). When a nodule demonstrates signal loss on out-of-phase images, a diagnosis of adenoma is made (**Fig. 3**).[22] In a large meta-analysis of 1280 adrenal nodules/masses, CSI showed a pooled sensitivity of 94% and a specificity of 95%, similar to adrenal CT.[23] However, the sensitivity and specificity of CSI diminishes as the CT number of the adrenal nodule increases.[24,25] For nodules 30 to 39 HU, the sensitivity of washout CT was 88.6% versus 39.5% for CSI MR imaging. For nodules greater than or equal to 40 HU, the sensitivity of CT was 87.5% compared with 9.1% for MR imaging. In a separate smaller series, only 62% of nodules measuring greater than 10 HU could be

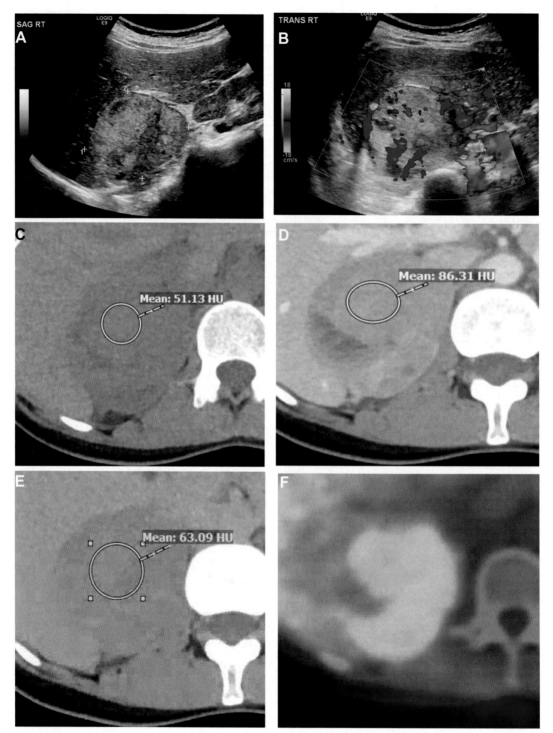

Fig. 2. A 36-year-old woman with hypertension resistant to medications, palpitations, and unintentional weight loss. Initial abdominal ultrasound demonstrates a heterogenous 6.8-cm solid right suprarenal mass (*A, B*). Subsequent adrenal protocol CT (*C–E*) demonstrates the mass to be heterogeneously enhancing with areas of peripheral necrosis. It measures 51 HU on noncontrast CT (*C*), 86 HU on portal venous phase, and 63 HU on 15-minute delay for an absolute washout of 65.7%. Although washout was greater than 60%, heterogeneity and size make the diagnosis of adenoma unlikely. PET/CT revealed that the mass was DOTATATE-avid except for the areas of peripheral necrosis (*F*). Clinical and imaging features were very consistent with pheochromocytoma, a diagnosis that was confirmed at subsequent adrenalectomy.

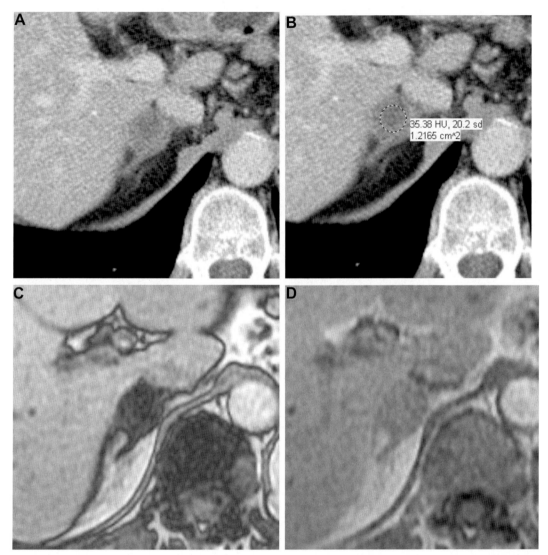

Fig. 3. An 80-year-old man with a 2.0-cm incidental right adrenal nodule (*A*). The nodule measured 35 HU on IV contrast-enhanced CT and was therefore indeterminant (*B*). Subsequently performed abdominal MR imaging demonstrates diffuse signal loss on out-of-phase (*C*) compared with in-phase images (*D*), diagnostic of a lipid-rich adenoma.

definitively characterized as adenomas based on CSI.[26] When dynamic IV contrast-enhancement with gadolinium is combined with CSI, performance of adrenal MR imaging is improved, with a sensitivity of 94% and a specificity of 98% in a series of 239 adrenal masses.[27]

As with washout CT, HCC and RCC metastases are difficult to diagnose with CSI MR imaging, because both tumors can demonstrate loss of signal on out-of-phase imaging owing to the presence of microscopic fat.[28] However, this is only a dilemma in the setting of a patient with known HCC or RCC. The presence of microscopic fat with RCC metastases does not correlate with the presence of microscopic fat in the primary RCC.[17]

In addition to lower test performance characteristics, MR imaging is generally less cost effective than CT. In a study from Europe, the cost-to-accuracy ratio was 1.46 for nonenhanced CT and 4.89 for MR imaging.[29] Given that a combined approach with nonenhanced CT followed by washout if necessary is superior to nonenhanced CT alone, the cost-to-accuracy ratio for CT is likely even lower.

MR imaging can readily depict macroscopic fat within a nodule. Macroscopic fat demonstrates diffuse signal loss following fat saturation techniques or shows chemical shift artifact of the second kind (India ink) at the interface between the fat and surrounding tumor.[11] Similar to CT, when macroscopic fat is identified within most of a mass, a diagnosis of myelolipoma is made.

PET/Computed Tomography

Typically, PET/CT and other nuclear medicine examinations are reserved for patients with a history of primary malignancy who present with an enlarging or otherwise indeterminate mass where there is a high suspicion for metastatic disease. Whole-body PET/CT allows for characterization of the adrenal nodule/mass, and whole-body staging to detect other sites of metastatic disease. In a large meta-analysis consisting of 1391 adrenal abnormalities, PET/CT demonstrated a sensitivity of 97% and a specificity of 91% for differentiating benign from malignant adrenal masses.[30] Some adenomas may be mildly fluorodeoxyglucose (FDG) avid, leading to an overlap with malignant disease. However, it is unlikely for a benign adrenal process to be markedly FDG avid.

ADVANCED IMAGING TECHNIQUES
Dual-Energy Computed Tomography

Dual-energy CT allows for the possibility of tissue characterization based on the creation of virtual noncontrast images (VNC), virtual monoenergic images, and material density images from an IV contrast-enhanced data set. Because most incidental adrenal nodules are identified on IV contrast-enhanced examinations, if the examination is obtained with dual-energy techniques, it may be possible to obtain an accurate diagnosis without requiring additional imaging examinations (**Figs. 4** and **5**).[31] Most commonly, VNC images are used to measure the native attenuation of the nodule.[32,33] As with single-energy CT, a VNC attenuation of less than or equal to 10 HU is diagnostic of a benign adenoma. This approach has been validated with single-source, dual-source, and spectral dual-energy CT platforms.[34–36] Besides measuring VNC, others have proposed using material density images to characterize adrenal nodules, although this approach requires a separate workstation and is thus less useful in regular clinical practice.[37] Recently, a series of 149 patients demonstrated that a combined approach using VNC and material density images is likely most accurate at distinguishing adenomas from metastases (sensitivity of 95% and specificity of 95%).[36]

As with other imaging techniques, there are limitations of dual-energy CT. The primary issue is that VNC images derived from an IV contrast-enhanced data set tend to overestimate the native attenuation of tissue (see **Fig. 1**). For adrenal nodules, this is a substantial limitation, and leads to decreased sensitivity of the technique. For

single-source dual-energy CT, VNC images typically overestimate attenuation by 5 to 9 HU.[38] A similar difference in attenuation was also noted for spectral dual-energy CT.[36]

Computed Tomography Histogram Analysis

CT histogram analysis is an imaging technique that allows for calculation of the distribution of tissue attenuation within a mass. This technique relies on the presence of microscopic fat within adenomas (<0 HU) to distinguish benign from other types of adrenal nodules and masses. Initial results of this technique were limited by low sensitivity and need for a separate workstation.[39,40] More recent advances in image processing (Gaussian model-based algorithm) have led to improvements in the technique when modern dose reduced imaging methods are used.[41] Additionally, there is an open-source software platform for CT histogram analysis, such that a separate workstation is no longer needed.[42] However, the sensitivity and specificity of this technique is not adequate at present to replace standard CT or MR imaging.[43]

RECOMMENDATIONS FOR MANAGEMENT OF INCIDENTALLY DETECTED ADRENAL NODULES

The American College of Radiology (ACR) has published an algorithm for the work-up of incidentally detected adrenal masses.[5] This algorithm distinguishes recommendations for further work-up/imaging based on nodule size and clinical history, and applies to adult patients who are asymptomatic and imaged for reasons unrelated to adrenal pathology. If benign imaging features are present (attenuation ≤10 HU, macroscopic fat, signal loss on CSI, or no enhancement), then no further imaging is needed. If the nodule is greater than or equal to 1 cm and less than 4 cm, then the next steps depend on clinical history and availability of prior imaging.

If prior imaging is available and a nodule is stable for greater than or equal to 1 year, it is considered benign, and no further follow-up is necessary. If it is new or enlarging, then adrenal CT (if no history of cancer) or biopsy or PET/CT (if history of cancer) are the recommended next steps. If prior imaging is not available and the nodule is between 1 and 2 cm, then the nodule is probably benign, but a 12-month follow-up adrenal CT is optional. If the nodule is greater than 2 cm and less than 4 cm, then an adrenal CT should be performed for more definitive diagnosis. If the nodule continues to remain indeterminate following adrenal CT, then further work-up with PET-CT, biopsy,

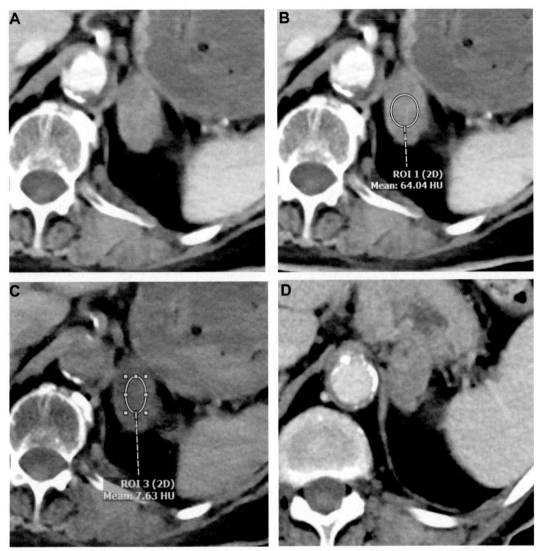

Fig. 4. A 76-year-old man presented to the emergency department following a fall and was found to have an incidental left adrenal mass. The mass measured 64 HU on an IV contrast-enhanced portal venous phase CT (*A, B*), which was indeterminant, although in the absence of known malignancy is still most likely an adenoma. Virtual noncontrast images obtained from the same examination on this dual-energy CT showed that the nodule measured less than 10 HU in attenuation (*C*), diagnostic of a benign, lipid-rich adenoma. Benign cause was confirmed, because the nodule was unchanged with greater than 1 year of follow-up imaging (*D*).

resection, or follow-up is indicated. Lastly, for masses greater than 4 cm surgical consultation for potential resection is recommended in the absence of a history of prior malignancy. In patients with a cancer history, biopsy, or PET/CT are the next tests.

Because imaging tests cannot address the functional status of a mass, biochemical work-up and endocrinology referral are now recommended by the ACR and have been previously recommend by multiple endocrine societies.[3,5,6,44,45] This allows for diagnosis of subclinical Cushing syndrome, hyperaldosteronism, and pheochromocytomas. However, some authorities consider this recommendation to be controversial and cost-ineffective, given the commonality of adrenal nodules. A recent multicenter study concluded that biochemical evaluation for possible pheochromocytoma was not needed for adrenal nodules with a nonenhanced attenuation of less than or equal to 10 HU.[46] The cost implications of the updated ACR guidelines to recommend routine biochemical evaluation is unknown, to our knowledge. A cost-

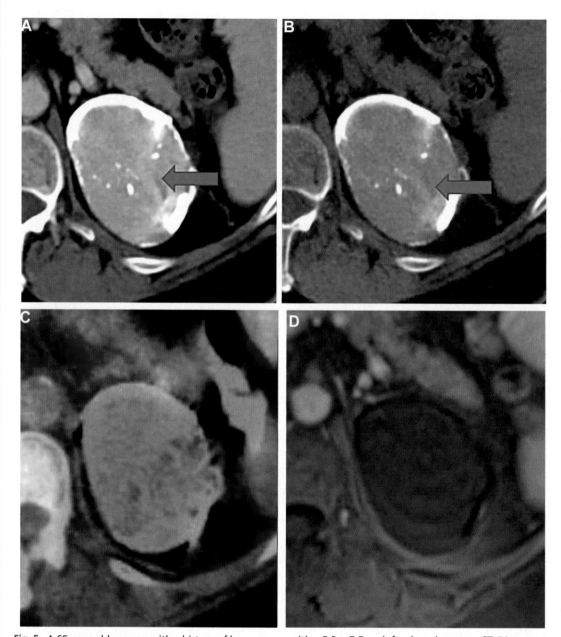

Fig. 5. A 65-year-old woman with a history of lung cancer, with a 5.3 × 7.5 cm left adrenal mass on CT. IV contrast-enhanced portal venous phase axial CT image (*A*) demonstrated a heterogenous mass with areas of peripheral mineralization and possible central enhancement (*arrow*). Axial virtual noncontrast image from the same dual-energy CT examination (*B*) demonstrated the areas of increased attenuation (*arrow*) to be calcification and not solid enhancement. This mass demonstrated no uptake on FDG-PET CT (*C*), and no internal enhancement on MR imaging (*D*). These imaging features were diagnostic of prior adrenal hemorrhage.

effectiveness analysis from Europe that predated the ACR changes concluded that screening urine metanephrines is the most cost-effective strategy and that full hormonal analysis should be reserved for larger masses or if the patient is symptomatic.[47]

In contrast to the approach taken by the ACR, the American Association of Clinical Endocrinologists and American Association of Endocrine Surgeons has taken a more conservative approach and recommend imaging evaluation 3 to 6 months after the initial diagnosis, and then annually for 1 to 2 years for all nodules less than 4 cm, even those with benign characteristics.[6] The European Society of Endocrinology and the European Network for the Study of

Adrenal Tumors has taken a simpler approach and recommend no further follow-up imaging for nodules less than 4 cm with a nonenhanced attenuation of less than 10 HU (ie, those that can be diagnosed as lipid-rich adenomas).[3] A single cost-effectiveness analysis comparing four surveillance strategies for incidental nonfunctional nodules less than 4 cm (no surveillance, single 1-year follow-up, annually for 2 years, and annually for 5 years) concluded that one-time follow-up noncontrast CT and biochemical evaluation were the most effective and additional imaging increased cost without benefit.[48] This suggests that the ACR and European society recommendations are likely most cost-effective.

The purpose of follow-up imaging is to assess for interval growth. Although benign and malignant adrenal masses can grow, malignant masses grow faster.[49] Approximately one-third of adenomas may grow, but at a rate of less than 3 mm per year. In one study, all malignant adrenal nodules grew, and at a rate of greater than 5 mm per year. This suggests that when performing follow-up adrenal CT at 1 year, growth of less than 3 mm should be considered a benign pattern. However, growth on a yearly basis is small so that with only a single follow-up examination it may be difficult to reach a definitive diagnosis because the difference between a benign and malignant diagnosis is 2 mm, which could easily be caused by measuring error.[50] Thus, continued follow-up may be appropriate for slowly growing nodules.

SUMMARY

Incidentally detected adrenal nodules are common, and prevalence increases with patient age. Although almost all are benign, it is important for the radiologist to be able to accurately determine which nodules require further testing and which are safely left alone. The most recent ACR incidental adrenal White Paper provides a structured algorithm based on expert consensus for management of incidental adrenal nodules. If further diagnostic testing is indicated, adrenal CT is the most appropriate test in patients for all nodules less than 4 cm regardless of cancer history. In addition to imaging, biochemical testing and endocrinology referral may be warranted to exclude a functioning mass (which should then be resected regardless of imaging features).

CLINICS CARE POINTS

- Most incidental adrenal nodules are benign.
- If further testing is required, adrenal CT is the recommended imaging test.
- Biochemical testing should be considered per current guidelines for patients with an incidentally detected adrenal nodule.

DISCLOSURE

Authors have nothing to disclose.

REFERENCES

1. Bovio S, Cataldi A, Reimondo G, et al. Prevalence of adrenal incidentaloma in a contemporary computerized tomography series. J Endocrinol Invest 2006; 29(4):298–302.
2. Young WF. Clinical practice. The incidentally discovered adrenal mass. N Engl J Med 2007;356(6): 601–10.
3. Fassnacht M, Arlt W, Bancos I, et al. Management of adrenal incidentalomas: European Society of Endocrinology Clinical Practice Guideline in collaboration with the European Network for the Study of Adrenal Tumors. Eur J Endocrinol 2016;175(2):G1–34.
4. Song JH, Chaudhry FS, Mayo-Smith WW. The incidental adrenal mass on CT: prevalence of adrenal disease in 1,049 consecutive adrenal masses in patients with no known malignancy. AJR Am J Roentgenol 2008;190(5):1163–8.
5. Mayo-Smith WW, Song JH, Boland GL, et al. Management of incidental adrenal masses: a white paper of the ACR incidental findings committee. J Am Coll Radiol 2017;14(8):1038–44.
6. Zeiger MA, Thompson GB, Duh QY, et al. The American Association of Clinical Endocrinologists and American Association of Endocrine Surgeons medical guidelines for the management of adrenal incidentalomas. Endocr Pract 2009;15(Suppl 1):1–20.
7. Corwin MT, Chalfant JS, Loehfelm TW, et al. Incidentally detected bilateral adrenal nodules in patients without cancer: is further workup necessary? AJR Am J Roentgenol 2018;210(4):780–4.
8. Boland GW, Goldberg MA, Lee MJ, et al. Indeterminate adrenal mass in patients with cancer: evaluation at PET with 2-[F-18]-fluoro-2-deoxy-D-glucose. Radiology 1995;194(1):131–4.
9. Song JH, Grand DJ, Beland MD, et al. Morphologic features of 211 adrenal masses at initial contrast-enhanced CT: can we differentiate benign from malignant lesions using imaging features alone? AJR Am J Roentgenol 2013;201(6):1248–53.
10. Kahramangil B, Kose E, Remer EM, et al. A modern assessment of cancer risk in adrenal

incidentalomas: analysis of 2219 patients. Ann Surg 2020. https://doi.org/10.1097/SLA.00000000 00004048.

11. Schieda N, Davenport MS, Pedrosa I, et al. Renal and adrenal masses containing fat at MRI: proposed nomenclature by the society of abdominal radiology disease-focused panel on renal cell carcinoma. J Magn Reson Imaging 2019;49(4):917–26.

12. Kenney PJ, Wagner BJ, Rao P, et al. Myelolipoma: CT and pathologic features. Radiology 1998; 208(1):87–95.

13. Schieda N, Al Dandan O, Kielar AZ, et al. Pitfalls of adrenal imaging with chemical shift MRI. Clin Radiol 2014;69(11):1186–97.

14. Shaaban AM, Rezvani M, Tubay M, et al. Fat-containing retroperitoneal lesions: imaging characteristics, localization, and differential diagnosis. Radiographics 2016;36(3):710–34.

15. Ranathunga DS, Cherpak LA, Schieda N, et al. Macroscopic fat in adrenocortical carcinoma: a systematic review. AJR Am J Roentgenol 2020;214(2): 390–4.

16. Choi YA, Kim CK, Park BK, et al. Evaluation of adrenal metastases from renal cell carcinoma and hepatocellular carcinoma: use of delayed contrast-enhanced CT. Radiology 2013;266(2):514–20.

17. Schieda N, Krishna S, McInnes MDF, et al. Utility of MRI to differentiate clear cell renal cell carcinoma adrenal metastases from adrenal adenomas. AJR Am J Roentgenol 2017;209(3): W152–9.

18. Patel J, Davenport MS, Cohan RH, et al. Can established CT attenuation and washout criteria for adrenal adenoma accurately exclude pheochromocytoma? AJR Am J Roentgenol 2013;201(1):122–7.

19. Boland GW, Lee MJ, Gazelle GS, et al. Characterization of adrenal masses using unenhanced CT: an analysis of the CT literature. AJR Am J Roentgenol 1998;171(1):201–4.

20. Caoili EM, Korobkin M, Francis IR, et al. Adrenal masses: characterization with combined unenhanced and delayed enhanced CT. Radiology 2002;222(3):629–33.

21. Woo S, Suh CH, Kim SY, et al. Pheochromocytoma as a frequent false-positive in adrenal washout CT: a systematic review and meta-analysis. Eur Radiol 2018;28(3):1027–36.

22. Adam SZ, Nikolaidis P, Horowitz JM, et al. Chemical shift MR imaging of the adrenal gland: principles, pitfalls, and applications. Radiographics 2016; 36(2):414–32.

23. Platzek I, Sieron D, Plodeck V, et al. Chemical shift imaging for evaluation of adrenal masses: a systematic review and meta-analysis. Eur Radiol 2019; 29(2):806–17.

24. Park BK, Kim CK, Kim B, et al. Comparison of delayed enhanced CT and chemical shift MR for

evaluating hyperattenuating incidental adrenal masses. Radiology 2007;243(3):760–5.

25. Seo JM, Park BK, Park SY, et al. Characterization of lipid-poor adrenal adenoma: chemical-shift MRI and washout CT. AJR Am J Roentgenol 2014;202(5): 1043–50.

26. Israel GM, Korobkin M, Wang C, et al. Comparison of unenhanced CT and chemical shift MRI in evaluating lipid-rich adrenal adenomas. AJR Am J Roentgenol 2004;183(1):215–9.

27. Rodacki K, Ramalho M, Dale BM, et al. Combined chemical shift imaging with early dynamic serial gadolinium-enhanced MRI in the characterization of adrenal lesions. AJR Am J Roentgenol 2014; 203(1):99–106.

28. Sydow BD, Rosen MA, Siegelman ES. Intracellular lipid within metastatic hepatocellular carcinoma of the adrenal gland: a potential diagnostic pitfall of chemical shift imaging of the adrenal gland. AJR Am J Roentgenol 2006;187(5):W550–1.

29. Lumachi F, Basso SM, Borsato S, et al. Role and cost-effectiveness of adrenal imaging and image-guided FNA cytology in the management of incidentally discovered adrenal tumours. Anticancer Res 2005;25(6C):4559–62.

30. Boland GW, Dwamena BA, Jagtiani Sangwaiya M, et al. Characterization of adrenal masses by using FDG PET: a systematic review and meta-analysis of diagnostic test performance. Radiology 2011; 259(1):117–26.

31. Hindman NM, Megibow AJ. One-stop shopping: dual-energy CT for the confident diagnosis of adrenal adenomas. Radiology 2020;296(2):333–4.

32. Ho LM, Marin D, Neville AM, et al. Characterization of adrenal nodules with dual-energy CT: can virtual unenhanced attenuation values replace true unenhanced attenuation values? AJR Am J Roentgenol 2012;198(4):840–5.

33. Gnannt R, Fischer M, Goetti R, et al. Dual-energy CT for characterization of the incidental adrenal mass: preliminary observations. AJR Am J Roentgenol 2012;198(1):138–44.

34. Morgan DE, Weber AC, Lockhart ME, et al. Differentiation of high lipid content from low lipid content adrenal lesions using single-source rapid kilovolt (peak)-switching dual-energy multidetector CT. J Comput Assist Tomogr 2013;37(6):937–43.

35. Kim YK, Park BK, Kim CK, et al. Adenoma characterization: adrenal protocol with dual-energy CT. Radiology 2013;267(1):155–63.

36. Nagayama Y, Inoue T, Oda S, et al. Adrenal adenomas versus metastases: diagnostic performance of dual-energy spectral CT virtual noncontrast imaging and iodine maps. Radiology 2020;296(2): 324–32.

37. Mileto A, Nelson RC, Marin D, et al. Dual-energy multidetector CT for the characterization of

incidental adrenal nodules: diagnostic performance of contrast-enhanced material density analysis. Radiology 2015;274(2):445–54.

38. Kaza RK, Raff EA, Davenport MS, et al. Variability of CT attenuation measurements in virtual unenhanced images generated using multimaterial decomposition from fast kilovoltage-switching dual-energy CT. Acad Radiol 2017;24(3):365–72.

39. Remer EM, Motta-Ramirez GA, Shepardson LB, et al. CT histogram analysis in pathologically proven adrenal masses. AJR Am J Roentgenol 2006;187(1): 191–6.

40. Bae KT, Fuangtharnthip P, Prasad SR, et al. Adrenal masses: CT characterization with histogram analysis method. Radiology 2003;228(3):735–42.

41. Clark TJ, Hsu LD, Hippe D, et al. Evaluation of diagnostic accuracy: multidetector CT image noise correction improves specificity of a Gaussian model-based algorithm used for characterization of incidental adrenal nodules. Abdom Radiol (NY) 2019;44(3):1033–43.

42. RadDecisionSupport.com. Available at: http://raddecisionsupport.com/. Accessed May 22, 2020.

43. Glazer DI, Mayo-Smith WW. Letter to the editor response. Abdom Radiol (NY) 2020. https://doi.org/10.1007/s00261-020-02666-5.

44. Lee JM, Kim MK, Ko SH, et al. Clinical guidelines for the management of adrenal incidentaloma. Endocrinol Metab (Seoul) 2017;32(2):200–18.

45. Sherlock M, Scarsbrook A, Abbas A, et al. Adrenal incidentaloma. Endocr Rev 2020;41(6). https://doi.org/10.1210/endrev/bnaa008.

46. Canu L, Van Hemert JAW, Kerstens MN, et al. CT characteristics of pheochromocytoma: relevance for the evaluation of adrenal incidentaloma. J Clin Endocrinol Metab 2019;104(2):312–8.

47. Kievit J, Haak HR. Diagnosis and treatment of adrenal incidentaloma. A cost-effectiveness analysis. Endocrinol Metab Clin North Am 2000;29(1): 69–90. viii-ix.

48. Chomsky-Higgins K, Seib C, Rochefort H, et al. Less is more: cost-effectiveness analysis of surveillance strategies for small, nonfunctional, radiographically benign adrenal incidentalomas. Surgery 2018; 163(1):197–204.

49. Corwin MT, Navarro SM, Malik DG, et al. Differences in growth rate on CT of adrenal adenomas and malignant adrenal nodules. AJR Am J Roentgenol 2019;213(3):632–6.

50. Zhao B, James LP, Moskowitz CS, et al. Evaluating variability in tumor measurements from same-day repeat CT scans of patients with non-small cell lung cancer. Radiology 2009;252(1):263–72.

Incidental Splenic Findings on Cross-Sectional Imaging

Pei-Kang Wei, MD, Karen S. Lee, MD, Bettina Siewert, MD*

KEYWORDS

• Spleen • Mass • CT • MRI • Management • Incidental finding

KEY POINTS

- Despite overlapping imaging features among benign and malignant splenic processes, certain splenic focal findings have unique imaging features that can lead to a definitive diagnosis or appropriate differential diagnosis.
- Incidental indeterminate splenic findings in patients with a history of malignancy or symptoms (epigastric or left upper quadrant pain, type B symptoms, immunocompromised) require further imaging follow-up or evaluation by MR imaging, PET/computed tomography, or tissue sampling.
- Incidental indeterminate splenic findings in patients without a history of malignancy or symptoms pose an exceedingly low risk for malignancy (1%). Patients with an incidental malignant mass in the spleen almost always have additional imaging findings that allow for a diagnosis of malignancy to be made. Therefore, no follow-up or evaluation is required if no additional concurrent imaging findings worrisome for malignancy are detected.

INTRODUCTION

With the increased use of cross-sectional imaging for the evaluation of a wide spectrum of clinical presentations, the discovery of incidental findings has become more common. Previously reported rates of incidental findings within the abdomen and pelvis range from 35% to 56% on computed tomography (CT) performed in the emergency department in the setting of trauma.[1,2] These findings include focal processes in the spleen, which frequently present a diagnostic dilemma as imaging features of benign and malignant entities demonstrate substantial overlap.[3,4] Consequently, the evaluation of incidentally discovered splenic focal findings relies heavily on clinical context as opposed to being primarily imaging based. Fortunately, most incidentally detected splenic focal findings are benign and of no clinical significance. Unwarranted workup or inappropriate follow-up for such findings, however, can lead to increased health care costs and expose patients to unnecessary procedures, and result in both physical risk and emotional stress.[5-7]

In this article, we focus on incidental focal splenic findings that radiologists may encounter in their usual clinical practice. A practical and simplified approach to the management of incidental splenic focal findings discovered on CT or MR imaging are described, incorporating both imaging features and clinical context.

INCIDENTAL FOCAL SPLENIC FINDINGS

A number of focal splenic findings can be seen incidentally on CT or MR imaging. These can be broadly grouped into non-neoplastic and neoplastic, which can be further subdivided into benign and malignant entities. Understanding the typical imaging features of more commonly encountered focal splenic processes can help

Department of Radiology, Beth Israel Deaconess Medical Center, 330 Brookline Avenue, Boston, MA 02215, USA
* Corresponding author.
E-mail address: bsiewert@bidmc.harvard.edu

Radiol Clin N Am 59 (2021) 603–616
https://doi.org/10.1016/j.rcl.2021.03.009
0033-8389/21/© 2021 Elsevier Inc. All rights reserved.

guide the need for further assessment or follow-up imaging.

Non-neoplastic Masses

Nonparasitic cyst

Splenic cysts can be either congenital (true cyst) or false (posttraumatic or secondary cyst). Congenital cysts are lined by epithelial cells that are thought to derive from peritoneal mesothelial cells.[8,9] False cysts, on the other hand, contain a fibrous lining and are more common than true cysts, representing 80% of all nonparasitic splenic cysts.[10] False cysts tend to be smaller and more commonly exhibit mural calcifications compared with true cysts.[10] Both types of cysts may be asymptomatic at the time of discovery, but a prior history of trauma can be extremely helpful in diagnosing a false cyst.

On imaging, splenic cysts typically present as well-circumscribed, homogeneous, simple fluid-containing masses. They are hypodense on CT (<10 HU) without internal or rim enhancement. Similarly, splenic cysts are homogeneously hypo-intense on T1-weighted images, and hyperintense on T2-weighted MR images, without enhancement on postcontrast sequences. Although the presence of thick rim calcification can differentiate a false cyst from a true cyst on imaging[10] (Fig. 1), distinction between these 2 entities is often of no clinical significance.

Abscess

Bacterial infection in the spleen can lead to development of a pyogenic abscess. Hematogenous spread from infection of other organs is the most common cause for splenic pyogenic abscess.[10,11] Patients with a pyogenic abscess tend to be symptomatic with fever, leukocytosis, and left upper quadrant pain and, hence, these are usually not truly incidental. On both CT and MR imaging, a pyogenic abscess may present as a single cystic process, or be multiple, usually unilocular with internal fluid attenuation or signal intensity with a thick, irregular and enhancing wall. Similar to pyogenic abscesses in other organs, a splenic pyogenic abscess can contain air (Fig. 2) and various amount of internal debris, resulting in increased internal heterogeneity.

Compared with bacterial infections, mycobacterial and fungal infections usually appear as multifocal or miliary abscesses within the spleen.[12] Patients with splenic mycobacterial or fungal infection may be immunocompromised and exhibit moderate splenomegaly with multiple to innumerable nodules that are smaller than 1 cm, although micronodules may not be apparent on imaging. These foci are usually hypodense on CT without substantial internal or rim enhancement. On MR imaging, mycobacterial nodules are typically isointense on precontrast T1-weighted images and hypointense on T2-weighted images, with peripheral enhancement. Fungal microabscesses appear hypointense on T1-weighted sequences and hyperintense on T2-weighted images, and may demonstrate peripheral enhancement.[12]

Parasitic cyst

Parasitic infection of the spleen by echinococcus can present with distinct imaging features that

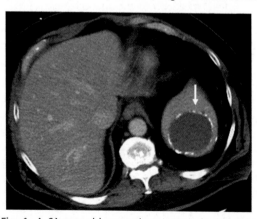

Fig. 1. A 61-year-old man who presented with right upper quadrant pain. Axial postcontrast CT image shows an incidental well-circumscribed homogeneously hypodense round splenic mass with thick rim calcification and without internal enhancement (*arrow*). Imaging findings are highly consistent with a posttraumatic cyst, and no further follow-up is needed.

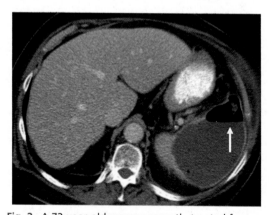

Fig. 2. A 72-year-old woman recently treated for urosepsis who presented with new malaise and general weakness. Axial IV contrast-enhanced CT image demonstrates a well-circumscribed fluid collection containing gas (*arrow*) within the spleen, which is highly consistent with an abscess. Fluid cultures grew *Escherichia coli.*

aid in its diagnosis. On both CT and MR imaging, hydatid cysts present as well-circumscribed cysts that may contain multiple peripheral smaller daughter cysts. The cyst contents are usually of fluid density or signal intensity. Hydatid sand and debris within the cyst may cause the cyst to be hyperdense on CT and hypointense on T2-weighted MR images.[10] On MR imaging, daughter cysts tend to have lower signal intensity than the mother cyst on T1-weighted images.[13] A thick hypointense rim on T2-weighted images surrounding the mother cyst can be seen, and is thought to represent collagen-rich material deposited by the host's response to the cyst.[13,14] Both the mother cyst wall (pericyst) and the collapsed internal parasitic membrane can calcify.[10,15] The cysts do not demonstrate enhancement after intravenous (IV) contrast administration.

Sarcoidosis

In patients with sarcoidosis, splenic involvement can be seen in 24% to 59% based on studies using fine needle splenic aspiration.[16,17] Patients with splenic sarcoidosis are usually asymptomatic, but can present with abdominal pain, fever, malaise, or rarely even splenic rupture. On imaging, splenic sarcoidosis can manifest with splenomegaly and diffuse homogeneous or nodular involvement. Abdominal lymphadenopathy is frequently visualized. Although the presence of intrathoracic findings of sarcoidosis can substantially aid in establishing the diagnosis of splenic sarcoidosis, chest radiographs have been reported to be normal in a quarter of patients with sarcoidosis presenting with splenomegaly or splenic nodules.[18] Sarcoidosis nodules are hypodense and hypoenhancing on CT. On MR imaging, these nodules are hypointense on all sequences, with minimal enhancement on postcontrast images[19,20] (Fig. 3).

Neoplastic Masses

Benign masses

Hemangioma Hemangioma is the most common primary neoplasm of the spleen, with incidence ranging from 0.3% to 14% on autopsy series.[21–23] The mass is characterized as a focal proliferation of blood vessels ranging from capillary to cavernous in size.[24] Splenic hemangiomas can be solitary or multiple. Most patients are asymptomatic with the hemangioma or hemangiomas found incidentally; however, large hemangiomas may rarely cause hemorrhage, rupture, anemia, thrombocytopenia, or high-output heart failure.

The appearance of splenic hemangiomas on noncontrast CT depends on the size of the blood vessels within, ranging from homogeneously hypodense or isodense in capillary hemangiomas, to heterogeneously hypodense and isodense in cavernous hemangiomas.[3,25] After intravenous contrast administration, capillary hemangiomas demonstrate avid homogeneous enhancement, whereas cavernous hemangiomas demonstrate heterogeneous enhancement on late to delayed-phase images.[3,25] Calcifications also can be seen.[3,25]

On MR imaging, splenic hemangiomas are hyperintense on T2-weighted images and hypointense on precontrast T1-weighted images compared with splenic parenchyma. On postcontrast T1-weighted images, splenic hemangiomas demonstrate either homogeneous early and persistent enhancement or early peripheral enhancement that progresses centripetally or homogeneously on delayed phases[3,26,27] (Fig. 4). The classic peripheral nodular centripetal enhancement seen in hepatic hemangiomas may be difficult to appreciate in splenic hemangiomas due to the avidly enhancing background splenic parenchyma.[3]

Hamartoma Splenic hamartoma is an abnormal growth of histologically normal cells in the spleen. It consists almost entirely of red pulp. Previous autopsy series demonstrate an incidence of 0.024% to 0.13%.[28] Similar to splenic hemangiomas, hamartomas rarely cause symptoms[29] and may present as a solitary mass or multiple masses.

Splenic hamartoma demonstrates imaging characteristics similar to focal nodular hyperplasia in the liver. On CT, it appears hypodense to isodense on noncontrast CT. Rarely, calcification within a splenic hamartoma has been reported.[30,31] On IV contrast-enhanced CT, splenic hamartomas demonstrate heterogeneous avid hyperenhancement on the early arterial phase.[32] The enhancement may become more uniform on delayed postcontrast phases, blending in with background splenic parenchyma. On MR imaging, splenic hamartomas are isointense on precontrast T1-weighted images, and isointense or mildly hyperintense on T2-weighted images compared with background splenic parenchyma[33] (Fig. 5). Appearance on postcontrast T1-weighted images is similar to postcontrast CT.

Lymphangioma Lymphangioma is a benign malformation of lymphatic channels, generally more common in children, with reported 10% of pediatric lymphangiomas involving visceral organs.[34] Lymphangiomas in other organs are frequently present when splenic lymphangioma is identified. Differentiation among capillary, cavernous, or

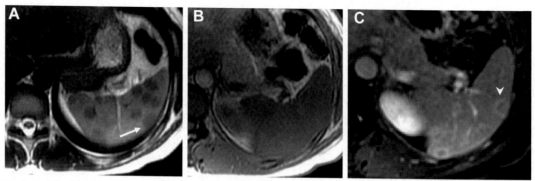

Fig. 3. A 31-year-old woman with a history of ovarian borderline mucinous tumor who presented with focal splenic findings initially discovered on CT performed during workup for acute onset nausea and vomiting (not shown). Follow-up MR imaging obtained after 18 months demonstrated interval growth. Biopsy confirmed isolated extrapulmonary splenic sarcoidosis. (A) Axial T2-weighted MR image demonstrates multiple small hypointense nodules (*arrow*). (B) On an axial T1-weighted MR image, these nodules are not discernible, appearing isointense to the background splenic parenchyma. (C) Axial postcontrast fat-suppressed T1-weighted MR image demonstrates rim enhancement and central hypoenhancement (*arrowhead*).

cystic subtypes is based on the size of the lymphatic channels.[35]

Splenic lymphangiomas present as a solitary cystic mass or as multiple well-circumscribed cystic masses, which may be multilocular with multiple thin septations. On precontrast CT, splenic lymphangiomas measure simple fluid density. Density of the fluid may increase as proteinaceous or hemorrhagic contents accumulate. On noncontrast MR imaging, lymphangiomas are typically homogeneously hypointense on T1-weighted imaging and hyperintense on T2-weighted imaging (**Fig. 6**). The signal intensity of lymphangiomas, however, can vary on T1-weighted and T2-weighted images depending on the presence of proteinaceous and hemorrhagic contents, which

may increase the signal intensity on T1-weighted images, and correspondingly decrease the signal intensity on T2-weighted images. On postcontrast CT and MR imaging, splenic lymphangiomas demonstrate no or minimal enhancement of the cyst wall or of the septations.

Littoral cell angioma Littoral cell angioma is a rare, benign neoplasm of the spleen that consists of numerous nodules that are made of various-sized vascular channels.[24] These vascular channels contain blood products of various ages,[36] resulting in red to brown color on gross pathologic examination. Littoral cells, which line the splenic sinuses of the red pulp and demonstrate immunohistochemical features for both endothelial and

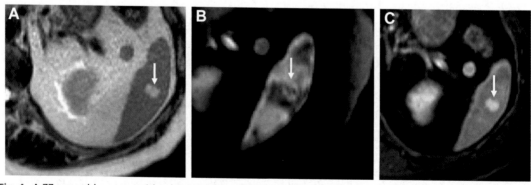

Fig. 4. A 77-year-old woman with a history of thyroid cancer who presented with an incidental splenic mass that was compatible with a hemangioma on MR imaging performed for evaluation of intraductal papillary mucinous neoplasm of the pancreas. The hemangioma remained stable for all available follow-up imaging (6 years). (A) Axial T2-weighted MR image demonstrates a small, lobulated, homogeneously hyperintense single splenic mass (*arrow*). (B) On an axial late arterial-phase postcontrast fat-suppressed T1-weighted MR image, the mass demonstrates peripheral enhancement (*arrow*). (C) On an axial delayed-phase postcontrast fat-suppressed T1-weighted MR image, the mass centripetally enhances, demonstrating homogeneous hyperenhancement (*arrow*).

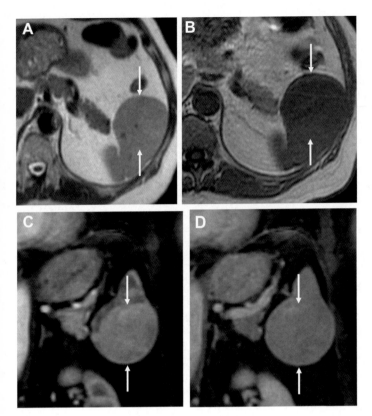

Fig. 5. A 60-year-old woman presented with an incidental splenic mass discovered during evaluation for a right renal mass. MR imaging features were consistent with a splenic hamartoma, and no further imaging follow-up was needed. (*A*) Axial T2-weighted MR image demonstrates a subtle hyperintense lobulated mass (*arrows*). (*B*) On an axial T1-weighted in-phase MR image, the mass is isointense to the background splenic parenchyma (*arrows*). (*C*) On a coronal late arterial-phase postcontrast fat-suppressed T1-weighted MR image, the mass is avidly enhancing (*arrows*). (*D*) On a coronal delayed-phase postcontrast fat-suppressed T1-weighted MR image, enhancement within the mass fades, appearing slightly hyperintense relative to the background splenic parenchyma (*arrows*).

histiocytic cells, are thought to give rise to the mass.[37] Clinically, littoral cell angioma may present as an incidental finding or with splenomegaly. No gender predilection has been reported. Association with other neoplasms has been reported despite the benignity of littoral cell angioma.[38]

On CT, littoral cell angioma may appear as a solitary mass or multiple, usually similar-sized masses ranging from smaller than a centimeter, to 6 cm. Although it is a circumscribed mass, littoral cell angioma is not encapsulated. The mass appears isodense to the splenic parenchyma on noncontrast CT,[37] and is hypoattenuating on the portal

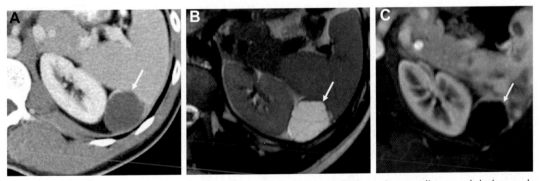

Fig. 6. A 37-year-old woman presented with an incidental complex splenic cystic mass discovered during evaluation for appendicitis. Imaging features were highly compatible with a splenic lymphangioma, and no further follow-up was necessary. (*A*) Axial contrast-enhanced CT image during the portal venous phase demonstrates a multilobular, homogeneous, fluid density mass (*arrow*). (*B*) On an axial T2-weighted MR image, the cystic mass (*arrow*) is uniformly hyperintense with multiple thin smooth internal septations. (*C*) On an axial postcontrast fat-suppressed T1-weighted MR image, the cystic mass (*arrow*) demonstrates no appreciable internal or peripheral enhancement.

venous phase. On MR imaging, it may manifest as marked hypointense masses on both precontrast T1-weighted and T2-weighted images due to hemosiderin deposition within the nodules,[3] although signal intensity on T2-weighted images may be heterogeneously hyperintense.[32] Peripheral arterial hyperenhancement with delayed centripetal filling on postcontrast MR images has been reported[39] (**Fig. 7**).

Sclerosing angiomatoid nodular transformation
Sclerosing angiomatoid nodular transformation (SANT) is a rare splenic neoplasm first described in 2004 by Martel and colleagues,[40] and is often incidentally found. On gross pathologic examination, SANT presents as a well-circumscribed mass containing multiple nodules separated by fibrous stroma that radiates from the center to the periphery, resulting in a stellate appearance.[41,42]

In limited reported cases, SANT presents as a solitary hypoattenuating mass compared with splenic parenchyma on precontrast CT. After IV contrast administration, the mass can demonstrate peripheral hyperenhancement on early phase. On portal venous and delayed phases, enhancement may demonstrate filling in toward the center in a stellate fashion, giving rise to a "spoke-wheel" appearance,[41] which has been

reported to be present in 88% of SANTs on a retrospective study by Lewis and colleagues.[43] The central fibrous scar is typically hypodense, reflecting the fibrotic nature. On MR imaging, SANT typically demonstrates central hypointensity on T2-weighted images, corresponding to the central fibrous stroma. The mass is homogeneously or heterogeneously hypointense on precontrast T1-weighted MR images. Hemosiderin deposition, if present, will demonstrate susceptibility artifact on longer echo-time in-phase imaging compared with out-of-phase imaging. On postcontrast MR imaging, the mass demonstrates peripheral hypoenhancing radiating lines during arterial and portal venous phase sequences, and isointensity or hyperintensity compared with splenic parenchyma on delayed phases[43] (**Fig. 8**).

Malignant tumors
Lymphoma Primary lymphoma accounts for fewer than 1% of splenic lymphoma.[44] Secondary involvement of the spleen, however, is the most common splenic malignancy, and splenic involvement frequently occurs for both Hodgkin lymphoma and non-Hodgkin lymphoma. Involvement of lymph nodes outside of splenic hilum differentiate secondary involvement from primary splenic lymphoma. Presenting symptoms include left upper quadrant pain, fever, weight loss, and malaise.

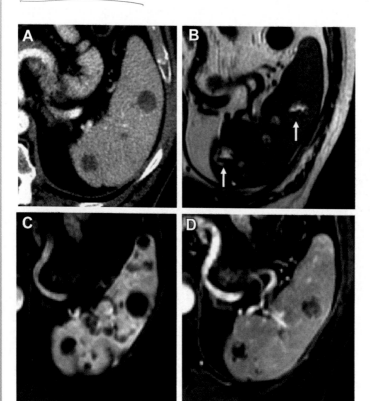

Fig. 7. A 64-year-old man with history of papillary urothelial carcinoma and multiple enlarging splenic masses. Biopsy confirmed the diagnosis of littoral cell angioma. (*A*) Axial contrast-enhanced CT image in the portal venous phase demonstrates several round hypodense masses in the spleen. (*B*) On an axial T2-weighted MR images, these masses are hyperintense with internal hypointense foci (*arrow*). (*C*) On an axial arterial-phase postcontrast fat-suppressed T1-weighted MR image, these masses are hypoenhancing. (*D*) On an axial delayed-phase postcontrast fat-suppressed T1-weighted MR image, there is progressive centripetal enhancement.

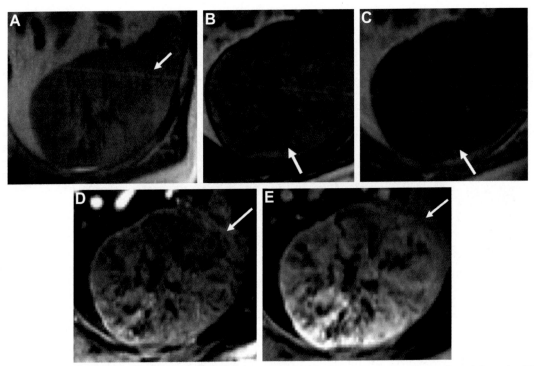

Fig. 8. A 76-year-old man presented for evaluation of splenomegaly. A new splenic mass was found since the CT from 10 years prior. Biopsy-confirmed SANT. (*A*) Axial T2-weighted MR image demonstrates an isointense mass with central hypointensity (*arrow*) compared with the splenic parenchyma. (*B*) On an axial gradient-echo out-of-phase MR image compared with (*C*) an in-phase image, several linear areas of signal dropout are noted on the in-phase image, which is consistent with susceptibility artifact from hemosiderin deposition (*arrow*). (*D*) Axial postcontrast fat-suppressed T1-weighted MR image in the arterial phase shows heterogeneous peripheral enhancement of the mass. (*E*) Axial postcontrast fat-suppressed T1-weighted MR image in portal venous phase shows progressive enhancement of the mass in a "spoke-wheel" pattern.

Several different patterns of lymphomatous involvement of the spleen have been reported, regardless of primary or secondary splenic lymphoma. These include (1) a large solitary mass (**Fig. 9**); (2) multiple discrete small nodules (**Fig. 10**); (3) diffuse miliary nodules; and (4) splenomegaly without a discrete nodule(s) or mass(es).[45] On CT, splenic lymphoma appears hypoattenuating, and is most conspicuous on late phases after IV contrast adminstration.[45,46] Splenic lymphoma may appear slightly hypointense on precontrast T1-weighted images, and slightly hypointense on T2-weighted MR images, compared with the normal splenic parenchyma. Frequently, however, the tumoral foci may also appear isointense to splenic parenchyma on both precontrast T1-weighted and T2-weighted MR images, making detection on noncontrast MR imaging difficult. These may become more conspicuous on postcontrast MR imaging sequences, as they are typically hypoenhancing.[47] Similar to lymphoma in other organs, splenic lymphoma is hyperintense on diffusion-weighted images, with corresponding hypointense signal on apparent diffusion coefficient maps.

Angiosarcoma Splenic angiosarcoma is an extremely rare aggressive primary splenic malignancy, with an incidence of approximately 0.14 to 0.25 cases per million persons.[48] The mass is composed of neoplastic nodules derived from endothelial cells, and contains various degrees of hemorrhage and necrosis.[24] The spleen is usually enlarged by the mass. Patients may exhibit abdominal pain, weight loss, anemia, left upper quadrant mass, and consumptive coagulopathy. Spontaneous splenic rupture has also been reported, with an incidence as high as 30% in a small number of cases.[49] The prognosis is poor, as metastases are common at the time of presentation, most frequently involving the liver, lung, and bones.

On both CT and MR imaging, angiosarcoma appears as a heterogeneous mass or masses on noncontrast images due to the presence of hemorrhage and necrosis, which correspond to various

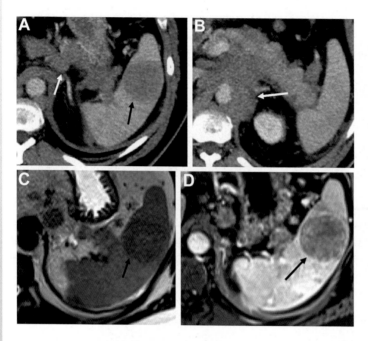

Fig. 9. A 48-year-old man presented with a solitary splenic mass and extensive retroperitoneal lymphadenopathy during evaluation for abdominal pain. Biopsy of the retroperitoneal lymphadenopathy confirmed lymphoma. Follow-up imaging after treatment demonstrates decrease in size of the splenic mass. (*A, B*) Axial IV contrast-enhanced CT images during the portal venous phase demonstrate a solitary round hypoenhancing splenic mass (*black arrow*), as well as an extensive retroperitoneal nodal conglomerate (*white arrows*). (*C*) Axial T2-weighted MR image shows the splenic mass is hypointense (*black arrow*) to splenic parenchyma. (*D*) Axial postcontrast fat-suppressed T1-weighted MR image shows the mass is hypoenhancing relative to the splenic parenchyma (*black arrow*).

densities on CT, and different signal intensities on precontrast T1-weighted and T2-weighted MR images. After administration of IV contrast, the mass or masses enhance(s) heterogeneously on both CT and MR imaging[33,44] (**Fig. 11**). Given the propensity of angiosarcoma to bleed, hemoperitoneum may be present[48] (**Fig. 12**).

Metastasis Metastases to the spleen primarily occurs due to hematogenous spread, but also can be due to direct invasion or peritoneal involvement. Although the reported incidence of splenic metastasis based on autopsy series is 3% to 9% in patients with a primary malignancy, one-third to one-half of these metastases were seen only on microscopic examination (87 of 92 cases, 5.3%).[50-52] Isolated splenic metastases is highly unusual, as one study showed that in all cases of splenic metastasis, at least 2 other concurrent metastatic locations were present.[50] Lung and breast carcinomas are the most common primary malignancies to metastasize to the spleen, with less common malignancies being tumors of gastrointestinal origin (stomach and colon), melanoma, and ovarian neoplasms.

No imaging patterns are specific for splenic metastasis. Solitary, multiple, and diffusely infiltrating metastases have been reported. On CT, splenic metastases tend to appear hypoattenuating and hypoenhancing. On MR imaging, metastases in the spleen may appear similar to normal splenic parenchyma, or occasionally can be hypointense on precontrast T1-weighted and slightly hyperintense on T2-weighted MR images

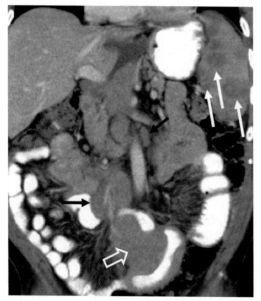

Fig. 10. A 65-year-old man presented with diffuse large B-cell lymphoma involving abdominal lymph nodes, small bowel, and spleen. Coronal contrast-enhanced CT during the portal venous phase demonstrates multiple hypoenhancing splenic masses (*white arrows*), and extensive retroperitoneal and mesenteric lymphadenopathy (*black arrows*), as well as lymphoma involvement of the small bowel (*white open arrow*) without obstruction, a specific feature of bowel lymphoma.

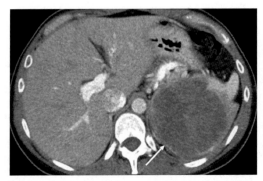

Fig. 11. A 46-year-old woman presented with a splenic mass during evaluation for left upper quadrant pain. Splenectomy confirmed a high-grade angiosarcoma. Axial portal venous phase contrast-enhanced CT image demonstrates a heterogeneously enhancing splenic mass with ill-defined borders (*white arrow*).

(**Fig. 13**). Various enhancement patterns may be observed depending on the nature of the primary malignancy. A cystic or necrotic appearance also can be seen, although calcifications are rare.[32,33]

Management Approach to Incidental Splenic Findings

For incidentally discovered splenic findings in asymptomatic patients, the 2013 American College of Radiology (ACR) "White Paper" established an initial algorithm for evaluation and follow-up based on cross-sectional imaging features and the presence or absence of a malignancy history.[53] Based on the "White Paper" recommendations, any splenic cyst with clearly benign imaging features or any splenic mass that demonstrates imaging stability for more than 1 year does not require further follow-up. All other focal abnormalities require further evaluation with MR imaging, PET/CT, and/or biopsy, or follow-up MR imaging in 6 to 12 months,

depending on malignancy history, size, or lack of imaging stability (**Fig. 14**).

Since these recommendations were published, however, our group retrospectively evaluated 379 patients presenting with incidental splenic masses on CT, and found that only 1% of patients who were asymptomatic and had no prior history of malignancy had a malignant splenic process.[54] These patients had additional imaging findings and a diagnosis of malignancy was made prospectively. Therefore, in an appropriately selected group of patients whose splenic findings are truly incidental, follow-up imaging or tissue sampling may be unnecessary. Using data from the study by our group in conjunction with the ACR "White Paper," an alternative management strategy can be formulated based on specific imaging features and available clinical context that may further decrease the need for workup of these splenic findings (**Fig. 15**).

Benign imaging features

If a splenic finding found on CT or MR imaging meets strict imaging criteria for benignity, no further follow-up is required. These criteria include cysts with homogeneous low attenuation (<20 HU) on CT, or fluid signal intensity on MR imaging, with well-circumscribed and smooth borders, nonenhancing imperceptible walls or rim calcification, and no internal enhancement. Any splenic mass with imaging features compatible with a hemangioma is also considered benign.

Interval Stability

If prior CT or MR imaging examinations are available for comparison and demonstrate imaging stability of a focal splenic finding for 1 year or more, then no further workup is needed, even if the finding does not meet imaging criteria for benignity. Notably, the size does not need to be exactly identical on follow-up imaging to be considered a benign process. Because hepatic hemangiomas

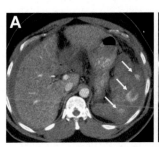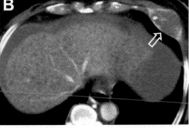

Fig. 12. A 64-year-old man presented with spontaneous hemoperitoneum secondary to splenic rupture. (*A*) Axial portal venous phase contrast-enhanced CT image demonstrates a heterogeneous-appearing spleen with indistinctness and obscuration of the lateral border by hemoperitoneum. Several foci of active extravasation are noted within the perisplenic hemoperitoneum (*white arrows*). Incidentally were noted innumerable punctate hypoattenuating foci in the liver, which are highly consistent with biliary hamartomas. (*B*) Axial portal venous phase contrast-enhanced CT image obtained of the lower chest shows an expansile and destructive process (*white open arrow*) in the left sixth rib. Biopsy confirmed metastatic angiosarcoma.

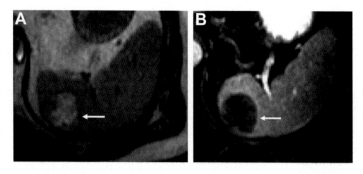

Fig. 13. A 51-year-old man with history of duodenal adenocarcinoma presented with an isolated splenic mass discovered during routine surveillance. Biopsy confirmed isolated metastatic duodenal adenocarcinoma. (*A*) On an axial T2-weighted MR image, a single hyperintense mass is seen in the posteromedial spleen (*arrow*). (*B*) An axial postcontrast fat-suppressed T1-weighted MR image in the portal venous phase shows mild and predominantly peripheral enhancement within the mass (*arrow*).

can grow up to 2 mm annually,[55] a splenic mass that demonstrates less than 2 mm annual growth can be regarded as benign; however, an additional 1-year follow-up could be considered.

Malignancy history

A history of malignancy is an important consideration in determining whether a splenic finding needs further assessment. Our group reported

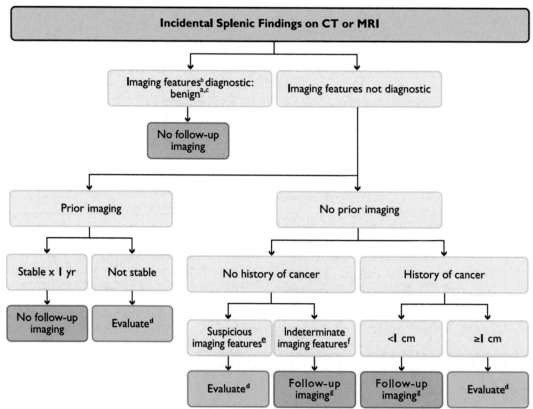

Fig. 14. ACR "White Paper" management of incidental splenic findings on CT or MR imaging. [a]Cyst: imperceptible wall, near-water attenuation (<10 HU), no enhancement. [b]Hemangioma: discontinuous, peripheral, centripetal enhancement (findings that are uncommon in splenic hemangiomas). [c]Benign imaging features: homogeneous, low attenuation (<20 HU), no enhancement, smooth margins. [d]Evaluate: PET versus MR imaging versus biopsy. [e]Suspicious imaging features: heterogeneous, enhancement, irregular margins, necrosis, splenic parenchymal or vascular invasion, substantial enlargement. [f]Indeterminate imaging features: heterogeneous, intermediate attenuation (>20 HU), enhancement, smooth margins. [g]Follow-up MR imaging in 6 and 12 months. (*From* J Am Coll Radiol, Vol. 10, Heller MT, Harisinghani M, Neitlich JD, Yeghiayan P, Berland LL, Managing incidental findings on abdominal and pelvic CT and MRI, Part 3: white paper of the ACR Incidental Findings Committee II on Splenic and Nodal Findings, pgs. 833-839, 2013, with permission.)

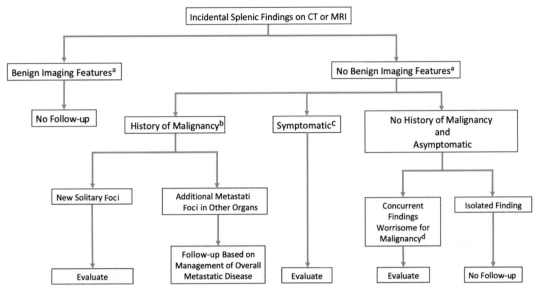

Fig. 15. Simplified management approach for incidental splenic findings on CT or MR imaging. [a]Benign imaging features: Cystic foci with homogeneous low attenuation (<20 HU) on CT or fluid signal intensity on MR imaging with well-circumscribed and smooth borders, nonenhancing imperceptible walls or rim calcification, and no internal enhancement. Any splenic mass with imaging features compatible with a hemangioma is also considered benign. [b]History of malignancy: further evaluation may not be needed, if patient has concomitant disease in other organs that require systemic treatment. [c]Symptomatic: Type B symptoms (fever, weight loss, night sweats), pain localized to the epigastrium or left upper quadrant, or immunocompromised with increased risk of infection. [d]Concurrent findings worrisome for malignancy: Suspicious imaging features, disease in other organs suspicious for metastasis or primary malignancy on imaging, or lymphadenopathy.

that approximately 34% of splenic masses on CT were malignant in patients with a history of malignancy.[54] Most of these were splenic metastatic foci from a nonlymphomatous primary malignancy (74%), with the remainder being lymphoma. All patients with splenic metastases from a nonlymphomatous primary malignancy had concomitant metastatic involvement of other organs in the abdomen and pelvis visible at the time of imaging, with 84% having 2 or more sites of metastatic disease noted outside of the spleen.

Solitary metastasis in the spleen are exceedingly rare, but have been reported. Consequently, splenic findings that do not meet benign imaging criteria in patients with a history of malignancy cannot be ignored. Further evaluation with PET/CT, MR imaging, and/or biopsy may be required if management decisions are based on the determination of the presence of splenic involvement with metastatic disease, such as in a patient with a new solitary splenic finding (see **Fig. 14**). If the patient will be treated for extrasplenic metastatic disease, the splenic focal finding can be reevaluated on follow-up imaging. For focal findings smaller than 1 cm, the ACR "White Paper" recommends a follow-up MR imaging in 6 to 12 months.[53]

Symptomatic patients
Symptomatic patients are defined as having either type B symptoms (fever, weight loss, night sweats) or pain localized to the epigastrium or left upper quadrant. Our group found that in such symptomatic patients, incidental splenic findings were malignant in approximately 28%, all of which were lymphoma.[54] Among these patients with a malignant splenic focus or foci, 75% demonstrated concomitant lymphadenopathy in the abdomen and pelvis. In the small percentage of patients ultimately diagnosed with lymphoma presenting with an isolated splenic mass and constitutional symptoms, the splenic masses were typically large, larger than 7 cm. Therefore, if a splenic mass not meeting benign imaging characteristics is identified in a symptomatic patient, further evaluation is warranted, initially with MR imaging if not previously performed, or PET/CT or tissue sampling. Akin to the workup of splenic findings in patients with a history of cancer, the size can be considered in the management of symptomatic patients. After initial characterization with MR imaging, short interval follow-up MR imaging (3 months) may be appropriate for small splenic foci <1 cm in symptomatic patients, taking into account concern for possible infection.

Importantly, immunocompromised patients who are at risk for the development of splenic microabscesses should also be grouped within the symptomatic category, even if considered asymptomatic otherwise.

Asymptomatic patients

Splenic abnormalities detected in patients without a history of malignancy and without type B symptoms or epigastric or left upper quadrant pain can be considered to be truly incidental findings. The likelihood of malignancy in these patients is extremely low, and the incidence does not change significantly when splenic findings meeting criteria for cysts are excluded (1.1% vs 1.0%).[54] Thus, truly incidental splenic findings in asymptomatic patients without a history of malignancy do not require further evaluation unless other imaging findings worrisome for malignancy are noted concurrently in the abdomen and pelvis, including lymphadenopathy.

Options for further evaluation

Further evaluation for splenic findings that do not meet strict benign imaging criteria should start with MR imaging or PET with fludeoxyglucose F 18 (^{18}F-FDG PET)/CT before tissue sampling. Dhyani and colleagues[56] demonstrated that MR imaging can provide a definitive diagnosis in 75% of benign and indeterminate masses, whereas ^{18}F-FDG PET/CT demonstrated 100% of the malignant splenic patients with a history of ^{18}F-FDG-avid malignancy. In addition, in patients with a solid splenic mass with known ^{18}F-FDG-avid malignancy, ^{18}F-FDG PET/CT has a sensitivity and specificity of 100% and 100%, respectively, for the diagnosis of malignant splenic masses, and 100% and 80%, respectively, for benign findings, with a negative predictive value of 100%.[57]

All incidental findings detected on CT in patients without a history of malignancy that require further evaluation should undergo MR imaging with and without contrast initially. Those detected on CT in patients with history of ^{18}F-FDG-avid malignancy should undergo ^{18}F-FDG PET/CT initially. If the primary malignancy is not ^{18}F-FDG-avid, patients should undergo IV contrast-enhanced MR imaging. In symptomatic patients, those initially found on CT should undergo MR imaging. If MR imaging or ^{18}F-FDG PET/CT remains indeterminate, tissue sampling should be performed if definitive diagnosis is required or desired before establishment of a treatment plan.

For incidental indeterminate findings initially detected on IV contrast-enhanced MR imaging in patients without a known history of malignancy, further evaluation with either ^{18}F-FDG PET/CT or tissue sampling should be obtained if concurrent findings in the abdomen and pelvis that are concerning for malignancy are present. If the patient has a history of malignancy or is symptomatic, either ^{18}F-FDG PET/CT or tissue sampling should be pursued.

SUMMARY

Incidental splenic findings are commonly encountered on cross-sectional imaging during the evaluation for various clinical indications. Familiarity with unique imaging characteristics of these entities will enable a more accurate and focused differential diagnosis. A definitive diagnosis, however, may not be possible based on imaging findings alone, as benign and malignant entities share overlapping imaging features. Fortunately, most incidentally encountered splenic findings are benign. In particular, in patients without a history of malignancy and without symptoms, only 1% of these are malignant. A proposed algorithm for the management of incidentally detected splenic findings that incorporates both imaging characteristics along with clinical information (history of malignancy and symptoms) may allow for an efficient approach to evaluating these incidental findings, thereby potentially decreasing anxiety and health care costs.

CLINICS CARE POINTS

- Truly incidental splenic masses have a very low likelihood of malignancy and usually do not require further work-up.
- Patients with fever, weight loss, left upper quadrant and/or epigastric pain require further work-up of an indeterminate splenic mass.
- MRI is the preferred imaging modality for further evaluaton of a splenic mass.

DISCLOSURE

All authors have nothing to disclose.

REFERENCES

1. Thompson RJ, Wojcik SM, Grant WD, et al. Incidental findings on CT scans in the emergency department. Emerg Med Int 2011;2011. https://doi.org/10.1155/2011/624847.
2. Onwubiko C, Mooney DP. The prevalence of incidental findings on computed tomography of the

abdomen/pelvis in pediatric trauma patients. Eur J Trauma Emerg Surg 2018;44(1):15–8.

3. Abbott RM, Levy AD, Aguilera NS, et al. From the Archives of the AFIP: primary vascular neoplasms of the spleen: radiologic-pathologic correlation. Radio-Graphics 2004;24(4):1137–63.

4. Olpin JD. Current management of the splenic incidentaloma. Curr Radiol Rep 2017;5(6):23.

5. Keogan MT, Freed KS, Paulson EK, et al. Imaging-guided percutaneous biopsy of focal splenic lesions: update on safety and effectiveness. AJR Am J Roentgenol 1999;172(4):933–7.

6. Makrin V, Avital S, White I, et al. Laparoscopic splenectomy for solitary splenic tumors. Surg Endosc 2008;22(9):2009–12.

7. Morgan AE, Berland LL, Ananyev SS, et al. Extraurinary Incidental findings on CT for hematuria: the radiologist's role and downstream cost analysis. AJR Am J Roentgenol 2015;204(6):1160–7.

8. Bürrig KF. Epithelial (true) splenic cysts. Pathogenesis of the mesothelial and so-called epidermoid cyst of the spleen. Am J Surg Pathol 1988;12(4): 275–81.

9. Morgenstern L. Nonparasitic splenic cysts: pathogenesis, classification, and treatment1 1No competing interests declared. J Am Coll Surg 2002;194(3):306–14.

10. Urrutia M, Mergo P, Ros L, et al. Cystic masses of the spleen: radiologic-pathologic correlation. Radio-Graphics 1996;16(1):107–29.

11. Freeman JL, Jafri SZ, Roberts JL, et al. CT of congenital and acquired abnormalities of the spleen. RadioGraphics 1993;13(3):597–610.

12. De Backer AI, Vanhoenacker FM, Mortelé KJ, et al. MRI features of focal splenic lesions in patients with disseminated tuberculosis. AJR Am J Roentgenol 2006;186(4):1097–102.

13. Marani SA, Canossi GC, Nicoli FA, et al. Hydatid disease: MR imaging study. Radiology 1990;175(3): 701–6.

14. Pedrosa I, Saíz A, Arrazola J, et al. Hydatid disease: radiologic and pathologic features and complications. RadioGraphics 2000;20(3):795–817.

15. Sinner WNV, Stridbeck H. Hydatid disease of the spleen. Acta Radiol 1992;33(5):459–61.

16. Selroos O. Fine-needle aspiration biopsy of the spleen in diagnosis of sarcoidosis. Ann N Y Acad Sci 1976;278(1):517–21.

17. Taavitsainen M, Koivuniemi A, Helminen J, et al. Aspiration biopsy of the spleen in patients with sarcoidosis. Acta Radiol 1987;28(6):723–5.

18. Warshauer DM, Dumbleton SA, Molina PL, et al. Abdominal CT findings in sarcoidosis: radiologic and clinical correlation. Radiology 1994;192(1): 93–8.

19. Palmucci S, Torrisi SE, Caltabiano DC, et al. Clinical and radiological features of extra-pulmonary sarcoidosis: a pictorial essay. Insights Imaging 2016;7(4):571–87.

20. Gezer NS, Başara I, Altay C, et al. Abdominal sarcoidosis: cross-sectional imaging findings. Diagn Interv Radiol 2015;21(2):111–7.

21. Husni EA. The clinical course of splenic hemangioma: with emphasis on spontaneous rupture. Arch Surg 1961;83(5):681–8.

22. Garvin DF, King FM. Cysts and nonlymphomatous tumors of the spleen. Pathol Annu 1981;16(Pt 1): 61–80.

23. Ros PR, Moser RP, Dachman AH, et al. Hemangioma of the spleen: radiologic-pathologic correlation in ten cases. Radiology 1987;162(1):73–7.

24. Sangiorgio VFI, Arber DA. Vascular neoplasms and non-neoplastic vascular lesions of the spleen. Semin Diagn Pathol 2020. https://doi.org/10.1053/j.semdp. 2020.07.001.

25. Ferrozzi F, Bova D, Draghi F, et al. CT findings in primary vascular tumors of the spleen. AJR Am J Roentgenol 1996;166(5):1097–101.

26. Mortelé KJ. Imaging of tumoral conditions of the spleen. JBR-BTR. 2000;83(4):213–5.

27. Ramani M, Reinhold C, Semelka RC, et al. Splenic hemangiomas and hamartomas: MR imaging characteristics of 28 lesions. Radiology 1997;202(1): 166–72.

28. Lam KY, Yip KH, Peh WCG. Splenic vascular lesions: unusual features and a review of the literature. Aust N Z J Surg 1999;69(6):422–5.

29. Lee H, Maeda K. Hamartoma of the spleen. Arch Pathol Lab Med 2009;133(1):147–51.

30. Zissin R, Lishner M, Rathaus V. Case report: unusual presentation of splenic hamartoma; computed tomography and ultrasonic findings. Clin Radiol 1992;45(6):410–1.

31. Cystic hamartoma of the spleen: CT and sonographic findings. - Harvard University. Available at: https://hollis.harvard.edu. Accessed October 4, 2020.

32. Gaetke-Udager K, Wasnik AP, Kaza RK, et al. Multimodality imaging of splenic lesions and the role of non-vascular, image-guided intervention. Abdom Imaging 2014;39(3):570–87.

33. Elsayes KM, Narra VR, Mukundan G, et al. MR imaging of the spleen: spectrum of abnormalities. Radio-Graphics 2005;25(4):967–82.

34. Alqahtani A, Nguyen LT, Flageole H, et al. 25 Years' experience with lymphangiomas in children. J Pediatr Surg 1999;34(7):1164–8.

35. Ioannidis I, Kahn AG. Splenic lymphangioma. Arch Pathol Lab Med 2015;139(2):278–82.

36. Bhatt S, Huang J, Dogra V. Littoral cell angioma of the spleen. AJR Am J Roentgenol 2007;188(5): 1365–6.

37. Levy AD, Abbott RM, Abbondanzo SL. Littoral cell angioma of the spleen: CT features with

clinicopathologic comparison. Radiology 2004; 230(2):485–90.

38. Bisceglia M, Sickel JZ, Giangaspero F, et al. Littoral cell angioma of the spleen: an additional report of four cases with emphasis on the association with visceral organ cancers. Tumori 1998;84(5):595–9.

39. Shah S, Wasnik A, Pandya A, et al. Multimodality imaging findings in image-guided biopsy proven splenic littoral cell angioma: series of three cases. Abdom Imaging 2011;36(6):735–8.

40. Martel M, Cheuk W, Lombardi L, et al. Sclerosing Angiomatoid Nodular Transformation (SANT): report of 25 cases of a distinctive benign splenic lesion. J Surg Pathol 2004;28(10):1268–79.

41. Raman SP, Singhi A, Horton KM, et al. Sclerosing angiomatoid nodular transformation of the spleen (SANT): multimodality imaging appearance of five cases with radiology–pathology correlation. Abdom Imaging 2013;38(4):827–34.

42. Sangiorgio VFI, Arber DA. Non-hematopoietic neoplastic and pseudoneoplastic lesions of the spleen. Semin Diagn Pathol 2020. https://doi.org/10.1053/j.semdp.2020.06.004.

43. Lewis RB, Lattin GE, Nandedkar M, et al. Sclerosing angiomatoid nodular transformation of the spleen: CT and MRI features with pathologic correlation. AJR Am J Roentgenol 2013;200(4):W353–60.

44. Kaza RK, Azar S, Al-Hawary MM, et al. Primary and secondary neoplasms of the spleen. Cancer Imaging 2010;10(1):173–82.

45. Saboo SS, Krajewski KM, O'Regan KN, et al. Spleen in haematological malignancies: spectrum of imaging findings. Br J Radiol 2012;85(1009):81–92.

46. Fishman EK, Kuhlman JE, Jones RJ. CT of lymphoma: spectrum of disease. RadioGraphics 1991; 11(4):647–69.

47. Leite NP, Kased N, Hanna RF, et al. Cross-sectional imaging of extranodal involvement in abdominopelvic lymphoproliferative malignancies. RadioGraphics 2007;27(6):1613–34.

48. Thompson WM, Levy AD, Aguilera NS, et al. Angiosarcoma of the spleen: imaging characteristics in 12 patients. Radiology 2005;235(1):106–15.

49. Autry JR, Weitzner S. Hemangiosarcoma of spleen with spontaneous rupture. Cancer 1975;35(2): 534–9.

50. Schön CA, Görg C, Ramaswamy A, et al. Splenic metastases in a large unselected autopsy series. Pathol - Res Pract 2006;202(5):351–6.

51. Abrams HL. The incidence of splenic metastasis of carcinoma. Calif Med 1952;76(4):281–2.

52. Lam KY, Tang V. Metastatic tumors to the spleen. Arch Pathol Lab Med 2000;124:5.

53. Heller MT, Harisinghani M, Neitlich JD, et al. Managing incidental findings on abdominal and pelvic CT and MRI, part 3: white paper of the ACR Incidental Findings Committee II on Splenic and Nodal Findings. J Am Coll Radiol 2013;10(11):833–9.

54. Siewert B, Millo NZ, Sahi K, et al. The incidental splenic mass at CT: does it need further work-up? an observational study. Radiology 2018;287(1): 156–66.

55. Hasan HY, Hinshaw JL, Borman EJ, et al. Assessing normal growth of hepatic hemangiomas during long-term follow-up. JAMA Surg 2014;149(12):1266–71.

56. Dhyani M, Anupindi SA, Ayyala R, et al. Defining an imaging algorithm for noncystic splenic lesions identified in young patients. AJR Am J Roentgenol 2013; 201(6):W893–9.

57. Metser U, Miller E, Kessler A, et al. Solid splenic masses: evaluation with 18F-FDG PET/CT. J Nucl Med 2005;46(1):52–9.

Incidental Pancreatic Cysts on Cross-Sectional Imaging

Shannon M. Navarro, MD, MPH[a],*, Michael T. Corwin, MD[a],
Douglas S. Katz, MD, FASER, FSAR[b], Ramit Lamba, MD, FSAR[a]

KEYWORDS

• Incidental • Pancreatic cyst • MR imaging • CT • Radiology

KEY POINTS

- Incidental pancreatic cysts are commonly encountered in a radiology practice.
- Although some of these are benign, mucinous cystic lesions have a potential to undergo malignant transformation.
- Characterization of some incidental pancreatic cysts based on imaging alone is limited, and given that some pancreatic cysts have a malignant potential, guidelines exist to help determine management and follow-up based on current evidence and consensus agreements.

INTRODUCTION

Incidental pancreatic cysts (PCs) are commonly encountered in radiology practice. The prevalence rate of PCs is estimated at 2.5%.[1] There is a 9% reported incidence on computed tomography (CT) and a 27% incidence on MR imaging.[2] PCs are a heterogeneous group, including intraductal papillary mucinous neoplasm (IPMN), serous cystic neoplasm (SCN), and mucinous cystic neoplasm (MCN). Non-neoplastic PCs are pancreatic pseudocysts (common), epithelial cysts (uncommon), and lymphoepithelial cysts (rare). The significance in categorizing PCs lies in the potential of the mucinous varieties to develop malignancy. There is substantial variability in the malignant potential of the incidentally detected PC, particularly if they are too small or otherwise cannot be fully characterized by imaging. For this reason, multiple societies have published follow-up imaging guidelines and management plans aimed at detecting early malignant transformation. The guidelines have been complicated with concerns of imaging costs and over-screening.[3] The prevalence rate of pancreatic ductal adenocarcinomas (PDACs) arising in patients with PCs is very low, at 33.2 per 100000; the rate of malignant transformation increases linearly with age.[1] This review provides a practical understanding of PCs because they are commonly encountered in radiology practice. The radiologist has an important opportunity to work with pancreatic surgeons and gastroenterologists to provide optimal multidisciplinary care to the many patients with PCs.

IMAGING TECHNIQUE AND PROTOCOL

The American College of Radiology (ACR) Appropriateness Criteria for initial evaluation of an incidental PC without high-risk stigmata list MR imaging of the abdomen without and with contrast with MR cholangiopancreatography (MRCP) as "usually appropriate" and intravenous (IV) contrast-enhanced CT (CECT) as "may be appropriate"; cyst size cutoff of greater than 2.5 cm adds a recommendation for endoscopic ultrasound (EUS). For initial evaluation of an incidental PC

The authors acknowledge and thank Dr Shiro Urayama, MD, for providing endoscopic ultrasound images.
[a] Department of Radiology, UC Davis, 4860 Y Street, Suite 3100, Sacramento, CA 95817, USA; [b] Department of Radiology, NYU Winthrop, 259 First Street, Mineola, NY 11501, USA
* Corresponding author.
E-mail address: smnavarro@ucdavis.edu

Radiol Clin N Am 59 (2021) 617–629
https://doi.org/10.1016/j.rcl.2021.03.010

greater than 2.5 cm, with worrisome features or high-risk stigmata, EUS and MR imaging of the abdomen without and with IV contrast with MRCP fall into the usually appropriate categories.[4]

For an incidentally detected main pancreatic duct (MPD) dilated beyond 7 mm and suspicion for main duct (MD)-IPMN, EUS, and MR of the abdomen without and with IV contrast with MRCP are considered usually appropriate.

Computed Tomography Protocol

Pancreatic CT is performed in the pancreatic parenchymal and portal venous phases. The pancreatic phase represents peak pancreatic parenchymal enhancement, which occurs 40 seconds to 45 seconds following the IV injection of contrast. The portal venous phase is obtained 70 seconds to 75 seconds following the IV injection of contrast. Because the time of peak parenchymal enhancement can vary based on a patient's physiology, an accurate method for achieving this phase entails triggering imaging at 16 seconds following the acquisition of a threshold of 175 Hounsfield units in the upper abdominal aorta. At UC Davis, the pancreatic CT protocol involves injecting 125 mL of iodinated contrast (iohexol, 350 mg Iodine/mL) at an injection rate of 4 mL/s. This acquisition approach also yields a late arterial phase which can be used for surgical resection planning of PDAC. One set of axial reconstructions is obtained at a slice thickness of 1.0 mm to 1.5 mm, which allows for better evaluation of small mural nodules, side duct branches, and for creating a curved-planar reformation (CPR) along the path of the main pancreatic duct. CPRs can better depict communication of a cyst with the pancreatic ductal system, changes in duct caliber, or intraductal enhancing masses.

MR Protocol

The pancreatic MR imaging protocol consists of multiplanar T2-weighted images, MRCP images, and precontrast and postcontrast 3-dimensional (3-D) –T1-weighted images. Coronal and axial single-shot fast spin-echo T2-weighted images with and/or without fat suppression are acquired because they allow for an anatomic overview and delineation of PCs. Fast spin-echo T2-weighted images are optional. Steady-state free-precession images provide contrast determined by the ratio of T2/T1. Fluid is high signal intensity and can be used as an alternative to single-shot fast spin-echo imaging. MRCP images can be acquired as 2-dimensional, thick (40 mm), heavily T2-weighted slabs and/or high-resolution (1–2 mm) 3-D volumetric acquisitions. The latter can result

in superior assessment of the features of PCs and should be acquired routinely.[5] Diffusion-weighted imaging now is a routine part of abdominal MR imaging, although not specifically necessary for PC follow-up.

Nonenhanced T1-weighted MR images are acquired using 3-D fat-suppressed spoiled gradient-echo sequences. The use of IV gadolinium in the follow-up of PCs is controversial. Studies have shown the addition of contrast adds little value in the follow-up of PCs and rarely changes management.[6,7] Nonenhanced MR imaging is faster, entails review of fewer images, and avoids the risks of IV gadolinium, although rarely IV contrast may be helpful in identifying high-risk features. One approach is to selectively administer contrast for larger cysts, cysts with known high-risk features, or for the initial evaluation of cysts, leaving nonenhanced MR imaging for follow-up of cysts known to be small and without high-risk features.

ULTRASOUND

Ultrasound (US) of the pancreas has been limited by the pancreas' anatomic location as a retroperitoneal organ with overlying bowel. The utility of transabdominal US to assess PCs is inversely related to a patient's weight and abdominal diameter.[8]

Conventional US has a sensitivity of 94% for the differentiation of pseudocysts and cystic neoplasms but a relatively poor specificity, at 44%.[9] The use of IV US contrast agents can increase the specificity to 97%, by demonstrating perfusion to small nodules or septations. IV contrast significantly improves the area under the curve in receiver operating characteristic curve analysis but has not yet gained widespread use.[10]

ENDOSCOPIC ULTRASOUND

EUS utilizes endoscopy to access the upper digestive tract. The endoscope is equipped with a small US transducer with high frequency and corresponding high spatial resolution (**Fig. 1**). EUS has been shown to help differentiate pseudocysts from cystic neoplasms and guides fine-needle aspiration (FNA).[11] SCNs have a heterogeneous appearance on EUS. Mural nodules, thick cyst walls, or intracystic growth are found more commonly in mucinous neoplasms.[11,12] EUS has been shown to be very sensitive in the diagnosis of PDAC during the follow-up of IPMNs, outperforming MR imaging, CT, and US.[13] Variables most predictive of malignancy on EUS include mural nodules and MPD greater than or equal to 10 mm.[14] The interobserver agreement

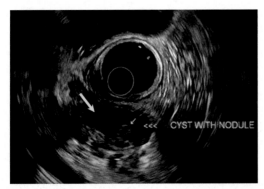

Fig. 1. EUS image of the pancreas shows a complex PC (*arrow*) with a mural nodule (annotated on the image), highly compatible with malignant degeneration. (*Courtesy of* S. Urayama, M.D., Sacramento, CA.)

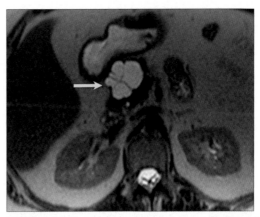

Fig. 2. SCN of the pancreas (macrocystic variant): axial T2-weighted MR image through the pancreatic head shows a multi-locular cystic mass (*arrow*) with thin septations. The largest cyst locule measures greater than 2 cm.

of EUS is low for differentiating neoplastic versus non-neoplastic, type of PC, and EUS features of a PC; EUS is limited in the differentiation of mucinous from nonmucinous cysts.[15,16] US contrast increases the accuracy of detection of mural nodules in branch duct (BD)-IPMNs from 72% to 98%.[17]

APPROACH TO THE INCIDENTAL PANCREATIC CYST

It is critical for radiologists to know if the PC actually is incidental. Any worrisome symptoms, such as pain, jaundice, or mass effect, should encourage further work-up, although PC signs and symptoms often are nonspecific. Clinical history, including patient age and gender as well as any known syndromes, may help in characterization.

DEFINITELY BENIGN
Serous Cystic Neoplasms

SCNs typically are described as having a honeycomb or multilocular appearance with or without a central scar. However, there can be variations in the morphologic appearance with polycystic, oligocystic, and solid patterns described[18,19] (**Figs. 2** and **3**). Microcystic morphology is more common in SCNs[19] (**Fig. 4**). The classic imaging features are a lobulated external contour and central scar with stellate calcification[18] (**Fig. 5**). SCNs rarely demonstrate peripheral enhancing capsule or mural nodules.[19]

The combination of morphologic features, such as location in the body or tail, size, and lobulated contour plus textural analysis, yields a high area under the receiver operator characteristic curve in differentiating SCNs from MCNs.[20] SCNs typically are isolated; however, patients with von Hippel-Lindau (VHL) disease may demonstrate multiple pancreatic masses in addition to cysts and tumors in other organ systems.[18]

Pancreatitis-Associated Fluid Collections

Pancreatitis is an inflammatory condition of the pancreas, which can result in fluid collections with a cystic appearance. The revised Atlanta classification for acute pancreatitis describes *acute peripancreatic fluid collections* (APFCs) as fluid collections associated with pancreatitis in the first 4 weeks of inflammation, with *acute necrotic fluid collections* (although the term is still used loosely in practice); used to denote any associated necrosis. Pseudocyst is restricted to evolving peripancreatic fluid collections, although the term is used loosely in practice. If an APFC persists beyond 4 weeks and develops an enhancing capsule the term pseudocyst is used (**Fig. 6**). If an acute necrotic collection lasts beyond 4 weeks and develops an enhancing capsule the term walled off necrosis is used.[21] It is important for the radiologist to consider pseudocyst in the differential given the high prevalence of pancreatitis.

Congenital or Syndromic Pancreatic Cysts

Congenital PCs with an epithelial lining are rare.[22] Pancreatic cystosis is a rare finding in cystic fibrosis in which the entire pancreatic parenchyma is replaced with macrocysts.[23]

Lymphoepithelial Cyst

Lymphoepithelial cysts are rare cysts lined with squamous epithelium and surrounded by

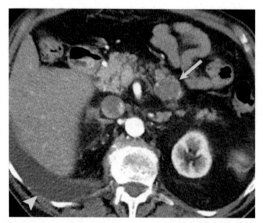

Fig. 3. SCN (solid appearing): IV CECT through the pancreatic tail shows a hypoenhancing cystic mass (*arrow*). The mass has attenuation greater than that of simple fluid compared with the simple right pleural effusion (*arrowhead*). Multiple tiny microcysts and enhancing septations can mimic a solid tumor.

lymphoid tissue. They typically affect men who are middle-aged or older and are exophytic with a higher CT attenuation compared with SCNs and MCNs.[24] The reference standard for diagnosis is excision.[25]

von Hippel-Lindau Disease

VHL disease is an autosomal dominant disorder with tumors affecting multiple organ systems. The pancreas is affected in VHL disease by PCs, endocrine tumors, and SCNs (**Fig. 7**).[26]

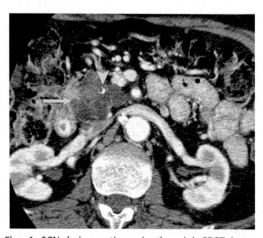

Fig. 4. SCN (microcystic variant): axial CECT image through the pancreatic head shows a cystic mass with multiple small cystic loculations (*arrow*). A focal area of calcification is seen centrally within a septation (*arrowhead*).

POTENTIALLY OR DEFINITELY MALIGNANT
Intraductal Papillary Mucinous Neoplasm

IPMNs are cystic neoplasms with variable degree of malignant potential. They may evolve into dysplasia or invasive carcinoma and are associated with a higher risk for the development of PDAC in the gland separate from the IPMN sites. The rate of progression increases with time.[27] Low-risk IPMNs have an approximately 8% chance of progression, whereas higher risk IPMNs have an approximately 25% chance of progression to PDAC in 10 years.[28] Even presumed low-risk BD-IPMNs may demonstrate growth after 5 years.[29]

IPMNs may be separated into BD-IPMNs, with a clear connection to the main duct; MD-IPMNs, in which there is either focal or diffuse ductal dilatation; or mixed types[30] (**Figs. 8–10**). Filling defects are worrisome for malignancy.[31] Variable MPD cutoff levels exist in the literature, with MPD dilatation between 5 mm and 15 mm reported as worrisome.[14,31] Other predictors of malignant IPMNs include an enhancing solid component/mural nodule(s) and thickened septae or walls.[14]

Mucinous Cystic Neoplasm

MCNs occur almost exclusively in women and more commonly are found in the pancreatic tail. MCNs are oval or round and can show septations, cyst wall calcifications, enhancing capsules, and occasionally mural nodules[19,32,33] (**Figs. 11** and **12**). MCNs typically do not cause dilatation of the biliary or pancreatic ductal system but can be associated with distal pancreatic atrophy.[34] They may be associated with lymphadenopathy but generally are not associated with peripancreatic fat infiltration or vascular involvement. Predictors

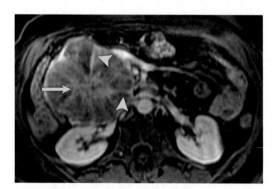

Fig. 5. SCN: axial IV contrast-enhanced MR image through the pancreatic head shows enhancement within the central scar of a SCN (*arrow*). Enhancing fibrous septations are seen radiating out from the central scar (*arrowheads*).

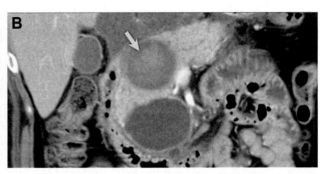

Fig. 6. Pseudocyst: (*A*) Axial CECT image in a patient with epigastric pain reveals peripancreatic fluid and pancreatic edema, compatible with acute edematous interstitial pancreatitis. (*B*) Coronal CECT image through the pancreas obtained 3 months later shows the development of 2 pseudocysts, 1 of which contains hemorrhagic material (*arrow*).

of high-grade dysplasia include size greater 8.5 cm.[32]

INDETERMINATE: REVIEW OF GUIDELINES

Many PCs are indeterminate by imaging and require imaging follow-up and/or EUS-FNA. The management of PCs is controversial and multiple societal guidelines exist (**Table 1**). It is important to work with gastroenterologists and pancreatic surgeons to ensure collaboration in regard to work-up and follow-up.

American Gastroenterological Association

The American Gastroenterological Association has published guidelines for diagnosis and management of PCs. Solid and pseudopapillary neoplasms (SPENs), cystic degeneration of adenocarcinomas, cystic neuroendocrine tumors,

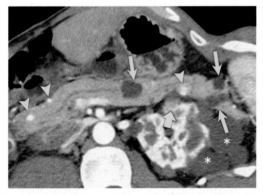

Fig. 7. VHL disease: CPR of a CECT through the pancreas shows cysts in the pancreatic body and tail (*arrows*). Hyperenhancing nodules are seen in the pancreas (*arrowheads*), compatible with neuroendocrine tumors. Cysts are seen in the left kidney (*asterisks*). An enhancing renal mass is in the anterior cortex of the left kidney (*short thick arrow*).

and MD-IPMNs were excluded. The guidelines call for involvement with the patient, and discussion of the goals and risks of PC surveillance.

Cysts with at least 2 high-risk features (size >3 cm, dilated MPD or solid component) should have EUS-FNA. After reassuring EUS-FNA, MR imaging surveillance is recommended after 1 year and then every 2 years; substantial changes in the cyst by imaging should result in repeat EUS-FNA. Cysts with solid components and a dilated MPD or concerning EUS-FNA should be offered surgery. After excision of cancer or a cystic/mucin-producing neoplasm with dysplasia, the residual pancreas should be examined using MR imaging surveillance every 2 years.[35]

Cyst surveillance may be ended after 5 years of stability or if a patient no longer is a surgical candidate. Surveillance cessation is controversial because risk of progression of PCs may increase after 5 years. This increased risk with time is reflected in the European Consensus Guidelines, which increased the follow-up time to every 6 months after 5 years.[27,36]

American College of Radiology

The initial guidelines published by the ACR incidental findings committee were released in 2010, in which they recommended PCs less than 2 cm undergo imaging at 1 year follow-up, and, if the PC is stable, to cease surveillance.[37] Subsequently, a study questioned the safety of stopping surveillance by demonstrating that 27% of PCs grow during the 1-year surveillance, and 11% grow after 1 year of stability.[38] The ACR published revised guidelines for the management of PCs in 2017, which takes a more conservative surveillance approach.[39] High-risk findings requiring EUS-FNA and surgical evaluation include mural nodularity, peripheral calcification, wall thickening, MPD greater than or equal to 7 mm, or

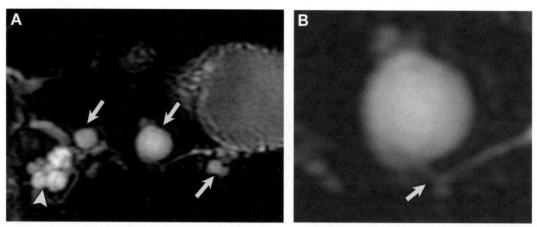

Fig. 8. BD-IPMN. (*A*) A 2-dimensional coronal MRCP image shows multiple unilocular cysts in the pancreatic head, body, and tail (*arrows*). In addition, a multilocular cyst is seen in the pancreatic head (*arrowhead*). (*B*) Magnified image of the cyst in the mid pancreas shows communication of the unilocular cyst in the pancreas body with the MPD (*arrow*).

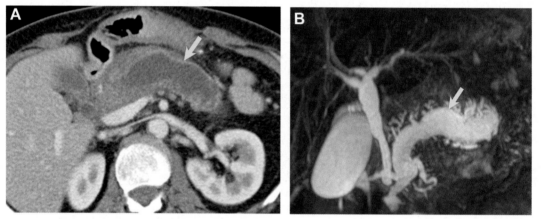

Fig. 9. MD-IPMN and BD-IPMN: (*A*) axial CECT image through the pancreas and (*B*) MRCP of the pancreas shows a markedly dilated pancreatic duct (*arrow*) with dilatation of multiple BD's.

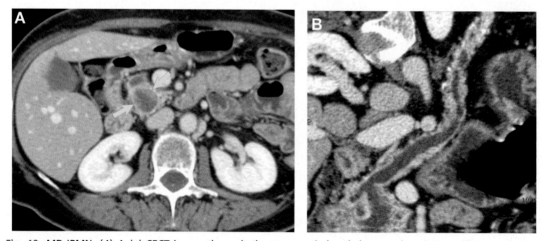

Fig. 10. MD-IPMN: (*A*) Axial CECT image through the pancreatic head shows enhancing papillary projections (*short arrows*) within the dilated pancreatic duct in the head. (*B*) CPR CECT image of the pancreatic duct shows the MPD to be dilated at 1 cm.

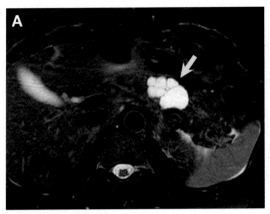
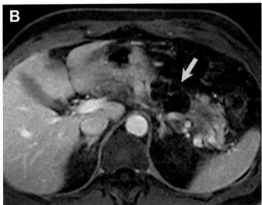

Fig. 11. MCN: (*A*) axial T2-weighted MR image through the pancreas and (*B*) axial contrast-enhanced MR image, show a multilocular cystic mass (*arrow*) in the pancreatic tail without a solid component or ductal dilatation.

extrahepatic biliary obstruction. Imaging follow-up is recommended using either a CT pancreas protocol or contrast-enhanced MR image. Growth is defined as 20% increase in the longest axis diameter on axial or coronal imaging. At the threshold of 1.5 cm to 2.5 cm, or with growth, EUS-FNA may be considered in the evaluation. Surveillance is ended at 10 years or after a patient is greater than 80 years of age, depending on the patient's health status and preferences.

Special consideration has been given to very small (<5 mm) PCs. A 2017 ACR white paper refers to these as white-dots and suggests a single follow-up MR imaging in 2 years with cessation of follow-up if stable. Pandey and colleagues[40] showed that 100% PCs with a baseline size of less than 5 mm were stable at 3 years, although 13% did demonstrate growth with a longer follow-up period. These findings

support less frequent follow-up of very small PCs, although the appropriate duration remains controversial.

International Association of Pancreatology

In 2010, in Fukuoka, Japan, a consensus symposium was held in which management of IPMNs and MCNs of the pancreas was established. For PCs larger than 1 cm, a CT or MR imaging/MRCP is recommended to establish high-risk stigmata, including a solid component, enhancement, and MPD greater than or equal to 10 mm, which yield a recommendation for surgery. Worrisome features include cyst size greater than or equal to 3 cm, thickened enhancing cyst walls, mural nodules, MPD 5 mm to 9 mm, change in MPD caliber with distal atrophy, and lymphadenopathy, which yield a recommendation for EUS-FNA.

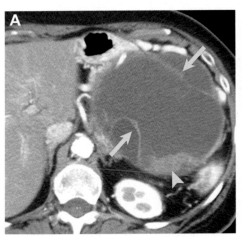
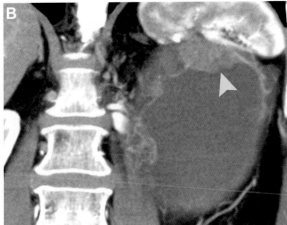

Fig. 12. MCN with malignant degeneration: (*A*) axial CECT image and (*B*) coronal reformation in a middle-aged woman show a cystic mass in the pancreatic tail. Septations (*arrows*) and enhancing solid components are seen (*arrowheads*).

Table 1
Summary of guidelines for follow-up of incidental pancreatic cysts

	High-Risk Criteria	Initial Work-up	Follow-up Modality	Follow-up Interval	Cessation
American Gastroenterological Association	At least 2 of the following: • Size >3 cm • Dilated main duct • Solid component	EUS-FNA	MR imaging	1 y, then every 2 y	After 5 y of stability or when patient is not a surgical candidate
ACR	• Mural nodularity • Peripheral calcifications • Wall thickening • Main duct >7 mm • Extrahepatic biliary obstruction	EUS-FNA and surgical consultation	CT pancreas protocol or IV contrast-enhanced MR imaging	Dependent on cyst size	After 10 y of stability or after patient is >80 y
International Association of Pancreatology (Fukuoka)	• Size >3 cm • Thick/enhancing wall • Mural nodule • Main duct 5–9 mm • Change in duct caliber with distal atrophy • Obstruction • Lymphadenopathy	EUS-FNA and surgical consultation	CT/MR imaging or EUS alternating with MR imaging	Dependent on cyst size	When patient is not a surgical candidate

If the initial imaging examination shows no high-risk stigmata or worrisome features, patients should undergo MR imaging/MRCP or CT after 3 months to 6 months, followed by annual follow-up clinically and by imaging.[41]

The Fukuoka guidelines were revised in regard to the follow-up of IPMNs.[30] Worrisome features now include rate of PC growth and imaging follow-up rate was stratified by size, with continuation until a patient no longer is a surgical candidate or elects to stop.

DIAGNOSTICS

FNA with fluid analysis of viscosity, cytology, and DNA molecular analysis can aid in the diagnostic work up of PC. Cytologic analysis of mucinous neoplasms shows clusters of columnar epithelial cells containing mucin in their cytoplasm.[16] There is low interobserver agreement in cytologic analysis of mucinous neoplasms.[42] A major problem with FNA of PCs is that many samples are limited in their cellularity; in a study of 618 samples, 53% of samples were either "less than optimal" or "unsatisfactory" for cytologic analysis. A majority (98%) of samples, however, were able to undergo molecular analysis.[43]

A combination of carcinoembryonic antigen (CEA) level greater than or equal to 192 ng/mL and molecular analysis, including DNA concentration, K-RAS mutations, and allelic imbalances, improves sensitivity in diagnosing mucinous from nonmucinous neoplasms, although CEA cutoff levels may be specific to the individual laboratory.[16,44] CA 19-9 analysis of cyst aspirate is not useful.[12] Large amounts of PC fluid DNA, high-amplitude mutations, and specific mutation acquisition sequences are predictors of malignancy.[45]

Genes associated with IPMNs include KRAS, GNAS, RNF43, TP53, PIK3CA, PTEN, CDKN2A, and SMAD4.[46] MCNs are associated with genetic alterations in KRAS, RNF43, TP53, PIK3CA, PTEN, CDKN2A, and SMAD4.[46] SCNs have a typical CEA fluid analysis of less than 5 ng/mL and low viscosity and are associated with mutations in the VHL gene.[46–48]

Fluid viscosity can be used to differentiate between mucinous and nonmucinous cysts.[49] The string sign is measured by the maximal length of mucus string between the thumb and index finger of the examiner; a positive string sign is if the mucus measures at least 3 mm.[16]

Given the limitations in adequately obtaining cells by FNA, molecular analysis likely is the direction forward in diagnostic analysis of aspirates of PCs.

POTENTIAL PITFALLS

There are several pancreatic masses in particular that may appear cystic and which are potential pitfalls to consider when assessing a PC mass.

Solid and Pseudopapillary Epithelial Neoplasms

SPENs are relatively rare low-grade malignant tumors that typically affect young women. These tumors can be solid, cystic, or mixed and frequently develop internal hemorrhage (**Fig. 13**). A well-defined thick enhancing capsule is typical. These usually are large (average 9 cm) and more often in the tail.[50]

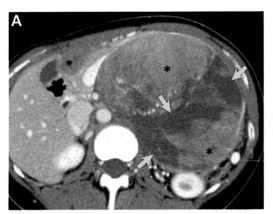
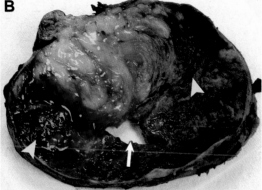

Fig. 13. SPEN. (*A*) Axial CECT image shows a large pancreatic mass with enhancing solid components (*asterisks*) and areas of cystic degeneration (*arrows*). (*B*) The gross resected specimen reveals areas of hemorrhage (*arrowheads*) and cystic degeneration (*arrow*).

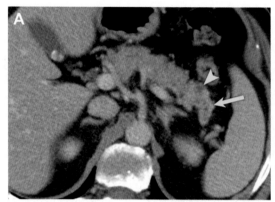
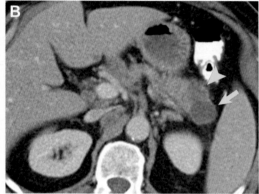

Fig. 14. PDAC with cystic component. (*A*) Axial CECT image shows focal dilatation of the MPD in the tail (*arrow*). A hypoenhancing focus (*arrowhead*) is seen proximally (*B*) Axial CECT image 3 months later shows a hypoenhancing mass in the pancreatic tail (*arrowhead*). Distal to this mass a cystic mass (*arrow*) is present that represents a cystic component of the adenocarcinoma and/or a pseudocyst after duct obstruction.

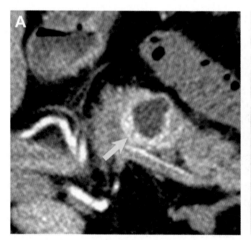
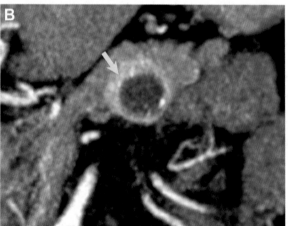

Fig. 15. (*A*) Neuroendocrine tumor with cystic degeneration: (*A*) Axial CECT image through the pancreatic neck with (*B*) coronal reformation shows a PC surrounded by peripheral enhancement (*arrows*). An arterial enhancing component almost always is present in a cystic neuroendocrine tumor.

Cystic Features of Pancreatic Ductal Adenocarcinoma

Although the classic appearance of PDAC is a solid, infiltrating mass, it may develop cystic features (**Fig. 14**), including large duct cysts, neoplastic mucinous cysts, colloid carcinomas, and degenerative cystic change. An obstructing mass can cause retention cysts or pseudocysts from pancreatitis.[51] There rarely can be a combination of these processes with the same patient, that is, areas of cystic degeneration/necrosis, as well as cystic changes related to secondary pancreatitis. Clear ductal obstruction should raise concern for PDAC. Careful assessment of the pancreas for a hypoattenuating infiltrative mass or clear ductal obstruction should raise concern for cystic degeneration of PDAC.

Cystic Neuroendocrine Tumor

Although typically solid and hyperenhancing, pancreatic neuroendocrine tumors can be mixed cystic and solid and, rarely, almost entirely cystic with a thick hyperenhancing rim or mural nodularity[52] (**Fig. 15**). These tumors can be multifocal, and, although they usually are sporadic, they can be associated with neurofibromatosis 1, multiple endocrine neoplasia type 1, or VHL disease. There is a relatively high degree of metastatic disease, either to lymph nodes or liver.[52]

SUMMARY

Incidental PCs commonly are encountered in a radiology practice. Some cystic masses of the pancreas, in particular pseudocysts, usually can be characterized accurately and adequately by a combination of imaging, history, and follow-up. Other PCs require further evaluation with EUS with FNA. Because some have malignant potential, many PCs require clinical and imaging follow-up. There are several available societal guidelines to help plan patient follow-up, with recent updates. The care of patients with PCs ideally is a multidisciplinary effort among radiologists, pathologists, surgeons, and gastroenterologists for optimal patient management.

CLINICS CARE POINTS

- Imaging alone cannot always differentiate benign pancreatic cysts from pancreatic cysts with malignant potential.
- Small indeterminate pancreatic cysts need to be followed-up, since invasive testing and resections are typically reserved for larger or growing cysts or definitively malignant cysts.

DISCLOSURE

The authors have nothing to disclose.

ACKNOWLEDGMENTS

The authors acknowledge and thank Dr Shiro Urayama, MD, for providing the endoscopic ultrasound images.

REFERENCES

1. Gardner TB, Glass LM, Smith KD, et al. Pancreatic cyst prevalence and the risk of mucin-producing adenocarcinoma in US adults. Am J Gastroenterol 2013;108(10):1546–50.
2. Mella JM, Gómez EJ, Omodeo M, et al. Prevalence of incidental clinically relevant pancreatic cysts at diagnosis based on current guidelines. Gastroenterol Hepatol 2018;41(5):293–301.
3. Rosenkrantz AB, Xue X, Gyftopoulos S, et al. Downstream costs associated with incidental pancreatic cysts detected at MRI. AJR Am J Roentgenol 2018;211(6):1278–82.
4. Fabrega-Foster K, Kamel IR, Horowitz JM, et al. ACR Appropriateness Criteria Pancreatic cyst. Available at: https://acsearch.acr.org/docs/3127236/Narrative/. American College of Radiology. Accessed August 3, 2020.
5. Liu K, Xie P, Peng W, et al. Magnetic resonance cholangiopancreatography: Comparison of two- and three-dimensional sequences for the assessment of pancreatic cystic lesions. Oncol Lett 2015;9(4):1917–21.
6. Macari M, Lee T, Kim S, et al. Is gadolinium necessary for MRI follow-up evaluation of cystic lesions in the pancreas? Preliminary results. AJR Am J Roentgenol 2009;192(1):159–64.
7. Pozzi-Mucelli RM, Rinta-Kiikka I, Wünsche K, et al. Pancreatic MRI for the surveillance of cystic neoplasms: comparison of a short with a comprehensive imaging protocol. Eur Radiol 2017;27(1):41–50.
8. Sun MRM, Strickland CD, Tamjeedi B, et al. Utility of transabdominal ultrasound for surveillance of known pancreatic cystic lesions: prospective evaluation with MRI as reference standard. Abdom Radiol (New York) 2018;43(5):1180–92.
9. Beyer-Enke SA, Hocke M, Ignee A, et al. Contrast enhanced transabdominal ultrasound in the characterisation of pancreatic lesions with cystic appearance. Jop 2010;11(5):427–33.
10. Chen F, Liang JY, Zhao QY, et al. Differentiation of branch duct intraductal papillary mucinous neoplasms from serous cystadenomas of the pancreas using contrast-enhanced sonography. J Ultrasound Med 2014;33(3):449–55.
11. Song MH, Lee SK, Kim MH, et al. EUS in the evaluation of pancreatic cystic lesions. Gastrointest Endosc 2003;57(7):891–6.
12. Leung KK, Ross WA, Evans D, et al. Pancreatic cystic neoplasm: the role of cyst morphology, cyst fluid analysis, and expectant management. Ann Surg Oncol 2009;16(10):2818–24.
13. Kamata K, Kitano M, Kudo M, et al. Value of EUS in early detection of pancreatic ductal adenocarcinomas in patients with intraductal papillary mucinous neoplasms. Endoscopy 2014;46(01):22–9.
14. Choi SY, Kim JH, Yu MH, et al. Diagnostic performance and imaging features for predicting the malignant potential of intraductal papillary mucinous neoplasm of the pancreas: a comparison of EUS, contrast-enhanced CT and MRI. Abdom Radiol (New York) 2017;42(5):1449–58.
15. Ahmad NA, Kochman ML, Brensinger C, et al. Interobserver agreement among endosonographers for the diagnosis of neoplastic versus non-neoplastic pancreatic cystic lesions. Gastrointest Endosc 2003;58(1):59–64.
16. Oh SH, Lee JK, Lee KT, et al. The Combination of Cyst Fluid Carcinoembryonic Antigen, Cytology and Viscosity Increases the Diagnostic Accuracy of Mucinous Pancreatic Cysts. Gut Liver 2017;11(2):283–9.

17. Harima H, Kaino S, Shinoda S, et al. Differential diagnosis of benign and malignant branch duct intraductal papillary mucinous neoplasm using contrast-enhanced endoscopic ultrasonography. World J Gastroenterol 2015;21(20):6252–60.

18. Kim HJ, Lee DH, Ko YT, et al. CT of serous cystadenoma of the pancreas and mimicking masses. AJR Am J Roentgenol 2008;190(2):406–12.

19. Manfredi R, Ventriglia A, Mantovani W, et al. Mucinous cystic neoplasms and serous cystadenomas arising in the body-tail of the pancreas: MR imaging characterization. Eur Radiol 2015;25(4): 940–9.

20. Yang J, Guo X, Zhang H, et al. Differential diagnosis of pancreatic serous cystadenoma and mucinous cystadenoma: utility of textural features in combination with morphological characteristics. BMC Cancer 2019;19(1):1223.

21. Thoeni RF. The revised Atlanta classification of acute pancreatitis: its importance for the radiologist and its effect on treatment. Radiology 2012;262(3):751–64.

22. Gerscovich EO, Jacoby B, Field NT, et al. Fetal true pancreatic cysts. J Ultrasound Med 2012;31(5): 811–3.

23. van Rijn RR, Schilte PP, Wiarda BM, et al. Case 113: pancreatic cystosis. Radiology 2007;243(2): 598–602.

24. Kim WH, Lee JY, Park HS, et al. Lymphoepithelial cyst of the pancreas: comparison of CT findings with other pancreatic cystic lesions. Abdom Imaging 2013;38(2):324–30.

25. Osiro S, Rodriguez JR, Tiwari KJ, et al. Is preoperative diagnosis possible? A clinical and radiological review of lymphoepithelial cysts of the pancreas. Jop 2013;14(1):15–20.

26. Mortelé KJ, Rocha TC, Streeter JL, et al. Multimodality imaging of pancreatic and biliary congenital anomalies. Radiographics 2006;26(3):715–31.

27. Del Chiaro M, Ateeb Z, Hansson MR, et al. Survival analysis and risk for progression of intraductal papillary mucinous neoplasia of the pancreas (IPMN) under surveillance: a single-institution experience. Ann Surg Oncol 2017;24(4):1120–6.

28. Choi SH, Park SH, Kim KW, et al. Progression of unresected intraductal papillary mucinous neoplasms of the pancreas to cancer: a systematic review and meta-analysis. Clin Gastroenterol Hepatol 2017;15(10):1509–20.e4.

29. Kayal M, Luk L, Hecht EM, et al. Long-term surveillance and timeline of progression of presumed low-risk intraductal papillary mucinous neoplasms. AJR Am J Roentgenol 2017;209(2):320–6.

30. Tanaka M, Fernández-Del Castillo C, Kamisawa T, et al. Revisions of international consensus Fukuoka guidelines for the management of IPMN of the pancreas. Pancreatology 2017;17(5):738–53.

31. Irie H, Honda H, Aibe H, et al. MR cholangiopancreatographic differentiation of benign and malignant intraductal mucin-producing tumors of the pancreas. AJR Am J Roentgenol 2000;174(5): 1403–8.

32. Garces-Descovich A, Beker K, Castillo-Angeles M, et al. Mucinous cystic neoplasms of the pancreas: high-resolution cross-sectional imaging features with clinico-pathologic correlation. Abdom Radiol (New York) 2018;43(6):1413–22.

33. Lee JH, Kim JK, Kim TH, et al. MRI features of serous oligocystic adenoma of the pancreas: differentiation from mucinous cystic neoplasm of the pancreas. Br J Radiol 2012;85(1013):571–6.

34. Lv P, Mahyoub R, Lin X, et al. Differentiating pancreatic ductal adenocarcinoma from pancreatic serous cystadenoma, mucinous cystadenoma, and a pseudocyst with detailed analysis of cystic features on CT scans: a preliminary study. Korean J Radiol 2011;12(2):187–95.

35. Vege SS, Ziring B, Jain R, et al. American gastroenterological association institute guideline on the diagnosis and management of asymptomatic neoplastic pancreatic cysts. Gastroenterology 2015;148(4):819–22 [quize: 12-3].

36. Del Chiaro M, Verbeke C, Salvia R, et al. European experts consensus statement on cystic tumours of the pancreas. Dig Liver Dis 2013;45(9):703–11.

37. Berland LL, Silverman SG, Gore RM, et al. Managing incidental findings on abdominal CT: white paper of the ACR incidental findings committee. J Am Coll Radiol 2010;7(10):754–73.

38. Brook OR, Beddy P, Pahade J, et al. Delayed Growth in Incidental Pancreatic Cysts: Are the Current American College of Radiology Recommendations for Follow-up Appropriate? Radiology 2016;278(3):752–61.

39. Megibow AJ, Baker ME, Morgan DE, et al. Management of Incidental Pancreatic Cysts: A White Paper of the ACR Incidental Findings Committee. J Am Coll Radiol 2017;14(7):911–23.

40. Pandey P, Pandey A, Luo Y, et al. Follow-up of incidentally detected pancreatic cystic neoplasms: do baseline MRI and CT Features Predict Cyst Growth? Radiology 2019;292(3):647–54.

41. Tanaka M, Fernández-del Castillo C, Adsay V, et al. International consensus guidelines 2012 for the management of IPMN and MCN of the pancreas. Pancreatology 2012;12(3):183–97.

42. Sigel CS, Edelweiss M, Tong LC, et al. Low interobserver agreement in cytology grading of mucinous pancreatic neoplasms. Cancer Cytopathol 2015; 123(1):40–50.

43. Nikiforova MN, Khalid A, Fasanella KE, et al. Integration of KRAS testing in the diagnosis of pancreatic cystic lesions: a clinical experience of 618 pancreatic cysts. Mod Pathol 2013;26(11):1478–87.

44. Sawhney MS, Devarajan S, O'Farrel P, et al. Comparison of carcinoembryonic antigen and molecular analysis in pancreatic cyst fluid. Gastrointest Endosc 2009;69(6):1106–10.

45. Khalid A, Zahid M, Finkelstein SD, et al. Pancreatic cyst fluid DNA analysis in evaluating pancreatic cysts: a report of the PANDA study. Gastrointest Endosc 2009;69(6):1095–102.

46. Theisen BK, Wald AI, Singhi AD. Molecular Diagnostics in the Evaluation of Pancreatic Cysts. Surg Pathol Clin 2016;9(3):441–56.

47. Elta GH, Enestvedt BK, Sauer BG, et al. ACG clinical guideline: diagnosis and management of pancreatic cysts. Am J Gastroenterol 2018;113(4):464–79.

48. Farrell JJ. Pancreatic Cysts and Guidelines. Dig Dis Sci 2017;62(7):1827–39.

49. Khamaysi I, Abu Ammar A, Vasilyev G, et al. Differentiation of pancreatic cyst types by analysis of rheological behavior of pancreatic cyst fluid. Sci Rep 2017;7:45589.

50. Buetow PC, Buck JL, Pantongrag-Brown L, et al. Solid and papillary epithelial neoplasm of the pancreas: imaging-pathologic correlation on 56 cases. Radiology 1996;199(3):707–11.

51. Youn SY, Rha SE, Jung ES, et al. Pancreas ductal adenocarcinoma with cystic features on cross-sectional imaging: radiologic-pathologic correlation. Diagn Interv Radiol 2018;24(1):5–11.

52. Kawamoto S, Johnson PT, Shi C, et al. Pancreatic neuroendocrine tumor with cystlike changes: evaluation with MDCT. AJR Am J Roentgenol 2013;200(3):W283–90.

The Incidental Renal Mass-Update on Characterization and Management

John J. Hines Jr, MD[a],*, Katherine Eacobacci, BS[b], Riya Goyal, MD[c]

KEYWORDS

- Renal mass imaging • Renal mass management • Renal cell carcinoma • Cystic renal mass
- Oncocytoma • Angiomyolipoma • Renal mass active surveillance

KEY POINTS

- Incidental renal masses and other processes are commonly encountered on routine cross-sectional imaging examinations. Most will be benign cysts; a minority are indeterminate and will require a dedicated renal mass imaging. Renal cell carcinoma (RCC) is now most commonly discovered as an incidental imaging finding.
- Changes to the existing Bosniak classification for cystic renal masses in the 2019 proposed revision include incorporation of MR imaging findings, eliminating the need for further imaging in likely benign cystic masses, and definitions of structural components within a cyst.
- Despite gains in knowledge regarding imaging features of renal masses, there are still no reliable criteria to our knowledge that can be used to determine whether a soft tissue mass in the kidney is benign or malignant, with the differential diagnosis including RCC, lipid-poor angiomyolipoma, and oncocytoma. Machine learning with attention to radiomics shows promise in identifying features that can provide a more specific and accurate diagnosis.
- Intravenous contrast-enhanced computed tomography (CT) and MR imaging continue to be the primary modalities for characterization of the indeterminate or suspicious renal mass; however, other modalities will likely take on a greater role in renal mass imaging, including contrast-enhanced ultrasound and dual-energy CT.

INTRODUCTION

Incidental findings on abdominal cross-sectional imaging examinations are frequently encountered in solid organs, bowel, blood vessels, bone, and the abdominal and pelvic wall. The kidney is one of the more common locations for encountering an incidental finding. Most kidney masses and other incidental findings, for example, scarring and calculi, can be either safely ignored or confidently diagnosed on routine cross-sectional imaging. A small percentage will need further imaging with a specific renal mass imaging examination, or referral for urologic management. The purpose of this article is to outline the spectrum of incidental renal masses in the kidney, both common and uncommon, to inform the reader on data and guidelines that can help to diagnose and triage these findings, and to discuss recent developments and future directions in renal imaging.

[a] Department of Radiology, Huntington Hospital, Northwell Health, 270 Park Avenue, Huntington, NY 11743, USA; [b] Donald and Barbara Zucker School of Medicine at Hofstra/Northwell, 500 Hofstra Boulevard, Hempstead, NY 11549, USA; [c] Department of Radiology, Donald and Barbara Zucker School of Medicine at Hofstra/Northwell, 500 Hofstra Boulevard, Hempstead, NY 11549, USA
* Corresponding author.
E-mail address: jhinesmd@gmail.com

Radiol Clin N Am 59 (2021) 631–646
https://doi.org/10.1016/j.rcl.2021.03.011
0033-8389/21/© 2021 Elsevier Inc. All rights reserved.

COMMONLY ENCOUNTERED RENAL MASSES AND CHARACTERIZATION WITH IMAGING
Renal Cysts

Renal cysts are ubiquitous in the adult population. Their prevalence increases with age, with cysts found in 30% to 50% of patients by the seventh decade.[1] Therefore, the most commonly encountered mass in the kidney will overwhelmingly be a benign renal cyst. Mensel and colleagues[2] showed a prevalence on MR imaging of 27%. O'Connor and colleagues[3] showed the prevalence of incidental renal masses on nonenhanced CT to be 17%.

Most simple renal cysts are easily diagnosed on conventional gray-scale ultrasound imaging. The ultrasound criteria for defining a simple, uncomplicated renal cyst include well-defined, thin, smooth walls, increased posterior acoustic enhancement, and no internal debris or septa.[4]

On computed tomography (CT), a simple cyst can be diagnosed in a homogeneous mass of variable size measuring −9 to 20 HU, as long as there is an imperceptible wall, and no septa, nodules, or calcifications.[4] Although in the past such cysts were considered to be incompletely evaluated on nonenhanced CT alone, recent literature supports the presumption that these masses are benign.[3]

A limitation in the diagnosis of small cysts on intravenous (IV) contrast-enhanced CT is "pseudoenhancement." Pseudoenhancement is an artifact that causes increased HU measurements adjacent to avidly enhancing tissue, such as renal parenchyma.[5,6] Pseudoenhancement introduces inaccuracy into the analysis of enhancement, and the potential to misdiagnose a benign, nonenhancing cyst as an enhancing mass. This phenomena may be more frequently encountered on newer generation multidetector CT scanners than on earlier scanners.

A minority (6%) of cysts are hemorrhagic or proteinaceous.[1] Although benign, hemorrhagic cysts may sometimes be difficult to characterize accurately on imaging examinations because of changes in echogenicity (ultrasound), attenuation (CT), and signal (MR).

On ultrasound, hemorrhagic cysts can have a complex appearance due to internal echoes from the presence of blood. Color and spectral Doppler can help in the evaluation of such a cyst by demonstrating lack of blood flow; however, a cystic mass with internal echoes often requires further evaluation with IV contrast-enhanced CT or MR imaging.[7]

The increased attenuation of a hemorrhagic cyst on CT often overlaps with that of a soft tissue mass, including renal cell carcinoma (RCC);

however if sufficiently dense enough, it can be confidently diagnosed as a benign cyst on nonenhanced CT alone. Jonisch and colleagues[8] in a study of 105 patients, 54 with renal cell carcinoma and 51 with high attenuation cysts showed a specificity of greater than 99.9% in the diagnosis of a hemorrhagic cyst in a homogeneous small renal mass uniformly measuring 70 HU or greater on nonenhanced CT (Fig. 1).

MR imaging can be used to accurately diagnose simple cysts, even subcentimeter cysts, by the presence of uniform high T2 signal equivalent to other fluid-containing structures.[9] Nonenhanced MR imaging also has utility for diagnosing a hemorrhagic or proteinaceous cyst. In a study looking at unenhanced T1-weighted MR images in 134 patients, 84 with hemorrhagic cysts and 50 with RCC, Davarpanah and colleagues[10] found that a homogeneous hyperintense renal mass with a smooth border and signal intensity ratio 2.5× greater than renal parenchyma was likely to be a benign hemorrhagic cyst, with a confidence level greater than 99.9% (Fig. 2).

Renal Cell Carcinoma

RCC now most often comes to attention as an incidental finding on abdominal cross-sectional imaging performed for other purposes. Clinical presentation with signs and symptoms of RCC is becoming less frequent.[11]

Eighty percent of RCCs are clear cell carcinomas (ccRCC). ccRCC has a more unfavorable prognosis than other RCC subtypes, with a higher frequency of metastatic disease and decreased survival.[12] ccRCC is a hypervascular tumor on

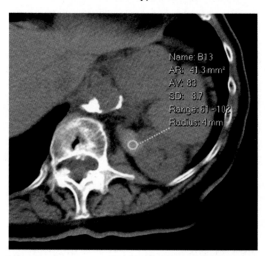

Fig. 1. Hemorrhagic cyst. An 85-year-old woman with abdominal pain. Axial nonenhanced CT image of the left kidney shows a uniformly high-density renal mass, measuring 83 HU.

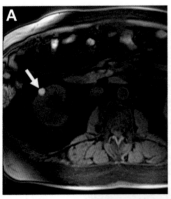
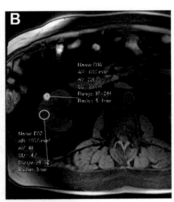
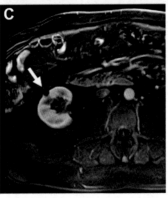

Fig. 2. Hemorrhagic cyst. A 72-year old man for evaluation of a renal mass. Axial T1-weighted fat-suppressed MR images obtained without (A) and with (B) region of interest measurements show a homogeneous hyperintense mass in the right kidney (arrow, A). The signal intensity is 220 (B), a value greater than 2.5 times that of the renal parenchyma (48). T1-weighted IV contrast-enhanced subtraction MR image (C) demonstrates lack of enhancement in the cyst (arrow, C).

imaging, and typically enhances rapidly and intensely, especially in the corticomedullary phase (Fig. 3).[13,14] On MR imaging, ccRCC frequently demonstrates high T2 signal, which is often heterogeneous because of necrosis, cystic degeneration, hemorrhage, or a combination of these findings.[15] Most ccRCCs will show drop out on chemical-shift imaging due to the presence of microscopic fat (Fig. 4).[16]

The second most common renal malignancy is papillary renal cell carcinoma (pRCC), comprising 10% to 15% of RCCs, including a typically indolent and slow-growing Type 1 pRCC and an aggressive Type 2.[17] pRCCs are typically hypovascular, demonstrating weak enhancement on CT and MR imaging, which can lead to the potential pitfall of misdiagnosis as a hemorrhagic or proteinaceous cyst on CT in a minority of cases.[18–21] pRCC tends to have lower T2 signal intensity than other RCC subtypes due to intratumoral hemorrhage and papillary architecture (Fig. 5).[22]

Chromophobe RCC (chrRCC) is the third most common RCC subtype, accounting for approximately 5% of RCC, and has the most favorable prognosis.[12] chrRCC has enhancement kinetics that are intermediate relative to ccRCC and pRCC (Fig. 6).[14]

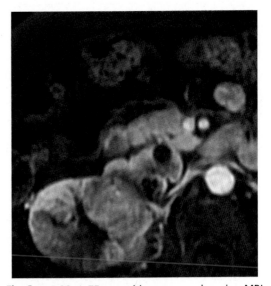

Fig. 3. ccRCC. A 75-year-old woman undergoing MRI for a known left renal mass. Axial T1-weighted IV contrast-enhanced MR image obtained in the corticomedullary phase shows an avidly enhancing left renal mass, a typical enhancement pattern for ccRCC.

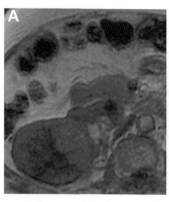
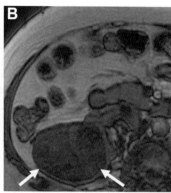

Fig. 4. ccRCC. A 71-year-old woman being evaluated for bilateral renal masses. Axial T1-weighted in-phase (A) and opposed-phase (B) axial MR images of the right kidney demonstrate a right renal mass showing loss of signal on the out-of-phase image (arrows), indicative of microscopic (intracellular) fat.

Malignant Renal Masses Other than Renal Cell Carcinoma

Malignant masses not of primary renal origin include transitional cell carcinoma, metastatic disease, and secondary lymphoma.

Transitional cell carcinoma (TCC) accounts for 10% of renal masses, and can mimic a centrally located RCC, especially when most of the tumor involves the renal parenchyma rather than the collecting system. Infiltrative TCCs tend to preserve the renal contour (**Fig. 7**), although less commonly can present as an eccentric tumor distorting the renal contour similar to RCC.[23]

Renal metastases account for only 0.9% of renal masses, but when they do occur they are mostly carcinomas (80.8%), typically solitary (77.5%), with lung cancer being the most common primary site.[24,25]

Renal lymphoma usually occurs in the setting of widespread nodal or extranodal lymphoma, has various presentations, and can be unilateral or bilateral, as well as solitary, multiple, or diffuse and ill defined.[26]

Benign Solid Renal Tumors

A limitation of all imaging modalities is the inability to differentiate RCC from a benign solid soft tissue attenuation renal mass. Approximately 40% of solid renal tumors smaller than 1 cm, and approximately 20% of tumors smaller than 3 cm, will be of

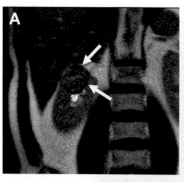
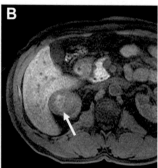
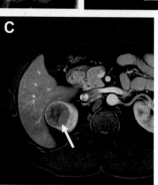

Fig. 5. pRCC. A 53-year-old man undergoing MR imaging for a renal mass found on ultrasound. Coronal T2-weighted (A) MR image of the right kidney demonstrates low signal within a right renal mass. Axial T1-weighted fat-suppressed MR image (B) shows mildly hyperintense signal within the center of the mass compatible with intratumoral hemorrhage. (C) Axial T1-weighted IV contrast-enhanced MR image shows mild enhancement of the mass (arrow).

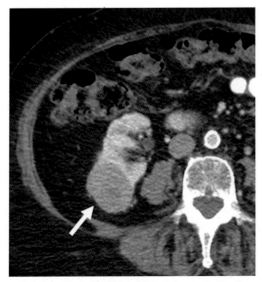

Fig. 6. chrRCC. An 85-year-old man. Axial contrast-image through the right kidney demonstrates a right renal mass with moderate diffuse enhancement (*arrow*). The mass was proven to be a chrRCC after resection and pathologic analysis.

a benign histology.[27] The most commonly encountered benign solid masses are angiomyolipoma (AML) and oncocytoma, which represented 44% and 35% of resected benign renal masses in one surgical series, respectively.[28]

AMLs are benign tumors composed of fat, smooth muscle, and vascular tissue in varying proportions. Most AMLs will contain fat in sufficient quantity for detection on CT and MR imaging, allowing for definitive diagnosis. Macroscopic fat is only rarely seen in RCC, and are often associated with calcifications, which are seldom seen in AMLs. Four percent to 5% of AMLs contain either minimal (3%–10% mature fat microscopically) or no fat, and

may resemble a nonspecific solid soft tissue mass on cross-sectional imaging (lipid-poor AML).[29]

An AML may be diagnosed by direct visualization of fat on CT (**Fig. 8**), or on MR imaging by loss of signal on frequency selective fat-suppressed sequences (**Fig. 9**), or the presence of an "India ink" artifact between the mass and normal renal parenchyma (**Fig. 10**). Loss of signal on out-of-phase (OOP) images may be seen in an AML due to small areas of fat within the tumor; however, this finding is not useful in differentiating from RCC, as OOP dropout can be seen in all renal cortical tumors, most frequently in ccRCC due to intracellular lipid.[30,31] More than 20% loss of signal intensity in a nodule without macroscopic fat has been shown to have high specificity for ccRCC.[16,30] However, individual pixel analysis of CT images is not useful for making the diagnosis, as ccRCC has been shown to have more pixels in the negative HU range than AML.[32]

Lipid-poor AMLs have attenuation similar to skeletal muscle on nonenhanced CT, and are more hyperattenuating than most RCCs; however, there is overlap between the density measurements of lipid-poor AMLs with chromophobe and other subtypes of RCC.[33] Low T2 signal on MR imaging is a feature suggestive of an AML, but is also commonly seen in papillary RCC. Therefore, although such findings are suggestive of a lipid-poor AML, they do not obviate the need for biopsy.

Oncocytomas account for approximately 7% of renal masses,[34] and more than half of all benign solid renal tumors smaller than 4 cm.[35] These tumors share a common progenitor cell with chrRCC, and therefore have overlapping histologic and imaging features. Characteristic imaging features of oncocytoma include peripheral location, lack of calcifications, well-circumscribed borders,

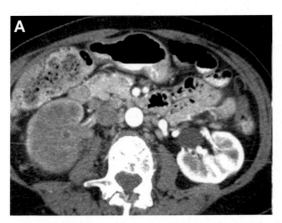
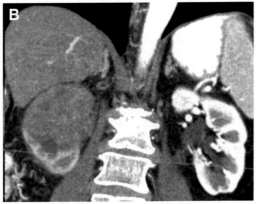

Fig. 7. TCC. A 62-year-old woman with gross hematuria. Axial (*A*) and coronal (*B*) IV contrast-enhanced CT images through the kidneys show a diffusely enhancing hypodense right renal mass that preserves the renal contour, a typical appearance of TCC.

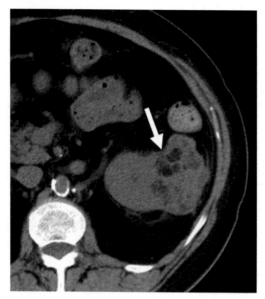

Fig. 8. Angiomyolipoma. A 45-year-old woman for follow-up of a known renal mass. Axial nonenhanced CT image of the left kidney demonstrates a left renal mass composed of soft tissue and macroscopic fat (*arrow*).

and heterogeneous T2 signal on MR imaging.[15] Enhancement is typically less than renal cortex at all phases of dynamic contrast-enhanced imaging.[36] Findings of a central stellate scar, seen in 50% to 61% of oncocytomas, typically with associated spoke-wheel enhancement, can suggest the diagnosis, but can also be seen in RCC, particularly in chrRCC.[36,37] Segmental contrast inversion, an interesting feature whereby portions of a tumor that enhance avidly on early-phase imaging washout on later phases, whereas areas that enhance weakly on early phase show increased enhancement on delayed images (**Fig. 11**), can be seen in oncocytomas, although the frequency of this observation greatly varies in the literature,

and segmental contrast inversion can also be seen in chrRCC.[36,38–40]

Despite the preceding advances in defining imaging characteristics of minimal-fat AML and oncocytomas, these tumors are currently unable to be reliably differentiated from RCC with any imaging modality, to our knowledge, and require either biopsy or surgical removal for definitive diagnosis.

Cystic Renal Masses

Cystic renal cancers account for 3% to 14% of renal cell carcinoma.[41] There is overlap in the imaging appearance of benign and malignant cystic renal masses, with the differential diagnosis including cystic degeneration of a usually solid RCC subtype, multilocular cystic renal cell carcinoma, multilocular cystic nephroma, mixed epithelial stromal tumor, hemorrhagic cysts, and atypical cysts, all of which may contain thickened, nodular septations, enhancing nodules, or a combination of these findings.[41,42]

Although portions of a cystic malignancy may measure less than 20 HU, in most cases cystic tumors will demonstrate some degree of heterogeneity, allowing for differentiation from a simple cyst. Rarely, necrosis within a papillary RCC may be extensive enough that it may resemble a cyst on imaging (**Fig. 12**). Corwin and colleagues[43] found that 2.8% of papillary RCCs were found to be homogeneous and less than 20 HU in attenuation on nonenhanced CT (**Fig. 13**). Fifteen percent of clear cell carcinomas may have cystic components, which can be due to multilocular cystic growth, origin from the wall of a preexisting cyst or cystic necrosis. Multilocular cystic renal carcinoma is a subtype of clear cell RCC and is a true cystic neoplasm, which is defined by strict pathologic criteria. These tumors exhibit benign behavior, and distant metastases have seldom, if

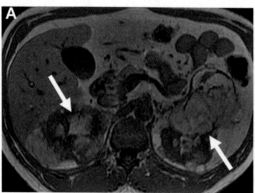
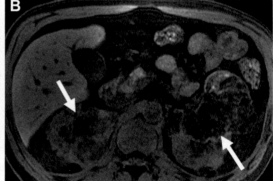

Fig. 9. Angiomyolipomas. A 28-year-old woman with tuberous sclerosis. Axial T1-weighted MR images obtained without (*A*) and with (*B*) fat suppression demonstrate bulk fat within multiple bilateral renal masses (*arrows*).

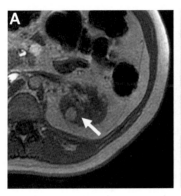
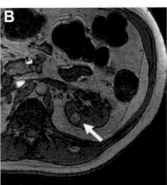

Fig. 10. Angiomyolipoma. A 70-year-old woman for follow-up of a left renal mass. Axial T1-weighted in-phase (A) and opposed-phase (B) MR images of the left kidney demonstrate a hyperintense mass. On the opposed-phase image, "India ink" artifact (arrow) is present along the border of the mass and the renal parenchyma, indicative of a fat-containing mass.

ever, been reported, to our knowledge.[9,44] Regardless of the exact tumor histology, cystic renal cancers tend to have less aggressive tumor biology and significantly improved survival compared with solid RCC.[41,42,45,46]

The Bosniak classification for cystic renal masses on CT has much practical value for assessing the malignant potential in a renal mass, and helps to guide management.[47] Although the original Bosniak classification was designed to be CT specific, it has been extrapolated to MR imaging over the years, and incorporation of MR imaging features is an important part of the 2019 proposed revision.[4] The Bosniak assessment is based on structural components of the cyst, including density of the cyst; number, thickness, and morphology of septae; and mural nodules, on CT. Calcification can be seen in both benign and malignant cystic masses, and is not a useful discriminator for cyst diagnosis. Bosniak 1 and 2 cystic masses are benign and require no further imaging follow-up. Bosniak 3 and 4 cystic masses have an intermediate (Bosniak 3) or high (Bosniak 4) probability of malignancy. Bosniak

2 F ("F" for follow-up) cysts demonstrate a minimally thickened wall, 1 or more minimally thick and enhancing septations, or many thin enhancing septations; such cystic masses, while likely benign, require imaging follow-up.

The overwhelming majority of incidentally encountered renal cystic masses are benign and can be classified as either Bosniak 1 or 2 cysts (Fig. 14). Surgery is usually indicated for Bosniak 3 and 4 category masses, unless the patient has comorbidities that would preclude resection. Features that are used to upgrade a cystic mass into higher categories include thick or irregular septations (Bosniak 3) (Fig. 15) and mural nodules (Bosniak 4) (Fig. 16), some or all of which are usually present in a cystic malignancy. There is a wide range in the malignancy rate for Bosniak 3 cystic masses, ranging from 25% to 82%[48]; this variability has led to an increasing role for renal biopsy.

A proposed update to the original Bosniak classification was recently published in 2019, as noted, with the overarching goals of decreasing follow-up imaging on cystic masses with a high likelihood of benignity, and decreasing the

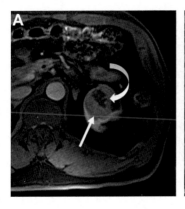
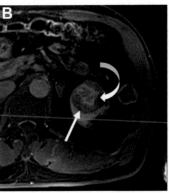

Fig. 11. Segmental contrast inversion. An 82-year-old man with lung cancer undergoing MR imaging for a renal mass found on chest CT (not shown). Axial T1-weighted IV contrast-enhanced MR images obtained in the corticomedullary (A) and nephrographic (B) phases demonstrate a left renal mass with an area of early avid enhancement that becomes less enhanced on the nephrographic-phase image (straight arrow), whereas an area showing weak early enhancement demonstrates increased enhancement on the nephrographic image (curved arrows).

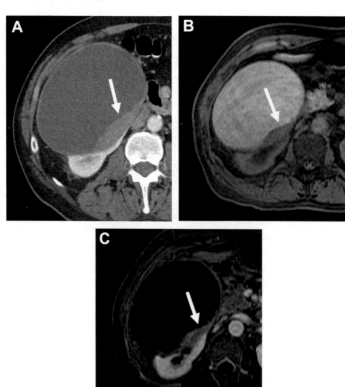

Fig. 12. Necrotic pRCC. A 58-year-old man with right flank pain. Axial IV contrast-enhanced CT image (*A*), axial T1-weighted fat-suppressed (*B*), and axial T1-weighted IV contrast-enhanced subtraction (*C*) MR images show a cystic mass with high T1 signal compatible with hemorrhage, and a plaquelike enhancing component medially (*arrows*).

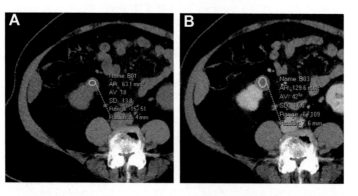

Fig. 13. RCC measuring less than 20 HU on nonenhanced CT. A 45-year-old man for evaluation of a renal mass found on ultrasound. Image from an axial nonenhanced CT (*A*) demonstrates an exophytic right homogeneous mass measuring 18 HU. (*B*) Axial IV contrast-enhanced CT image obtained at the same level as (*A*) demonstrates weak but unequivocal enhancement of the mass, which now measures 42 HU (an increase of 24 HU from the nonenhanced scan).

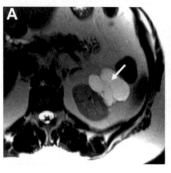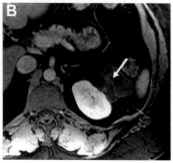

Fig. 14. Bosniak 2 cystic mass. A 39-year-old woman with a left renal mass incidentally found on CT (not shown) performed for epigastric pain. Axial T2-weighted (*A*) and T1-weighted IV gadolinium-enhanced (*B*) MR images show a cystic left renal mass (*arrows*) with a few thin enhancing septations.

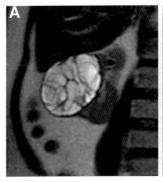 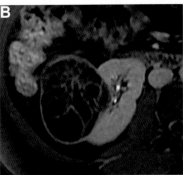

Fig. 15. Bosniak 3 cystic renal mass. A 31-year-old woman with known renal mass which has been stable for 5 years. Coronal T2-weighted (*A*) and T1-weighted IV gadolinium-enhanced (*B*) MR images of the right kidney show a cystic renal mass with a thick-wall and numerous thick enhancing septations.

frequency of surgical resection of benign cystic renal masses.[4]

Important changes in this proposal include the following:

1. Integration of MR imaging features into the classification scheme.
2. Precise characterization of cyst characteristics that were previously left to the judgment of the radiologist. These include quantitative definitions of a cystic mass; mural and septal enhancement; mural nodules; thickness of thin, thick, and irregular thickened septations; and number and type of septations specific for each category (**Table 1**).
3. Classification of cysts that are highly likely to be benign, but that previously were considered as needing further workup, now considered benign (Bosniak 2) cysts; these include:
   a. homogeneous cysts measuring between −9 and 20 HU on nonenhanced CT
   b. homogeneous hyperdense cysts measuring more than 70 HU on nonenhanced CT
   c. cysts measuring less than 30 HU on portal venous phase CT
   d. homogeneous hypodense cysts, which are too small to characterize on IV contrast-enhanced CT
   e. uniformly markedly T2 bright cysts on non-enhanced MR imaging
   f. uniformly markedly T1 bright cysts on non-enhanced MR imaging[4]

NON-NEOPLASTIC RENAL PROCESSES AND MIMICS

Non-neoplastic conditions may occasionally mimic a renal neoplasm, and include infectious, granulomatous, and vascular etiologies.

Developmental pseudotumors include hypertrophied columns of Bertin, splenic or dromedary humps, and persistent fetal lobulation. CT, MR imaging, and/or ultrasound can help to differentiate developmental pseudotumors from RCC; the corticomedullary phase is particularly useful in this regard.[49]

In the absence of clinical signs of infection, focal pyelonephritis may be difficult to differentiate from RCC. However, on CT, focal pyelonephritis will not demonstrate a well-defined wall or bulge on the renal surface, as is frequently seen with RCC.[49]

Granulomatous causes are uncommon, and include focal xanthogranulomatous pyelonephritis (XGP), sarcoidosis, and malakoplakia. A minority of cases of XGP, approximately 10%, will be isolated to a segment of an otherwise normal kidney.[50] The focality of the disease can be confused with a renal neoplasm.[51]

Vascular etiologies include congenital intraparenchymal or renal sinus arterial-venous malformation and acquired arteriovenous fistula, both of which demonstrate characteristic findings on

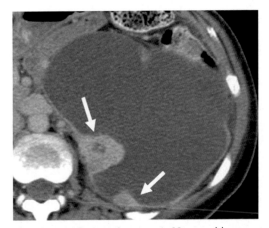

Fig. 16. Bosniak 4 cystic mass. A 66-year-old woman undergoing CT to evaluate bilateral renal masses. Axial IV contrast-enhanced CT image of the left kidney shows a large cystic mass in the left kidney with enhancing mural nodules (*arrows*).

Table 1
Definitions of renal mass features in 2019 proposed Bosniak revision

Term	Definition in the Proposed Bosniak Classification, Version 2019
Enhancement	Enhancement is either unequivocally perceived (ie, there is clear visible enhancement when noncontrast and contrast-enhanced images are compared) or is measurable by using established quantitative thresholds.
Homogeneous	Mass containing similar attenuation, signal intensity, or echogenicity throughout; a thin wall is allowed but there can be no septa or calcifications.
Simple fluid	Homogeneous attenuation −9 to 20 HU at noncontrast or contrast-enhanced CT. Homogeneous signal intensity similar to that of cerebrospinal fluid at T2-weighted MR imaging. Anechoic with increased posterior through-transmission at ultrasound.
Septum	Linear or curvilinear structure(s) in a cystic mass that connect 2 surfaces.
Number of septa	
Few	One to 3. For example, 1–3 thin enhancing septa is a feature of Bosniak II.
Many	Four or more. For example, 4 or more thin enhancing septa is a feature of Bosniak IIF.
Thickness	
Thin	≤2 mm in thickness.
Minimally thickened	3 mm in thickness.
Thick	≥4 mm in thickness.
Irregular thickening	≤3 mm focal or diffuse enhancing convex protrusion that has obtuse margins with the wall or septa.
Nodule	Focal enhancing convex protrusion of any size that has acute margins with the wall or septa, or a focal enhancing convex protrusion ≥4 mm that has obtuse margins with the wall or septa.
Cystic mass	Less than approximately 25% of the mass is composed of enhancing tissue.

color-flow Doppler[52] and multi-phasic CT or MR imaging.

Renal involvement occurs in 35% of patients with immunoglobulin (Ig)G-4 disease,[53] with 5 patterns being described, the most common of which is multiple bilateral hypoattenuating wedge-shaped or round cortical masses.[54] Involvement of other organs, particularly the pancreas, can help in suggesting the diagnosis (**Fig. 17**).

MANAGEMENT OF THE INCIDENTAL RENAL MASS

The diagnosis of most incidental renal masses is straightforward on routine CT, MR imaging, or ultrasound examination, and the great majority will not require any additional imaging. On nonenhanced CT, cystic processes with uniform low (<20 HU) or high attenuation (>70 HU) can be diagnosed as simple or hemorrhagic cysts, respectively. T1 hyperintense cysts (signal intensity >2.5 renal parenchyma) on nonenhanced MR imaging also meet criteria for hemorrhagic cysts. Visible fat is virtually diagnostic of a lipid-rich AML. A renal mass measuring less than 1 cm with uniform low attenuation can safely be ignored except in cases in which the radiologist identifies worrisome features, such as irregular and ill-defined borders.

A mass with HU measurements of between 20 to 70 on nonenhanced CT or greater than 30 HU on IV contrast-enhanced CT is indeterminate, and requires dedicated renal imaging. It is unusual for RCC to have density measurements of less than 30 HU on contrast-enhanced CT, and when present it is almost exclusively seen in pRCC. Corwin and colleagues[43] reported 1.8% (2 of 114) of

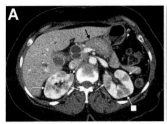

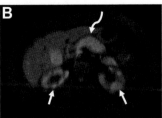

Fig. 17. IgG4-related disease. A 63-year-old man with jaundice. Axial IV contrast-enhanced CT image (*A*) shows bilateral hypoattenuating wedge-shaped kidney abnormalities (*white arrows*). Note the "sausage pancreas," representing associated autoimmune pancreatitis (*black arrows*). Axial diffusion-weighted MR image (*B*) shows diffusion restriction in the renal abnormalities (*white arrows*).

pRCC measured less than 30 HU in either the nephrographic or excretory phase, and 0 of 114 measuring less than 30 HU on portal venous phase. Cysts with pseudoenhancement likely account for the large majority of homogeneous masses measuring between 20 and 30 HU.[19,43]

WHAT TYPE OF FOLLOW-UP IMAGING SHOULD BE PERFORMED?

In cases in which definitive renal mass characterization is desired, CT or MR imaging are first-line modalities. Both modalities have been shown to be highly accurate in this setting. MR imaging is the preferred examination for evaluation of a small renal mass, due to lack of pseudoenhancement artifact and additional information obtained from nonenhanced T1 and T2 sequences. MR imaging is also preferred for evaluation of a hypovascular mass, due to the ability to depict mild contrast enhancement in cases in which enhancement is either insignificant or equivocal on CT, a scenario commonly encountered with pRCC.[20,21]

An alternative modality is IV contrast-enhanced ultrasound (CEUS), which has shown excellent diagnostic performance in renal mass characterization due to its high sensitivity for depiction of enhancement (**Fig. 18**). In a study by Barr and

colleagues,[55] which included 721 patients with 1018 indeterminate renal masses CEUS was used to correctly diagnose renal malignancy in 100% of cases (124 RCC, 1 TCC, 1 lymphoma).

Although CT is often the initial modality used for evaluation of a cystic renal mass, MR imaging can depict septae, nodules, and enhancement within a complex cystic mass in exquisite detail. CEUS has also shown excellent performance in the characterization of complex cystic renal masses, rivaling or even exceeding IV contrast-enhanced CT (**Fig. 19**).[56–58] CEUS was found to result in the assignment of a higher Bosniak classification in approximately one-quarter of cystic masses previously characterized at IV contrast-enhanced enhanced CT.[4]

GUIDANCE FROM PROFESSIONAL SOCIETIES ON MANAGEMENT OF THE INCIDENTAL RENAL MASS

Size is an important factor in renal mass management, with smaller masses being more likely to be benign. American College of Radiology guidelines suggest active imaging surveillance of solid renal masses smaller than 1 cm with semi-annual followed by annual CT or MR imaging.[59] A solid renal mass between 1 and 4 cm should be managed

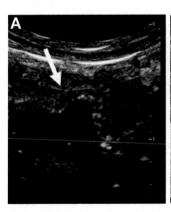

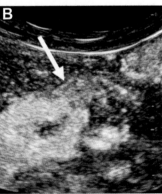

Fig. 18. Solid renal mass on CEUS. A 79-year-old man with chronic renal insufficiency and indeterminate renal mass found on nonenhanced CT. Sagittal CEUS images of the left kidney obtained before (*A*) and after IV contrast administration (*B*) show diffuse contrast enhancement of a solid renal mass (*arrows*). Neither biopsy nor surgical resection was performed; therefore pathology analysis is not available for this patient.

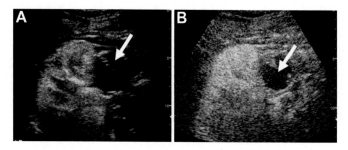

Fig. 19. Complex renal cyst on CEUS. A 71-year-old man with complex cystic mass found on conventional gray-scale ultrasound. Early-phase (*A*) and delayed (*B*) CEUS images of the left kidney obtained in the sagittal plane demonstrate enhancement of a thick septation and mural nodule within a renal cyst (*arrows*), compatible with a Bosniak 4 cystic renal mass. Neither biopsy nor surgical resection was performed; therefore pathology analysis is not available for this patient.

with either surgical resection or percutaneous ablation, if technically amenable. Active surveillance with CT, MR imaging, or ultrasound is also an option, particularly in patients with limited life expectancy or comorbidities putting them at higher risk for surgical complications.[18] This recommendation is in line with American Urologic Association and American Society of Clinical Oncology guidelines.[60,61] The upper limit of 4 cm was chosen based on the low likelihood of metastatic disease in tumors this size or less, and the increasing likelihood of malignancy in larger tumors, with approximately 90% of tumors exceeding 4 cm being malignant.[62] No differences in 7-year cancer-free survival have been found between patients with tumors ≤4 cm who underwent active surveillance versus intervention.[63]

Growth of a renal mass is defined as an increase of 4 mm or more in 1 year. A renal mass with a growth rate of *less than* 3 mm/y for 5 years is considered stable, and with an insignificant risk for metastatic disease. Unfortunately, there is no defined time interval of stability after which a renal mass can be declared benign, to our knowledge.[18]

There is great variation in the growth rate of small renal masses, and tumor biology can range between indolent and aggressive. Masses showing rapid growth are more likely to be higher-grade tumors, usually ccRCC, and rapid growth is also associated with a higher probability of metastatic disease. On the other end of the spectrum, slower growth rates of RCC overlap with those of benign masses such as oncocytoma, and there is less likelihood of metastatic disease. Note, however, there is no difference in the rate of malignancy of masses that have been stable for 2 years, versus tumors that have shown growth.[64]

Active surveillance with cross-sectional imaging and/or ultrasound every 3 to 6 months for 5 years is indicated for all Bosniak 2F cystic masses, as well as for a subset of Bosniak 3 and 4 cystic masses. Up to 12% of class 2F masses progress on imaging to class 3/4 within 5 years, with 85% of such masses being malignant.[65] Class 3 masses are historically surgical, but recent evidence shows that observing these masses may be a suitable option, even for those patients without a limited life expectancy or contraindications to surgery, to avoid unnecessary surgery for benign cysts (approximately 50% of class 3 masses). Schoots and colleagues[65] found that only 0.2% of Bosniak 3/4 masses progressed to metastatic disease during active surveillance. However, the most recent American Urologic Association guidelines (2019) still recommend surgery for Bosniak 3 and 4 masses 2 cm or larger in patients who are surgical candidates.[60]

RENAL MASS BIOPSY

There is a growing list of scenarios in which renal tumor biopsy can guide management and should be considered. These include patients in whom metastatic disease or lymphoma is suspected, as systemic therapy would be indicated rather than surgical resection.[61] Patients in whom a lipid-poor AML is a consideration, particularly in younger women, may also be biopsy candidates. Biopsy should also be considered if focal pyelonephritis is suspected as the cause of an apparent mass. In the case of unresectable disease or planned treatment with percutaneous ablation or stereotactic radiotherapy, biopsy may be used for histologic diagnosis. Patients with bilateral renal masses without a known familial syndrome or with syndromes that are associated with benign pathology also should be considered for renal biopsy. An additional indication for biopsy is in patients with a solitary kidney to avoid unnecessary nephrectomy and dialysis. There is also a role for biopsy in the case of a mass 4 cm or smaller if the patient is a candidate for active surveillance.[66] The utility of biopsy of Bosniak III cystic masses remains controversial, as there is a low negative predictive value due to the possibility of sampling error from failure to target the solid cellular component of the mass.

EVOLVING TECHNOLOGY
Dual-Energy Computed Tomography

Dual-energy CT (DECT) is an imaging modality that can potentially allow for characterization of incidentally discovered renal masses on routine IV contrast-enhanced abdominal CT, without the need for further imaging using a multiphasic protocol. The 2 main DECT techniques relevant to renal mass imaging are virtual noncontrast (VNC) images and iodine maps.

VNC images have been shown to have a sensitivity and specificity of 79% and 90% for differentiation of nonenhancing versus enhancing renal masses, which is slightly inferior to standard non-enhanced CT images (85% and 97%). A known pitfall is imprecise subtraction due to limitations in discriminating iodine from iron or calcium. This can lead to false positives due to a cystic mass containing hemorrhage or complex fluid being perceived as enhancing. On-going technical improvements in spectral separation, beam hardening correction, radiation tube output, and material decomposition all hold promise for increasing diagnostic performance.[67]

Iodine maps are created by isolating iodine from other organic and inorganic compounds with the use of material decomposition techniques. Iodine within a mass can be used as a surrogate for IV contrast enhancement, and can be assessed either qualitatively, by the presence of iodine signal, or quantitatively, by measurement of iodine content (in milligrams/gram).[68]

Artificial Intelligence

Machine learning is a rapidly growing body of research with the potential to improve the characterization of renal masses. Using radiomic features extracted from standard CT and MR images, machine learning has been shown to increase diagnostic as well as prognostic accuracy. Radiomics analysis allows for quantitative features, some imperceptible to the human eye, to be mathematically extracted, analyzed, and incorporated into a model.

Miskin and colleagues[69] classified benign from malignant cystic renal masses according to the Bosniak system based on CT texture features (mean, standard deviation, mean of positive pixels, entropy, skewness, and kurtosis) by using 3 different machine learning algorithms (random forest [RF], logistic regression [LR], and support vector machine [SVM]). Sensitivity, specificity,

positive predictive value, negative predictive value, and area under the curve of the RF model was 0.67, 0.91, 0.75, 0.88, and 0.88; of the LR model was 0.63, 0.93, 0.78, 0.86, and 0.90; and of the SVM model was 0.56, 0.91, 0.71, 0.84, and 0.89, respectively.

MR imaging radiomic features have also been shown to help in characterizing renal masses; Said and colleagues[70] studied a machine learning model, and achieved an area under the curve of 0.73 (confidence interval 0.5–0.96) for differentiating RCC from benign masses using a combination of qualitative radiologic evaluation and quantitative radiomics features.

Improvements in the areas of reproducibility and validation are necessary for radiomics to become generalizable enough to have broad clinical applications across different vendors and scanners.[71]

SUMMARY

The incidental renal mass is encountered with such high frequency that there is now a collective familiarity with diagnosis and management. There is also a growing body of literature defining relevant imaging features and the natural history of common renal masses, which has helped in guiding imaging and clinical management. Renal mass biopsy has become an increasingly important component in the diagnostic workup of a renal mass, prompted in part by the use of active surveillance for management of small and cystic renal masses. Technological advances in noninvasive imaging and machine learning will lead to further improvements in detection and diagnosis in the near future, and help to refine existing guidelines.

CLINICS CARE POINTS

- Incidental renal masses are commonly encountered on routine cross-sectional imaging examinations. Most will be benign cysts; a minority are indeterminate and will require a dedicated renal mass examination. Renal cell carcinoma (RCC) is now most commonly discovered as an incidental imaging finding.

- Changes to the existing Bosniak classification for cystic renal masses in the 2019 proposed revision include incorporation of MRI findings, eliminating the need for further imaging in likely benign cystic masses, and definitions of structural components within a cyst.

- Despite gains in knowledge regarding imaging features of renal masses, there is still no reliable criteria to our knowledge which can be used to determine whether a soft-tissue mass in the kidney is benign or malignant, with the differential diagnosis including RCC, lipid-poor angiomyolipoma, and oncocytoma. Machine learning with attention to radiomics shows promise in identifying features which can provide a more specific and accurate diagnosis.

- IV contrast-enhanced CT and MRI continue to be the primary modalities for characterization of the indeterminate or suspicious renal mass; however, other modalities will likely take on a greater role in renal mass imaging, including contrast-enhanced ultrasound and dual-energy CT.

DISCLOSURE

The authors have nothing to disclose.

REFERENCES

1. Eknoyan G. A clinical view of simple and complex renal cysts. J Am Soc Nephrol 2009;20:1874–6.
2. Mensel B, Kuhn JP, Kracht F, et al. Prevalence of renal cysts and association with risk factors in a general population: an MRI-based study. Abdom Radiol 2018;43(11):3068–74.
3. O'Connor SD, Silverman SG, Ip IK, et al. Simple cyst–appearing renal masses at unenhanced CT: Can they be presumed to be benign? Radiology 2013;269:793–800.
4. Silverman SG, Pedrosa I, Ellis JH, et al. Bosniak classification of cystic renal masses, version 2019: an update proposal and needs assessment. Radiology 2019;292(2):475–88.
5. Maki DD, Birnbaum BA, Chakraborty DP, et al. Renal cyst pseudoenhancement: beam-hardening effects on CT numbers. Radiology 1999;213:468–72.
6. Bae KT, Heiken JP, Siegel CL, et al. Renal cysts: is attenuation artifactually increased on contrast-enhanced CT images? Radiology 2000;216:792–6.
7. Hirai T, Ohishi H, Yamada R, et al. Usefulness of color doppler flow imaging in differential diagnosis of multilocular cystic lesions of the kidney. J Ultrasound Med 1995;14:771–6.
8. Jonisch AI, Rubinowitz AN, Mutalik PG, et al. Can high-attenuation renal cysts be differentiated from renal cell carcinoma at unenhanced CT? Radiology 2007;243:445–50.
9. Hindman NM. Approach to very small (< 1.5 cm) cystic renal lesions: ignore, observe, or treat? Am J Roentgenol 2015;204:1182–9.
10. Davarpanah A, Spektor M, Mathur M, et al. Homogeneous T1 hyperintense renal lesions with smooth borders: is contrast-enhanced MR imaging needed? Radiology 2016;280:128–36.
11. Mickisch G, Carballido J, Hellsten S, et al. Guidelines on renal cell cancer. Eur 2001;40:252–5.
12. Amin MB, Tamboli P, Javidan J, et al. Prognostic impact of histologic subtyping of adult renal epithelial neoplasms: an experience of 405 cases. Am J Surg Pathol 2002;26:281–91.
13. Young JR, Coy H, Kim HJ, et al. Performance of relative enhancement on multiphasic MRI for the differentiation of clear cell renal cell carcinoma (RCC) from papillary and chromophobe RCC subtypes and oncocytoma. Am J Roentgenol 2017;208:812–9.
14. Sun MR, Ngo L, Genega EM, et al. Renal cell carcinoma: dynamic contrast-enhanced MR imaging for differentiation of tumor subtypes—correlation with pathologic findings. Radiology 2009;250:793–802.
15. Vendrami CL, Parada Villavicencio C, DeJulio TJ, et al. Differentiation of solid renal tumors with multiparametric MR imaging. Radiographics 2017;37:2026–42.
16. Jhaveri KS, Elmi A, Hosseini-Nik H, et al. Predictive value of chemical-shift MRI in distinguishing clear cell renal cell carcinoma from non–clear cell renal cell carcinoma and minimal-fat angiomyolipoma. Am J Roentgenol 2015;205:W79–86.
17. Lopez-Beltran A, Carrasco JC, Cheng L, et al. 2009 update on the classification of renal epithelial tumors in adults. Int J Urol 2009;16:432–43.
18. Herts BR, Coll DM, Novick AC, et al. Enhancement characteristics of papillary renal neoplasms revealed on triphasic helical CT of the kidneys. Am J Roentgenol 2002;178:367–72.
19. Agochukwu N, Huber S, Spektor M, et al. Differentiating renal neoplasms from simple cysts on contrast-enhanced CT on the basis of attenuation and homogeneity. Am J Roentgenol 2017;208:801–4.
20. Dilauro M, Quon M, McInnes MDF, et al. Comparison of contrast-enhanced multiphase renal protocol CT versus MRI for diagnosis of papillary renal cell carcinoma. Am J Roentgenol 2016;206:319–25.
21. Egbert ND, Caoili EM, Cohan RH, et al. Differentiation of papillary renal cell carcinoma subtypes on CT and MRI. Am J Roentgenol 2013;201:347–55.
22. Oliva MR, Glickman JN, Zou KH, et al. Renal cell carcinoma: T1 and T2 signal intensity characteristics of papillary and clear cell types correlated with pathology. Am J Roentgenol 2009;192:1524–30.
23. Prando A, Prando P, Prando D. Urothelial cancer of the renal pelvicaliceal system: unusual imaging manifestations. Radiographics 2010;30:1553–66.
24. Patel U, Ramachandran N, Halls J, et al. Synchronous renal masses in patients with a non renal malignancy: incidence of metastasis to the kidney versus primary renal neoplasia and differentiating features on CT. Am J Roentgenol 2011;197:W680–6.
25. Zhou C, Urbauer DL, Fellman BM, et al. Metastases to the kidney: a comprehensive analysis of 151

patients from a tertiary referral centre. BJU Int 2016; 117:775–82.

26. Ganeshan D, Iyer R, Devine C, et al. Imaging of primary and secondary renal lymphoma. Am J Roentgenol 2013;201:W712–9.

27. Johnson DC, Vukina J, Smith AB, et al. Preoperatively misclassified, surgically removed benign renal masses: a systematic review of surgical series and United States population level burden estimate. J Urol 2015;193:30–5.

28. Kutikov A, Fossett LK, Ramchandani P, et al. Incidence of benign pathologic findings at partial nephrectomy for solitary renal mass presumed to be renal cell carcinoma on preoperative imaging. Urology 2006;68:737–40.

29. Jinzaki M, Tanimoto A, Narimatsu Y, et al. Angiomyolipoma: imaging findings in lesions with minimal fat. Radiology 1997;205:497–502.

30. Karlo CA, Donati OF, Burger IA, et al. MR imaging of renal cortical tumours: qualitative and quantitative chemical shift imaging parameters. Eur Radiol 2013;23:1738–44.

31. Outwater EK, Bhatia M, Siegelman ES, et al. Lipid in renal clear cell carcinoma: detection on opposed-phase gradient-echo MR images. Radiology 1997; 205:103–7.

32. Chaudhry HS, Davenport MS, Nieman CM, et al. Histogram analysis of small solid renal masses: differentiating minimal fat angiomyolipoma from renal cell carcinoma. Am J Roentgenol 2012;198:377–83.

33. Jeong CJ, Park BK, Park JJ, et al. Unenhanced CT and MRI parameters that can be used to reliably predict fat-invisible angiomyolipoma. Am J Roentgenol 2016;206:340–7.

34. Perez-Ordonez B, Hamed G, Campbell S, et al. Renal oncocytoma: a clinicopathologic study of 70 cases. Am J Surg Pathol 1997;21:871–83.

35. Sasaguri K, Takahashi N, Gomez-Cardona D, et al. Small (< 4 cm) renal mass: differentiation of oncocytoma from renal cell carcinoma on biphasic contrast-enhanced CT. Am J Roentgenol 2015;205: 999–1007.

36. Rosenkrantz AB, Hindman N, Fitzgerald EF, et al. MRI features of renal oncocytoma and chromophobe renal cell carcinoma. Am J Roentgenol 2010;195:W421–7.

37. Davidson AJ, Hayes WS, Hartman DS, et al. Renal oncocytoma and carcinoma: failure of differentiation with CT. Radiology 1993;186:693–6.

38. Kim JI, Cho JY, Moon KC, et al. Segmental enhancement inversion at biphasic multidetector CT: characteristic finding of small renal oncocytoma. Radiology 2009;252:441–8.

39. O'Malley ME, Tran P, Hanbidge A, et al. Small renal oncocytomas: is segmental enhancement inversion a characteristic finding at biphasic MDCT? Am J Roentgenol 2012;199:1312–5.

40. McGahan JP, Lamba R, Fisher J, et al. Is segmental enhancement inversion on enhanced biphasic MDCT a reliable sign for the noninvasive diagnosis of renal oncocytomas? Am J Roentgenol 2011;197:W674–9.

41. Jhaveri K, Gupta P, Elmi A, et al. Cystic renal cell carcinomas: do they grow, metastasize, or recur? Am J Roentgenol 2013;201:292–6.

42. Hindman NM, Bosniak MA, Rosenkrantz AB, et al. Multilocular cystic renal cell carcinoma: comparison of imaging and pathologic findings. Am J Roentgenol 2012;198:20–6.

43. Corwin MT, Loehfelm TW, McGahan JP, et al. Prevalence of low-attenuation homogeneous papillary renal cell carcinoma mimicking renal cysts on CT. Am J Roentgenol 2018;211:1259–63.

44. Koga S, Nishikido M, Hayashi T, et al. Outcome of surgery in cystic renal cell carcinoma. Urology 2000;56:67–70.

45. Onishi T, Oishi Y, Goto H, et al. Cyst-associated renal cell carcinoma: clinicopathologic characteristics and evaluation of prognosis in 27 cases. Int J Urol 2001;8:268–74.

46. Webster WS, Thompson RH, Cheville JC, et al. Surgical resection provides excellent outcomes for patients with cystic clear cell renal cell carcinoma. Urology 2007;70:900–4.

47. Bosniak MA. The current radiological approach to renal cysts. Radiology 1986;158:1–10.

48. Mousessian PN, Yamauchi FI, Mussi TC, et al. Malignancy rate, histologic grade, and progression of Bosniak category III and IV complex renal cystic lesions. Am J Roentgenol 2017;209:1285–90.

49. Bhatt S, MacLennan G, Dogra V. Renal pseudotumors. Am J Roentgenol 2007;188(5):1380–7.

50. Craig WD, Wagner BJ, Travis MD. Pyelonephritis: radiologic-pathologic review. RadioGraphics 2008; 28(1):255–76.

51. Pickhardt PJ, Lonergan GJ, Davis CJ Jr, et al. Infiltrative renal lesions: radiologic–pathologic correlation. Armed Forces Institute of Pathology. RadioGraphics 2000;20:215–43.

52. Cura M, Elmerhi F, Suri R, et al. Vascular malformations and arteriovenous fistulas of the kidney. Acta Radiologica 2010;51:144–9.

53. Takahashi N, Kawashima A, Fletcher JG, et al. Renal involvement in patients with autoimmune pancreatitis: CT and MR imaging findings. Radiology 2007; 242:791–801.

54. Martínez-de-Alegría A, Baleato-González S, García-Figueiras R, et al. IgG4-related disease from head to toe. Radiographics 2015;35:2007–25.

55. Barr RG, Peterson C, Hindi A. Evaluation of indeterminate renal masses with contrast-enhanced US: a diagnostic performance study. Radiology 2014; 271:133–42.

56. Park BK, Kim B, Kim SH, et al. Assessment of cystic renal masses based on Bosniak classification:

comparison of CT and contrast-enhanced US. Eur J Radiol 2007;61:310–4.

57. Ascenti G, Mazziotti S, Zimbaro G, et al. Complex cystic renal masses: characterization with contrast-enhanced US. Radiology 2007;243:158–65.

58. Quaia E, Bertolotto M, Cioffi V, et al. Comparison of contrast-enhanced sonography with unenhanced sonography and contrast-enhanced CT in the diagnosis of malignancy in complex cystic renal masses. Am J Roentgenol 2008;191: 1239–49.

59. Herts BR, Silverman SG, Hindman NM, et al. Management of the incidental renal mass on CT: a white paper of the ACR Incidental Findings Committee. JACR 2018;15(2):264–73.

60. Campbell SC, Novick AC, Belldegrun A, et al. Guideline for management of the clinical T1 renal mass. J Clin Oncol 2017;35:668–80.

61. Finelli T. Partial nephrectomy is not the proven standard for stage T1b renal cell carcinoma. Can Urol Assoc J 2012;6:131–3.

62. Umbreit EC, Shimko MS, Childs MA, et al. Metastatic potential of a renal mass according to original tumour size at presentation. BJU Int 2012;109: 190–4.

63. Alam R, Patel HD, Riffon MF, et al. Intermediate-term outcomes from the DISSRM registry: a prospective analysis of active surveillance in patients with small renal masses. J Clin Oncol 2017;35(6_suppl):430.

64. Kunkle DA, Crispen PL, Chen DY, et al. Enhancing renal masses with zero net growth during active surveillance. J Urol 2007;177(3):849–54.

65. Schoots IG, Zaccai K, Hunink MG, et al. Bosniak classification for complex renal cysts reevaluated: a systematic review. J Urol 2017;198:12–21.

66. Lim CS, Schieda N, Silverman SG. Update on indications for percutaneous renal mass biopsy in the era of advanced CT and MRI. Am J Roentgenol 2019;212:1187–96.

67. Meyer M, Nelson RC, Vernuccio F, et al. Virtual unenhanced images at dual-energy CT: influence on renal lesion characterization. Radiology 2019;291: 381–90.

68. Mileto A, Allen BC, Pietryga JA, et al. Characterization of incidental renal mass with dual-energy CT: diagnostic accuracy of effective atomic number maps for discriminating nonenhancing cysts from enhancing masses. Am J Roentgenol 2017;209: 221–30.

69. Miskin N, Qin L, Matalon SA, et al. Stratification of cystic renal masses into benign and potentially malignant: applying machine learning to the bosniak classification. Abdom Radiol 2020;46(1):311–8.

70. Said D, Hectors SJ, Wilck E, et al. Characterization of solid renal neoplasms using MRI-based quantitative radiomics features. Abdom Radiol 2020;25:1.

71. Kocak B, Durmaz ES, Erdim C, et al. Radiomics of renal masses: systematic review of reproducibility and validation strategies. Am J Roentgenol 2020; 214:129–36.

Spectrum and Relevance of Incidental Bowel Findings on Computed Tomography

John J. Hines Jr, MD[a],*, Mark A. Mikhitarian, DO[b], Ritesh Patel, MD[b], Andy Choy, MD[b]

KEYWORDS

- CT • Gastrointestinal tract • Bowel • Incidental findings

KEY POINTS

- Incidental bowel findings commonly are discovered on computed tomography (CT); most are benign and require no further work-up or management; however, some are clinically relevant. In particular, bowel wall thickening may reflect underlying neoplasm and should be brought to the attention of the referring clinician.
- There are a wide variety of causes of pneumatosis intestinalis, with clinical presentations ranging from asymptomatic to life-threatening bowel ischemia.
- Bowel dilatation most often is due to mechanical obstruction; however, the radiologist should be aware of the causes of acute and chronic nonobstructive bowel dilatation.
- Bowel intussusception in an adult should raise suspicion for a neoplasm acting as the lead point; however, a transient self-resolving intussusception can be suggested in the setting of a short segment intussusception with no upstream bowel dilatation or visible lead point.
- The fat halo sign can be a CT sign of inflammatory bowel disease; however, it probably is seen more frequently as an incidental and clinically insignificant finding.

INTRODUCTION

Incidental findings in the bowel commonly are encountered on CT examinations and encompass a diverse array of pathology, reflective of the unique spectrum of disease encountered in each segment of the intestine. Similar to incidental findings in other organ systems, most of these findings are benign and require no further work-up. Examples of benign disease covered in this chapter include diverticulosis, most cases of intramural fat, asymptomatic pneumatosis, nonobstructive bowel dilatation, and transient intussusception. A minority of incidental findings are clinically relevant or initially indeterminate, requiring further patient management and often necessitating additional imaging examinations and interventions. For example, malignant tumors of the gastrointestinal (GI) tract may have a long latency period before becoming symptomatic and frequently are detected on CT as incidental findings. Determination of the clinical relevance and optimal management of incidental findings often poses a dilemma for the radiologist. In recent years, there has been a proliferation of studies reviewing incidental findings on CT as well as position papers from the American College of Radiology written for the purpose of providing guidelines for management. Unfortunately, many of these articles do not include discussions or data regarding incidental bowel

[a] Donald and Barbara Zucker School of Medicine at Hofstra/ Northwell, Department of Radiology, Huntington Hospital, Northwell Health, 270 Park Avenue, Huntington, NY 11743, USA; [b] Department of Radiology, Northwell Health, Donald and Barbara Zucker School of Medicine at Hofstra/Northwell, North Shore University Hospital, 300 Community Drive, Manhasset, NY 11030, USA
* Corresponding author.
E-mail address: jhinesmd@gmail.com

Radiol Clin N Am 59 (2021) 647–660
https://doi.org/10.1016/j.rcl.2021.03.012

findings nor is there yet an American College of Radiology white paper dedicated to management of bowel findings. The goal of this article is to review the various incidental findings that can be detected on CT and MR imaging, discuss their clinical implications, and give examples from the literature in order to provide a perspective on management.

WALL THICKENING

Incidental bowel wall thickening (IBWT) is a relatively frequent finding and can be focal or regional. Although IBWT may be inflammatory, infectious, ischemic, or neoplastic in etiology, its clinical relevance when detected incidentally remains unclear, particularly when identified on CT (or occasionally on MR imaging or ultrasound [US]) performed for apparently unrelated reasons.[1] Furthermore, there is no consensus in the literature, to the authors' knowledge, on how to approach this finding.[2]

The first challenge for radiologists is to determine to the best of their ability whether the suspected wall thickening is truly pathologic, or spurious, due to under-distention. Trends toward decreased use of positive oral contrast at many centers can make evaluation of the bowel difficult, especially when under-distended (**Figs. 1–3**), and CT examinations performed without intravenous contrast do not allow for analysis of mural enhancement. Additionally, false-positive and false-negative results for an intestinal mass can result from stool or other intraluminal contents either obscuring or mimicking a mass.

The thickness of the wall of the GI tract varies between small bowel and large bowel and also is affected by multiple factors, including the degree of luminal distention.[2–4] Normal small bowel wall is thin, measuring between 1 mm and 2 mm, when the lumen is well distended.[4] When the bowel is partially collapsed, it can measure between 2 mm and 3 mm in thickness, which frequently is used as the upper limit of normal.[3–6] The jejunum commonly appears falsely thickened when under-distended due to a greater fold density than the ileum. The normal wall of the colon is very thin—often barely perceptible—and when distended should measure less than 3 mm.[4,7] The wall generally is considered abnormal if there is thickening greater than 5 mm.[3] Normal bowel wall also enhances predictably following intravenous contrast administration. Enhancement typically is uniform and symmetric and also usually is more pronounced in the mucosal layer.[4]

When bowel wall thickening is detected, additional CT findings need to be analyzed for complete assessment and to formulate an effective differential diagnosis. Salient features include degree of thickening, symmetry, length of affected segment, mural attenuation, and any associated perienteric abnormalities.[4,8]

The primary entity of concern in a patient with a short segment of thickened bowel is neoplasia, which is uncommonly but not rarely detected as a purely incidental finding on CT. For example, in a study of 1175 emergency department patients in whom abdominal/pelvic CT was performed, incidental findings were detected in 700, including 15 patients with colonic wall thickening, which yielded 4 colon cancers and 5 colorectal polyps. Additionally, 11 gastric lesions were detected, which yielded 1 gastric cancer.[9]

In studies that have investigated the significance of IBWT diagnosed on CT, there is a high

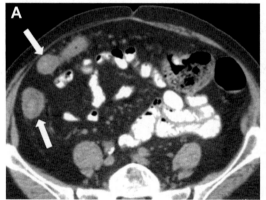
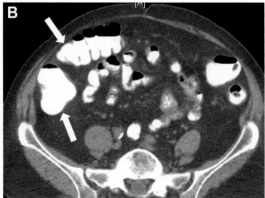

Fig. 1. Under-distended colon mimicking colitis. A 72-year-old woman with generalized abdominal pain. Axial CT image (*A*) shows apparent wall thickening of the under-distended right colon (*arrows*), which could erroneously raise concern for colitis. Image from repeat CT performed 1 hour later (*B*), however, demonstrates oral contrast progression into the right colon, which now is well opacified and with normal wall thickness (*arrows*).

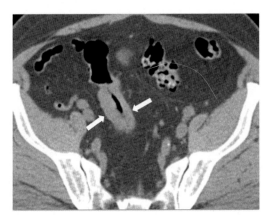

Fig. 2. Sigmoid colon cancer. A 69-year-old man with back pain and suspected abdominal aortic aneurysm. Axial image from a CT performed without oral or intravenous contrast. There is wall thickening of the sigmoid (*arrows*), which potentially could be difficult to detect due to bowel under-distention and lack of oral and intravenous contrast. The patient also had a liver metastasis visualized on this CT (not shown).

rate of disease found on endoscopic examination. A meta-analysis evaluating incidental colonic wall thickening on CT, and which included 9 studies and 1252 patients, found that 73% of patients had abnormalities at colonoscopy, with a cancer rate that ranged from 14% to 27%.[10] Eskaros and colleagues[11] found that 64% of patients with incidental colonic wall thickening on CT had a corresponding abnormality on colonoscopy. Colitis was the diagnosis in a majority of cases; however, in a subset of patients in which a mass was suspected on CT, this was confirmed

in 100% (12/12) of cases. Uzzaman and colleagues[12] found abnormalities on optical colonoscopy at the exact site of IBWT seen on CT in 58% of patients; in 36/95 of these patients, the abnormality was a malignancy. Documentation of the characteristics of the wall thickening would help in assessing the clinical relevance of IBWT in predicting the presence of a colonic neoplasm. Shorter segment of wall thickening, irregular or eccentric thickening, and greater degree of wall thickness all are factors that favor a neoplastic process; however, such analysis is lacking in most studies. Note that routine abdominal CT has been shown to be moderately sensitive for detection of colorectal neoplasia. Ozel and colleagues[13] found routine abdominal CT to be 72% sensitive and 84% specific in diagnosing invasive colorectal cancer.

There are fewer studies in the literature that have looked at the significance of esophageal or gastric wall thickening compared with colonic wall thickening on CT, to the authors' knowledge. Cai and colleagues[14] found endoscopic abnormalities in 22/27 patients with distal esophageal wall thickening on abdominal CT, with esophagitis, varices, and hiatal hernia diagnosed in approximately equal frequency. Tellez-Avila and colleagues[15] found abnormalities on endoscopy in 6/19 patients with incidental gastric wall thickening, all of which were adenocarcinomas.

The appendix also can be a site of incidental tumors, such as a neuroendocrine tumor (NET) (the appendix is the most common site in the GI tract for NET), mucinous tumor, or adenocarcinoma (**Fig. 4**).[16]

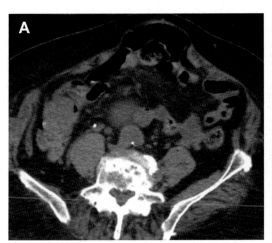
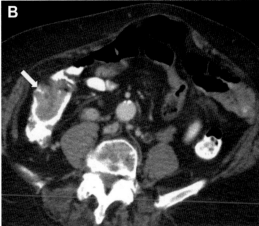

Fig. 3. Cecal cancer. An 81-year-old woman with failure to thrive. Axial image (*A*) from a CT performed without oral or intravenous contrast shows no detectable colonic abnormality. Image (*B*) from repeat CT examination performed a few days later with oral and intravenous contrast clearly shows a large cecal mass (*arrow*), confirmed to be adenocarcinoma on colonoscopy.

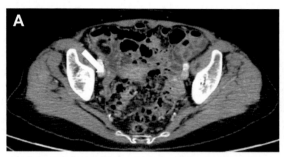
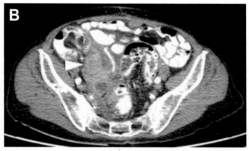

Fig. 4. Incidental appendiceal cancer. A 69-year-old woman with weight loss. Axial intravenous contrast-enhanced CT image (*A*) of the abdomen and pelvis demonstrates a subtle mass at the base of the appendix, which was overlooked by the interpreting radiologist (*arrow*). Two years later, the mass has increased in size (*B* [*arrowhead*]). The patient underwent right hemicolectomy with pathology revealing adenocarcinoma.

In contrast to the more infiltrative appearance of wall thickening commonly encountered with gastric or colonic adenocarcinoma, an incidentally found circumscribed masslike focal process suggests an alternative diagnosis on CT, such as a NET, or GI stromal tumor (GIST), which arises most commonly in the stomach (**Fig. 5**), followed by the small bowel.

Lipomas are benign submucosal tumors found throughout the GI tract, most commonly in the colon, and easily are diagnosed on CT as fat attenuation intramural or intraluminal masses. Although these generally can be ignored, lipomas occasionally can be the cause of complications, such as intussusception or bleeding. Tumors greater than 2 cm are more likely to ulcerate, leading to acute or chronic anemia.[17]

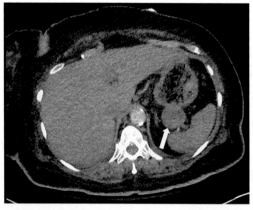

Fig. 5. GIST. A 52-year-old man with chest pain and dyspnea. Axial image from CT angiography performed to evaluate for pulmonary embolism incidentally shows an exophytic mass emanating from the posterior gastric fundus (*arrow*), which was strongly suggestive of a GIST. Patient underwent endoscopic ultrasound and biopsy with pathology confirming the diagnosis of GIST.

Non-neoplastic entities also can be the cause of an incidental mass or wall thickening in the GI tract. Bowel wall thickening from chronic diverticulosis is a common finding, particularly in the sigmoid colon on CT, and usually can be distinguished from cancer by the longer length of involvement and presence of diverticulosis. Wall thickening in the setting of cirrhosis can be due to portal hypertensive colopathy, a benign condition with no clinical relevance in and of itself. CT shows wall thickening, usually involving the right colon, indistinguishable from a colitis; diagnosis can be made based on the presence of findings indicative of cirrhosis and portal hypertension and lack of symptomatology.[18]

Heterotopic pancreas can occur in the stomach, duodenum, or jejunum and usually is discovered as an incidental small nodule or mass on CT or MR imaging, although rarely it can be the cause of acute pancreatitis (**Fig. 6**).[19]

In an estimated 12% to 37% of cases of endometriosis, endometriotic implants can involve the bowel, usually bowel segments in the dependent pelvis, involving in decreasing order of frequency, the rectosigmoid, appendix, cecum, and terminal ileum.[20] These implants appear as serosal masses and may be large enough to be visualized on cross-sectional imaging (**Fig. 7**). A diagnosis can be suggested when there is involvement of pelvic bowel loops and in the setting of a known history of endometriosis, although primary GI tract tumor and metastatic disease are in the differential diagnosis. Concurrent findings of endometriosis, such as complex adnexal cyst(s) or hydrosalpinx, if present, can assist the radiologist in arriving at the correct diagnosis.

Splenosis, a condition defined by heterotopic autotransplantation of splenic tissue due to traumatic or iatrogenic cause, can mimic a primary intestinal tumor in cases of an implant detected along the serosal surface of the bowel.[21]

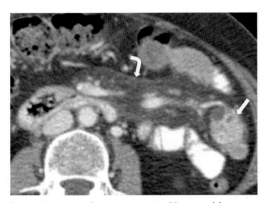

Fig. 6. Heterotopic pancreas. A 69-year-old woman with abdominal pain and bloating; clinical concern was for ovarian cancer. Axial CT image from a CT performed with oral and intravenous contrast demonstrates a circumscribed mass along the serosal surface of a jejunal loop (*arrow*), predominantly solid, but also containing a few cysts. Findings were thought to be most likely due to a GIST; however, intraoperative and pathologic findings revealed heterotopic pancreas, which was causing acute pancreatitis. Note fat stranding of the small bowel mesentery from acute inflammation (*curved arrow*).

PNEUMATOSIS INTESTINALIS

Pneumatosis intestinalis (PI) is a radiological finding that refers to gas in the subserosal or submucosal layers of the GI tract.[22,23] The etiology commonly is associated with serious underlying pathology, which may require immediate surgical intervention but also can be seen with benign conditions requiring no intervention.[24] With the widespread increase of imaging, the prevalence of PI,

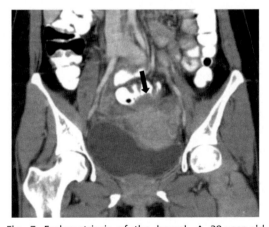

Fig. 7. Endometriosis of the bowel. A 38-year-old woman with a history of endometriosis, scanned for rectal bleeding. Axial coronal image from a CT performed with oral and intravenous contrast demonstrates a spiculated serosal soft-tissue mass involving the sigmoid colon (*arrow*), representing an endometriotic implant.

in particular benign pneumatosis, is higher than previously thought.[25] Given that incidental findings can prompt additional diagnostic and therapeutic intervention in some cases, which can be harmful to the patient, it is important to understand the differential diagnosis and associated clinical significance of PI.[25] Identifying which patients can be managed conservatively and which require urgent intervention requires an understanding of the various etiologies of PI, assessment of the clinical context, and the recognition of associated radiological findings.

PI is classified into primary PI and secondary PI. Primary PI, or pneumatosis cystoides intestinalis (pneumatosis coli), is less common (15%), is idiopathic, and has the morphology of well-circumscribed cysts or bubbles within the walls of the bowel. It has an incidence of approximately 0.03%.[26] A majority of cases (approximately 85%) of PI are secondary to an underlying disease process, including mesenteric ischemia, bowel necrosis, trauma, inflammatory bowel disease (IBD), malignancy, autoimmune conditions (scleroderma, dermatomyositis), infection (*Clostridium difficile*, human immunodeficiency virus, or cytomegalovirus), chronic obstructive pulmonary disease, postoperative changes (laparotomy, laparoscopy, peritoneal dialysis, and so forth), or medications (corticosteroids, immunosuppressants, and chemotherapeutic agents).[25,27,28] The pathogenesis of PI is not fully understood but likely is multifactorial and involves the disruption of mucosal integrity and the migration of gas either via direct dissection into the wall or through translocation of gas-producing bacteria from the lumen into the submucosal space, and/or increased thoracic pressure, causing alveolar rupture and gas diffusion via perivascular or perilymphatic routes.[24,27]

Benign PI appears as intramural cystic/bubble-like gas collections on CT (**Fig. 8**) is often and asymptomatic. Studies have shown that benign PI often is confined to the right colon. As a result, patients with PI confined to the right colon, without signs of peritonitis or sepsis, in the appropriate clinical context, and in the absence of worrisome imaging findings (discussed later) can be treated with supportive care.[24] A theory proposes that immunosuppressive or steroid therapies may induce lymphoid depletion in Peyer patches, which impairs the GI defense mechanism, reduces peristalsis, and compromises the intestinal wall integrity resulting in PI.[29,30] An association with tapering and discontinuation of steroids has been associated with improvement of PI.[29]

Worrisome features indicative of fulminant PI include linear or circumferential morphology of intramural gas (**Fig. 9**), bowel dilatation, bowel wall thickening, mesenteric stranding, hemorrhagic ascites, small bowel involvement, obstruction, ischemia, visceral infarction, portomesenteric venous gas, and perforation.[27,28,31,32]

To summarize, the finding of PI demands a multidisciplinary approach to identify its clinical relevance, and thoughtful assimilation of clinical, radiologic, and laboratory findings to determine appropriate management. This is best accomplished through direct communication between the radiologist and clinical provider(s).

DIVERTICULA

Diverticula of the GI tract are extremely common incidental imaging findings. Although radiologists are most familiar with colonic diverticulosis due to its very high incidence in the Western world, and the common occurrence of symptomatic colonic diverticulitis, diverticulosis frequently is found in other sites of the digestive tract, occurring in decreasing order of frequency in the colon, duodenum, esophagus, stomach, jejunum, and ileum.[33] Kelly and colleagues[9] found colonic diverticulosis to be the most commonly reported

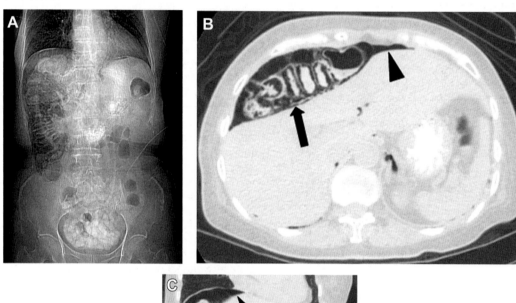

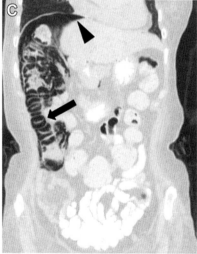

Fig. 8. Pneumatosis cystoides coli. A 66-year-old man with abdominal distention. Scout (*A*) and nonenhanced axial (*B*) and coronal (*C*) CT images performed for evaluation of intraperitoneal free air seen on radiographs. There is extensive pneumatosis along the wall of the ascending colon (*arrows*), which demonstrates cystic/bubble-like morphology, an appearance which supports a benign process. Lucency under the right diaphragm represents a combination of pneumatosis and pneumoperitoneum (*arrowheads*). The pneumoperitoneum likely is secondary to escaped intramural air.

incidental finding on abdominal CT. This study did not include data on diverticula in other regions of the bowel. Other than including the presence of a diverticulum or diverticulosis in the radiology report, there usually is no need for any further work-up or management of the patient, because only a minority manifest with any symptomatology. Common complications of diverticula include infection, perforation, abscess, obstruction, and hemorrhage. Typical signs of acute diverticular infection on CT are well known to the practicing radiologist and include focal wall thickening of the involved segment of bowel, stranding of the adjacent fat, and, in complicated cases, localized abscess formation.

Esophageal diverticula are classified as either pulsion or traction diverticula, with pulsion diverticula much more common and usually located in the mid to distal esophagus, whereas traction diverticula usually are found in the mid-esophagus. Epiphrenic diverticula are located within 10 cm of the gastroesophageal junction. These diverticula can grow to a large size and cause dysphagia due to compression of the true lumen of the esophagus. Regurgitation of contents of the diverticulum can lead to reflux symptoms and aspiration. Due to their location near the gastroesophageal junction, epiphrenic diverticula may be confused with a hiatal hernia on radiographs or on CT (**Fig. 10**).[34] Visualization of the entire stomach below the diaphragm and lack of gastric folds extending through the esophageal hiatus can help in making a correct diagnosis.

Gastric diverticula are uncommon and occur most frequently along the posterior wall of the fundus (**Fig. 11**). Their significance to the radiologist is for the potential to be misdiagnosed as a left adrenal nodule or exophytic gastric mass on CT, especially if there is no air in the lumen of the diverticulum.

Duodenal diverticula are found in up to 22% of patients in autopsy studies and usually are asymptomatic. Most arise along the medial wall of the second portion of the duodenum, within 2.5 cm of the ampulla of Vater. Infection of a duodenal diverticulum is an infrequent occurrence in comparison to diverticula of the colon, a fact attributed to their larger size and relatively sterile and liquid contents of the duodenum.[35] Periampullary diverticula can be the cause of recurrent pancreatitis, cholangitis, and common duct calculi due to obstruction of the ampulla. The abnormal anatomy created by the diverticulum can make it technically difficult for the endoscopist to perform a sphincterotomy, and it may be appropriate to state the presence of a periampullary diverticulum in the impression of the radiology report, if the patient

is being considered for such a procedure.[36] A potential pitfall is for a periampullary diverticulum to be mistaken for a pancreatic mass, whether a cystic process if its lumen is entirely fluid-filled, or a solid mass if the lumen is collapsed (**Fig. 12**).

Diverticulosis of the mesenteric small bowel is uncommon, occurring in 0.6% to 2.3% of the population. The jejunum is involved more often than the ileum. Diverticula often are multiple rather than solitary, and most are discovered incidentally during radiologic investigations. Bacterial overgrowth in jejunoileal diverticula can be symptomatic, although imaging findings may be absent. Use of multiplanar CT reformations, especially in the coronal plane, often facilitates visualization of jejunoileal diverticula.[37]

Meckel diverticulum is the most common congenital bowel anomaly, with a prevalence of 1% to 4% in autopsy studies. Most are asymptomatic, but a Meckel diverticulum can cause complications, including GI bleeding, obstruction, perforation, intussusception, and neoplasm. On CT, a Meckel diverticulum appears as a cystic or blind-ending tubular mass of variable size connected to the ileum. Wall thickening, intraluminal gas and fluid, and localized inflammatory changes may be present in the setting of Meckel diverticulitis.[38,39]

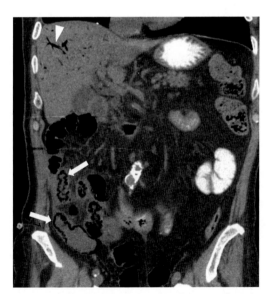

Fig. 9. Small bowel pneumatosis secondary to ischemic bowel. An 81-year-old man with severe abdominal pain and elevated serum lactate. Coronal image from CT performed without oral or intravenous contrast demonstrates linear submucosal gas collections (*arrows*) within the wall of right lower quadrant small bowel loops, representing pneumatosis from bowel ischemia. Note portal venous gas (*arrowhead*).

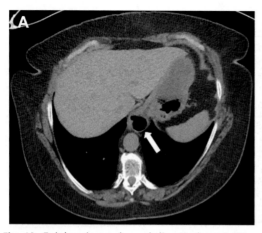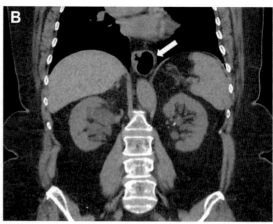

Fig. 10. Epiphrenic esophageal diverticulum. A 57-year-old man with suspected renal/ureteral calculi. Axial (*A*) and coronal (*B*) images from CT performed without oral or intravenous contrast shows an epiphrenic pulsion diverticulum of the distal esophagus (*arrows*). Although the imaging appearance can be similar, the finding should not be misinterpreted as a hiatal hernia.

Diverticular disease is the most common colonic disease in the Western world, present in 5% of the population before the age of 40% and in 33% to 50% of the population after the age of 50. This contrasts sharply with the low prevalence of diverticulosis (0.2%) in Asia and Africa. The sigmoid colon is involved in 95% of cases. Diverticula appear as small rounded outpouchings projecting from the colonic wall, typically measuring between 0.5 cm and 1.0 cm. Diverticulitis occurs in approximately 4% of patients with colonic diverticula.[40]

NON-OBSTRUCTIVE BOWEL DILATATION

Abnormally dilated bowel is an infrequent incidental finding on CT. Mechanical obstruction is far and away the most common cause of bowel dilatation and usually is symptomatic. Nonobstructive causes of bowel dilatation are neuromuscular dysfunction and are classified as adynamic ileus. Acute causes, which most often are symptomatic and not incidental, include recent laparotomy, intraperitoneal infection, ischemia, electrolyte imbalance and colonic pseudo-obstruction (Ogilvie syndrome). Chronically dilated small bowel and/or large bowel can be caused by various etiologies, including medications (eg, narcotics), endocrine disorders, such as diabetes and hypothyroidism, scleroderma, celiac disease, amyloidosis, lymphangiectasia, Parkinson disease, and Chagas disease.[41–44]

Classifying bowel dilatation as obstructive or nonobstructive is the most essential task of the radiologist in the setting of bowel dilatation on CT. Fundamental in making the diagnosis of a bowel obstruction is the detection of a transition point, or change in caliber of the bowel at the site of obstruction, whether in the small or large bowel. Chou and colleagues[45] found 4 criteria, which were statistically significant in the diagnosis of small bowel obstruction—continuous dilatation of proximal bowel, greater amount of fluid in bowel loops proximal to the obstruction, abrupt transition, and less intraluminal content in the colon. Prior abdominal radiographs or CT scans, if

Fig. 11. Gastric diverticulum. A 49-year-old man with shortness of breath. Axial image from chest CT performed without intravenous contrast reveals a gastric diverticulum (*arrow*) emanating from the posterior gastric fundus, a typical location for a gastric diverticulum. Layering hyperdense debris helps to distinguish the finding from other entities, such as an exophytic gastric mass.

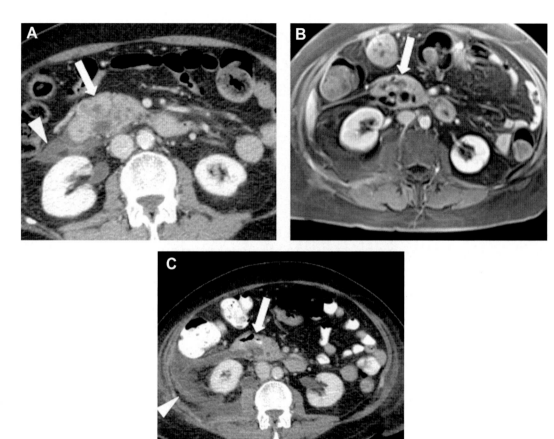

Fig. 12. Periampullary duodenal diverticulum. A 70-year-old woman with elevated liver function tests. Axial CT (*A*) and MR (*B*) images, both performed with intravenous contrast, demonstrate a heterogeneous focus adjacent to the pancreas head (*arrows*) which was mistaken for a mass. (*C*) Image from subsequent oral and intravenous contrast-enhanced CT shows air and oral contrast at the same site (*arrow*), diagnostic of a duodenal diverticulum. Peripancreatic and right-sided retroperitoneal fluid (*A, C [arrowheads]*) is secondary to acute pancreatitis.

available, may help in suggesting the diagnosis of chronic nonobstructive dilatation.

INTUSSUSCEPTION

Intussusception is a well-known medical condition characterized by the invagination of a bowel segment into an adjacent segment. Although a common entity in the pediatric population, only 5% of symptomatic intussusceptions occur in adults.[46] In the pediatric population, the cause of intussusception most frequently is idiopathic and thought to be the result of enlarged gut lymphoid tissue (Peyer patches) brought on by viral infection.[47] Classic symptoms in children have been described as abdominal pain, currant jelly stool, and a palpable sausage-like mass. Symptoms in adults, however, can be more nonspecific, if present at all, and can include abdominal pain, nausea, and vomiting.

In adults, an intussusception, particularly if it involves the colon, usually is a pathologic condition, with tumor serving as a lead point (**Fig. 13**). Neoplasm is the most common cause of adult intussusception.[48] Additional causes of intussusception in adults include benign tumors, feeding tubes, Meckel diverticulum, and foreign bodies. Symptoms of intussusception with a lead point include abdominal pain and nausea/vomiting. Intussusception can be divided into anatomic location: entero-enteric, colocolic, and ileocolic.

With the improving resolution and widespread adoption of CT, incidental entero-enteric transient intussusceptions have been detected with increasing frequency.[49] Transient intussusceptions usually are idiopathic and do not have a visible lead point. The mechanism of transient intermittent intussusceptions is not entirely established, to the authors' knowledge, but may involve dysrhythmic contractions that result in abnormal

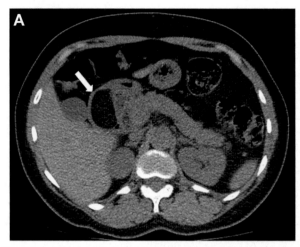
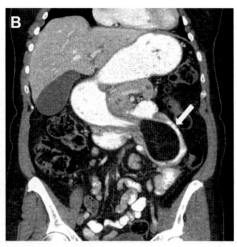

Fig. 13. Intussuscepting duodenal lipoma. A 63-year-old woman (on initial presentation). (*A*) Axial image from chest CT performed with intravenous contrast to evaluate for a possible lung mass demonstrates an incidental lipoma (*arrow*) within the duodenal bulb. (*B*) Coronal image from without intravenous contrast-enhanced abdominal CT 3 years later, after the patient presented with abdominal pain, now shows duodenal intussusception into the proximal jejunum with the lipoma increased in size, and now serving as lead point (*arrow*).

peristalsis.[49] The condition also has been described in patients with celiac disease and Crohn disease.[50] Unlike pathologic lead point cases, transient intussusceptions present without obstructive symptoms and may be asymptomatic.[51] Many studies have established that these cases can be treated with conservative management, even in the presence of GI symptoms.

In an extensive CT report search for cases of intussusception, Lvoff and colleagues[52] identified 37 patients with small bowel intussusception and found conservative management successful in 84% of cases. In another large review of CT reports, Rea and colleagues[53] identified 149 patients with entero-enteric intussusception and found fewer than 5% of those patients underwent operative intervention.

Intussusception is readily detectable on CT. The CT findings of intussusception are the classic targetoid bowel in bowel appearance. Predictive features of benign self-resolving intussusceptions include lack of visible lead point, absent

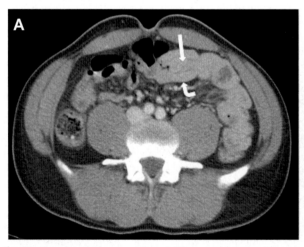
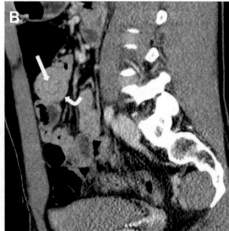

Fig. 14. Transient intussusception. A 32-year-old man with acute abdominal pain. Axial (*A*) and sagittal (*B*) images from CT performed with intravenous and without oral contrast, show an entero-enteric intussusception with the classic bowel in bowel appearance of the intussusceptum (*straight arrows*) within the receiving segment of small bowel, referred to as the intussuscipiens (*curved arrows*). This is a short segment intussusception without evidence of pathologic lead point, bowel obstruction, or inflammation. Therefore, findings are highly suggestive of a benign transient intussusception, a self-limiting condition. On follow-up CT 1 week later (not shown), the intussusception had resolved.

obstruction, proximal small bowel location, and length less than 3.5 cm (**Fig. 14**).[52]

Benign entero-enteric intussusception is a condition that is being diagnosed with increasing frequency on CT. CT plays a critical role not only in detection but also stratifying cases that are likely to respond to conservative treatment.

SUBMUCOSAL FAT DEPOSITION

Submucosal fat deposition within the bowel, also known as the fat halo sign on CT, describes a middle layer of submucosal fat (low attenuation (below −10 HU)), surrounded by an inner layer (mucosa) and outer layer (muscularis propria and serosa) of soft tissue attenuation.[5,54,55] The fat halo sign initially was described in the setting of chronic IBD (Crohn disease and ulcerative colitis) and formerly was thought to be pathognomonic for IBD.[4,5,55,56] With the advent of improved CT technology, however, including the capability for routine rapid acquisition of thinner slices, and the increased utilization of imaging, the presence of this finding now is known to be more common than previously reported and has been associated with a broader differential, including obesity and chronic steroid use. In a patient without signs or symptoms related to bowel disease, this finding can be treated as purely incidental and of no clinical significance. Analysis of the distribution of submucosal fat, and correlating with associated findings and clinical history, can assist in determining clinical significance.

According to published data, the presence of the fat halo sign has been reported in 61% of patients with ulcerative colitis and in only 8% of patients with Crohn disease.[54,55] When submucosal fat is noted in both the small bowel and large bowel, the sign is considered as suggestive of Crohn disease. Additional findings typical for Crohn disease, including fistula or stricture formation, skip areas, and proliferation of mesenteric fat, when present, increase the likelihood of Crohn disease. When only the colon is affected, these findings as well as the degree and geographic distribution of bowel wall thickness sometimes can be used to distinguish ulcerative colitis from Crohn disease (**Fig 15**).[4,5,56] Isolated fat deposition in the duodenum or the proximal jejunum in the setting of fatty stools is suggestive of celiac disease. Other uncommon causes of the fat halo sign include acute presentations in patients receiving cytoreductive therapy or patients with graft-versus-host disease.[55,57]

The fat halo sign in patients without GI symptoms or clinical or radiological evidence of GI disease is considered a normal variant and may be linked with obesity. Harisinghani and colleagues[58] conducted a retrospective review and identified submucosal fat deposition in 21 of 100 patients who had computed tomographs (CTs) ordered for suspected urolithiasis. Of these 21 patients, none had any prior or subsequently recorded history of GI disease compatible with IBD.[58] The increased prevalence of fat in collapsed/underdistended bowel, thin caliber of the fatty layer, and disappearance of the fat halo sign with additional distention should favor a normal variant rather than a pathologic cause (**Fig. 16**). In addition, the presence of a normal haustral pattern can provide reassurance.[54,55,58]

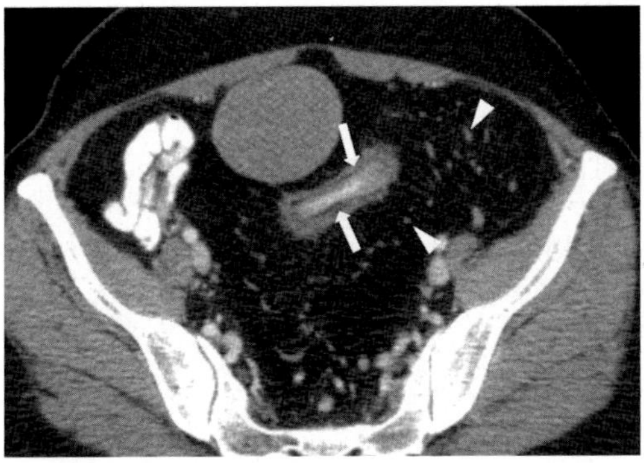

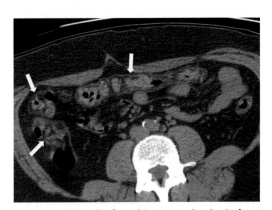

Fig. 15. Fat halo sign secondary to IBD. A 53-year-old woman with nausea and vomiting. Axial image through the pelvis from CT performed with oral and intravenous contrast demonstrates the fat halo sign in the rectosigmoid colon (*arrows*) as well as marked mesocolic fat proliferation and dilated vasa recta (*arrowheads*), findings highly compatible with IBD.

Fig. 16. Incidentally found intramural colonic fat. A 48-year-old woman undergoing CT in the prone position without oral or intravenous contrast for renal colic. The fat halo sign is seen at the hepatic flexure and in the transverse colon (*arrows*). The patient was obese and had no history of IBD or bowel-related symptoms; therefore, this finding is likely of no clinical significance.

SUMMARY

A variety of incidental findings in the bowel are seen with an overall relatively high frequency on CT. Typically, these scans are not performed to specifically optimize bowel visualization and characterization, for example, in the emergency setting. The role of the radiologist is to distinguish benign and clinically unimportant findings from findings needing further management. Knowledge pertaining to the specific CT appearances, pathophysiology, and clinical relevance associated with findings, including PI, diverticular disease, bowel dilatation, intussusception, and submucosal fat, can help the radiologist make the correct diagnosis. The radiologist also must be aware that neoplasms (both benign and malignant) of the GI tract occasionally can present as incidental findings, and conversely, that under-distention of the bowel, stool and other intraluminal contents, and the lack of intravenous contrast, can make accurate analysis of the bowel difficult, potentially obscuring or mimicking inflammatory or neoplastic disease.

CLINICS CARE POINTS

- Incidental bowel findings are commonly discovered on CT; most are benign and require no further workup or management, however some will be clinically significant. In particular, bowel wall thickening with suspicious features may reflect underlying neoplasm and should be brought to the attention of the referring physician.

- There are a wide variety of causes of pneumatosis intestinalis, with clinical presentation ranging from asymptomatic to life threatening bowel ischemia.

- Bowel dilatation is most often due to mechanical obstruction, however the radiologist should be aware of the causes of acute and chronic non obstructive bowel dilatation.

- Bowel intussusception in an adult should raise suspicion for a neoplasm acting as the lead point, however a transient self-resolving intussusception can be suggested in the setting of a short segment intussusception with no upstream bowel dilatation or visible lead point.

- The fat halo sign can be a CT sign of longstanding inflammatory bowel disease, however it is more frequently seen as an incidental and clinically insignificant finding.

DISCLOSURE

The authors have nothing to disclose.

REFERENCES

1. Troppmann M, Lippert E, Hamer OW, et al. Colonic bowel wall thickening: is there a need for endoscopic evaluation? Int J Colorectal Dis 2012;27(5): 601–4.
2. Bleibel W, Guerrero JE, Kim S, et al. The clinical significance of incidental computer tomography finding of gastrointestinal luminal wall thickening as evaluated by endoscopy. Dig Dis Sci 2007;52(7): 1709–12.
3. Desai RK, Tagliabue JR, Wegryn SA, et al. CT evaluation of wall thickening in the alimentary tract. Radiographics 1991;11(5):771–83 [discussion 784].
4. Macari M, Balthazar EJ. CT of bowel wall thickening: significance and pitfalls of interpretation. AJR Am J Roentgenol 2001;176(5):1105–16.
5. Gore RM, Balthazar EJ, Ghahremani GG, et al. CT features of ulcerative colitis and Crohn's disease. AJR Am J Roentgenol 1996;167(1):3–15.
6. James S, Balfe DM, Lee JK, et al. Small-bowel disease: categorization by CT examination. AJR Am J Roentgenol 1987;148(5):863–8.
7. Horton KM, Corl FM, Fishman EK. CT evaluation of the colon: inflammatory disease. Radiographics 2000;20(2):399–418.
8. Akcalar S, Turkbey B, Karcaaltincaba M, et al. Small bowel wall thickening: MDCT evaluation in the emergency room. Emerg Radiol 2011;(18):409–15.
9. Kelly ME, Heeney A, Redmond CE, et al. Incidental findings detected on emergency abdominal CT scans: a 1-year review. Abdom Imaging 2015; 40(6):1853–7.
10. Chandrapalan S, Tahir F, Kimani P, et al. Systematic review and meta-analysis: does colonic mural thickening on CT correlate with endoscopic findings at colonoscopy? Frontline Gastroenterol 2018;9(4): 278–84.
11. Eskaros S, Ghevariya V, Diamond I, et al. Correlation of incidental colorectal wall thickening at CT compared to colonoscopy. Emerg Radiol 2009; 16(6):473–6.
12. Uzzaman MM, Alam A, Nair MS, et al. Computed tomography findings of bowel wall thickening: its significance and relationship to endoscopic abnormalities. Ann R Coll Surg Engl 2012;94(1): 23–7.
13. Ozel B, Pickhardt PJ, Kim DH, et al. Accuracy of routine nontargeted CT without colonography technique for the detection of large colorectal polyps and cancer. Dis Colon Rectum 2010;53(6):911–8.
14. Cai Q, Baumgarten DA, Affronti JP, et al. Incidental findings of thickening luminal gastrointestinal organs

on computed tomography: an absolute indication for endoscopy. Am J Gastroenterol 2003;98(8):1734–7.

15. Tellez-Avila FI, García-Osogobio S, Chavez-Tapia NC, et al. Utility of endoscopy in patients with incidental gastrointestinal luminal wall thickening detected with CT. Surg Endosc 2009;23(10):2191–6.

16. Hines JJ, Paek GK, Lee P, et al. Beyond appendicitis; radiologic review of unusual and rare pathology of the appendix. Abdom Radiol (NY) 2016; 41(3):568–81.

17. Thompson WM. Imaging and findings of lipomas of the gastrointestinal tract. AJR Am J Roentgenol 2005;184(4):1163–71.

18. Ormsby EL, Duffield C, Ostovar-Sirjani F, et al. Colonoscopy findings in end-stage liver disease patients with incidental CT colonic wall thickening. AJR Am J Roentgenol 2007;189(5):1112–7.

19. Rezvani M, Menias C, Sandrasegaran K, et al. Heterotopic pancreas: histopathologic features, imaging findings, and complications. Radiographics 2017;37(2):484–99.

20. Woodward PJ, Sohaey R, Mezzetti TP Jr. Endometriosis: radiologic-pathologic correlation. Radiographics 2001;21(1):193–294.

21. Lake ST, Johnson PT, Kawamoto S, et al. CT of splenosis: patterns and pitfalls. AJR Am J Roentgenol 2012;199(6):W686–93.

22. Khalil PN, Huber-Wagner S, Ladurner R, et al. Natural history, clinical pattern, and surgical considerations of pneumatosis intestinalis. Eur J Med Res 2009;14(6):231–9.

23. Heng Y, Schuffler MD, Haggitt RC, et al. Pneumatosis intestinalis: a review. Am J Gastroenterol 1995; 90(10):1747–58.

24. Sassi C, Pasquali M, Facchini G, et al. Pneumatosis intestinalis in oncologic patients: when should the radiologist not be afraid? BJR Case Rep 2016;3(1): 20160017.

25. Hoot NR, Pfennig CL, Johnston MN, et al. An incidental finding? Pneumatosis intestinalis after minor trauma. J Emerg Med 2013;44(2):e145–7.

26. Wang YJ, Wang YM, Zheng YM, et al. Pneumatosis cystoides intestinalis: six case reports and a review of the literature. BMC Gastroenterol 2018;18(1):100.

27. Lassandro G, Picchi SG, Romano F, et al. Intestinal pneumatosis: differential diagnosis [published online ahead of print, 2020 Jul 31]. Abdom Radiol (NY) 2020. https://doi.org/10.1007/s00261-020-02639-8.

28. Ho LM, Paulson EK, Thompson WM. Pneumatosis intestinalis in the adult: benign to life-threatening causes. AJR Am J Roentgenol 2007;188(6): 1604–13.

29. Ezuka A, Kawana K, Nagase H, et al. Improvement of pneumatosis cystoides intestinalis after steroid tapering in a patient with bronchial asthma: a case report. J Med Case Rep 2013;7:163.

30. Nakagawa S, Akimoto T, Takeda S, et al. Antineutrophil cytoplasmic antibody-associated glomerulonephritis complicated by pneumatosis intestinalis. Clin Med Insights Case Rep 2015;8:65–70.

31. Kwon HJ, Kim KW, Song GW, et al. Pneumatosis intestinalis after liver transplantation. Eur J Radiol 2011;80(3):629–36.

32. Lee KS, Hwang S, Hurtado Rúa SM, et al. Distinguishing benign and life-threatening pneumatosis intestinalis in patients with cancer by CT imaging features. AJR Am J Roentgenol 2013;200(5): 1042–7.

33. Ceuppens AS, Dhont S, Sneyers B, et al. Jejuno-ileal diverticulosis: a review of literature. Acta Gastroenterol Belg 2018;81(4):517–9.

34. Levine M. Miscellaneous abnormalities of the esophagus. In: Gore RM, Levine MS, editors. Textbook of gastrointestinal radiology. 3rd edition. Philadelphia: Saunders Elsevier; 2008. p. 475–9.

35. Coulier B, Maldague P, Bourgeois A, et al. Diverticulitis of the small bowel: CT diagnosis. Abdom Imaging 2007;32(2):228–33.

36. Shuck JM, Stallion A. Duodenal diverticula. In: Holzheimer RG, Mannick JA, editors. Surgical treatment: evidence-based and problem-oriented. Munich (Germany): Zuckschwerdt; 2001.

37. Hines J, Rosenblat J, Duncan DR, et al. Perforation of the mesenteric small bowel: etiologies and CT findings. Emerg Radiol 2013;20(2):155–61.

38. Bennett GL, Birnbaum BA, Balthazar EJ. CT of Meckel's diverticulitis in 11 patients. AJR Am J Roentgenol 2004;182(3):625–9.

39. Elsayes KM, Menias CO, Harvin HJ, et al. Imaging manifestations of Meckel's diverticulum. AJR Am J Roentgenol 2007;189(1):81–8.

40. Gore RM, Yaghmai V. Diverticular disease of the colon. In: Gore RM, Levine MS, editors. Textbook of gastrointestinal radiology. 3rd edition. Philadelphia: Saunders Elsevier; 2008. p. 1019.

41. Rubesin SE, Gore RM. Small bowel obstruction. In: Gore RM, Levine MS, editors. Textbook of gastrointestinal radiology. 3rd edition. Philadelphia: Saunders Elsevier; 2008. p. 871.

42. Katz DS, Scheirey CD, Bordia R, et al. Computed tomography of miscellaneous regional and diffuse small bowel disorders. Radiol Clin North Am 2013; 51(1):45–68.

43. Choi JS, Lim JS, Kim H, et al. Colonic pseudoobstruction: CT findings. AJR Am J Roentgenol 2008; 190(6):1521–6.

44. Gore RM. Colon: differential diagnosis. In: Gore RM, Levine MS, editors. Textbook of gastrointestinal radiology. 3rd edition. Philadelphia: Saunders Elsevier; 2008. p. 1248.

45. Chou CK, Mak CW, Huang MC, et al. Differentiation of obstructive from non-obstructive small bowel dilatation on CT. Eur J Radiol 2000;35(3):213–20.

46. Azar T, Berger DL. Adult intussusception. Ann Surg 1997;226(2):134–8.

47. Waseem M, Rosenberg HK. Intussusception. Pediatr Emerg Care 2008;24(11):793–800.

48. Marinis A, Yiallourou A, Samanides L, et al. Intussusception of the bowel in adults: a review. World J Gastroenterol 2009;15(4):407–11.

49. Kim YH, Blake MA, Harisinghani MG, et al. Adult intestinal intussusception: CT appearances and identification of a causative lead point. Radiographics 2006;26(3):733–44.

50. Napora TE, Henry KE, Lovett TJ, et al. Transient adult jejunal intussusception. J Emerg Med 2003; 24(4):395–400.

51. Gayer G, Apter S, Hofmann C, et al. Intussusception in adults: CT diagnosis. Clin Radiol 1998;53(1):53–7.

52. Lvoff N, Breiman RS, Coakley FV, et al. Distinguishing features of self-limiting adult small-bowel intussusception identified at CT. Radiology 2003;227(1): 68–72.

53. Rea JD, Lockhart ME, Yarbrough DE, et al. Approach to management of intussusception in adults: a new paradigm in the computed tomography era. Am Surg 2007;73(11):1098–105.

54. Ahualli J. The fat halo sign. Radiology 2007;242(3): 945–6.

55. Philpotts LE, Heiken JP, Westcott MA, et al. Colitis: use of CT findings in differential diagnosis. Radiology 1994;190(2):445–9.

56. Jones B, Fishman EK, Hamilton SR, et al. Submucosal accumulation of fat in inflammatory bowel disease: CT/pathologic correlation. J Comput Assist Tomogr 1986;10(5):759–63.

57. Muldowney SM, Balfe DM, Hammerman A, et al. "Acute" fat deposition in bowel wall submucosa: CT appearance. J Comput Assist Tomogr 1995;19(3): 390–3.

58. Harisinghani MG, Wittenberg J, Lee W, et al. Bowel wall fat halo sign in patients without intestinal disease. AJR Am J Roentgenol 2003;181(3): 781–4.

Incidental Ovarian and Uterine Findings on Cross-sectional Imaging

Margarita V. Revzin, MD, MS, FSRU, FAIUM[a,]*, Anne Sailer, MD[a],
Mariam Moshiri, MD, FSAR, FSRU[b]

KEYWORDS

- Incidentaloma • CT • Adnexa • Uterine leiomyoma • Uterine arteriovenous malformation
- Endometrial cancer • Displaced IUD • Cervical cancer

KEY POINTS

- Although CT detection of many incidental ovarian and uterine findings may not warrant further investigation, a substantial number of findings may require prompt management and additional imaging and follow-up. To avoid unnecessary imaging or potentially a missed critical diagnosis, radiologists must be familiar with the management of the incidentally discovered findings.
- Utilization of established management algorithm for adnexal cysts is based on CT features, which allows subcategorization of these cysts into three main groups: simple cysts, cystic mostly benign masses, and masses suspicious for malignancy (solid, cystic or both).
- A number of vascular gynecologic disorders may be incidentally discovered on CT. These include but not limited to pelvic vein phlebitis, deep pelvic veins or ovarian vein thrombosis, pelvic congestion syndrome, pelvic arteriovenous malformation and or fistula.
- Degenerating fibroids; endometrial, uterine, cervical or vaginal malignancies are pathologies that when discovered incidentally on CT, should warrant further evaluation with MRI or tissue sampling.
- Various nongynecologic pelvic processes may mimic gynecological disorders and should be considered in the differential diagnosis when discovered incidentally. These entities include but not limited to Tarlov and duplication cysts, nerve sheath tumors and bowel tumors. Recognition of their key features can help to avoid misinterpretations and mismanagement.

INCIDENTAL GYNECOLOGIC FINDINGS ON COMPUTED TOMOGRAPHY

Summary

In nonpregnant postmenarchal patients imaged with computed tomography (CT), various incidental findings, also called incidentalomas, encompass a potential broad spectrum of pelvic gynecologic disorders.[1] A knowledge of the management recommendations for incidental findings is critical to avoid unnecessary imaging and surgical interventions, as well as to avoid failure in diagnosis and management of some of these conditions. Detection of some of these incidental findings may not warrant further investigation; however, a substantial number of findings may require prompt management and additional imaging. This article reviews this spectrum of adnexal, ovarian, and uterine incidental disorders discovered on CT, describes their characteristic imaging features, and provides an algorithm for their

Grant funding and financial support: None.
[a] Department of Radiology and Biomedical Imaging, Abdominal Imaging and Emergency Radiology, Yale School of Medicine, 333 Cedar Street, PO Box 208042, Room TE-2, New Haven, CT 06520, USA;
[b] Department of Radiology, University of Washington Medical Center, 1959 NE Pacific Street, Box 357115, Seattle, WA 98195, USA
* Corresponding author.
E-mail address: margarita.revzin@yale.edu

Radiol Clin N Am 59 (2021) 661–692
https://doi.org/10.1016/j.rcl.2021.03.013

Table 1
Computed tomography findings of incidental adnexal cystic adnexal masses: simple and mostly benign

CT Findings of Adnexal Cystic Adnexal Masses	
Simple-appearing cystic adnexal masses: oval or round unilocular masses of uniform fluid signal attenuation, with a regular or imperceptible wall, without solid components or mural nodules, and measuring <10 cm in maximum diameter	
Corpus luteum	• Intraovarian location of the cyst with a visible rim of ovarian parenchyma around its margins • Crenulated hyperenhancing rim sign around its margins that corresponds to peripheral hypervascularity or a ring-of-fire sign seen on color Doppler US • Size typically <3 cm • Hypodense on both nonenhanced and enhanced CT measuring fluid density (−10 to 20 HU) • Small to moderate amount of simple-appearing free fluid may be seen in the ipsilateral adnexa and cul-de-sac if ruptured • Hemorrhagic corpus luteum may be hyperdense
Paraovarian and paratubal cysts	• Findings on CT are nonspecific because they may not be definitively identified as nonovarian in origin • Do not enhance and may show a barely perceptible wall • May become particularly large, especially paratubal cysts
Mostly benign-appearing cystic adnexal masses: do not meet the criteria for a benign-appearing cyst because of issues such as angulated margins, nonround or oval shapes, and/or portions that are obscured on examination or poorly imaged because of technical limitations that result in suboptimal evaluation of the cyst	
PIC	• Unilocular or multilocular septated complex cyst that conforms to the shape of the pelvis and pelvic organs • CT characteristics may be nonspecific; however, patients usually have a history of prior pelvic surgery, inflammation, infection, endometriosis, peritoneal dialysis, IBD, and so forth • Unilocular appearance of the mass on CT, associated with either centrally or eccentrically positioned spider-in-web appearance on US and MR imaging • Normal ovary: absence of complex features differentiates from peritoneal disease such as lack of solid components, nodularity, or thick septations, all of which are more characteristic in malignant processes
Hydrosalpinx	• Fluid-filled round or tubular structure with a waist sign and evidence of incomplete septations, located separate from the ovary and bowel (in the presence of enteric contrast present). Same risk factors as PIC
Hematosalpinx	• Relatively hyperdense dilated tubular structure with incomplete septa, interposed between the uterus and the ovary • Mildly enhancing not thickened wall • The folded appearance of the tube in hematosalpinx may mimic a complex cystic adnexal mass
Endometriosis	• Appearance of endometriomas on CT is nonspecific and CT plays no major role in its diagnosis • The cysts can appear as nonenhancing hypodense or hyperdense masses or solid masses, either within or outside of the ovary

(continued on next page)

Table 1 (continued)
CT Findings of Adnexal Cystic Adnexal Masses
<ul><li>DIE: complex adnexal mass or masses, mimicking pelvic inflammatory disease. Nodular peritoneal plaques can mimic peritoneal metastases</li><li>Endometriosis in cesarean section scar: nonspecific soft tissue mass that may show mild contrast enhancement and irregular or lobulated borders</li></ul>

Abbreviations: DIE, deep infiltrating endometriosis; IBD, inflammatory bowel disease; PIC, peritoneal inclusion cyst US, ultrasonography.

management that can serve as a guide for radiologists and clinicians.

INTRODUCTION

CT scanning is an extremely informative diagnostic technique with a wide range of clinical applications. Because of the rapid imaging time compared with other techniques such as magnetic resonance (MR) imaging, CT scanning is generally appropriate for many indications in all age groups. In the United States, more than 70 million CT scans are performed every year.[2] The widespread use of CT not only allows quick and accurate diagnosis pertaining to the reason the examination was ordered but also results in the depiction and then detection by the interpreting radiologist of various incidental findings, including in the female pelvis.[3–5] Detection of many of these incidental findings may not warrant further investigation; however, a substantial number of findings may require prompt management and additional imaging and follow-up. Radiologists must be familiar with the management of these incidentally discovered findings and recognize the impact of incorrect interpretation, which may result in either unnecessary imaging (causing anxiety for the patient, and potentially also for the referring clinician who ordered the imaging examination) or potentially a missed critical diagnosis. This article reviews adnexal, ovarian, and uterine incidental findings discovered on CT in nonpregnant postmenarchal patients for whom no gynecologic disorder is clinically known or suspected (**Table 1**). It reviews general findings associated with various pelvic incidentalomas and discusses the main management recommendations, with the assumption that these patients are presenting with symptoms not related to the adnexal regions and without positive pelvic examinations findings. An algorithm describing management of various adnexal and uterine disorders is provided, which can serve as a guide for radiologists and general practitioners.

DISCUSSION
Incidental Findings of Adnexal Disorder

Development of a dominant follicle followed by a corpus luteum is an expected physiologic change in a premenopausal woman and may be incidentally detected on imaging.[6] Asymptomatic small uncomplicated adnexal and ovarian cysts are also common findings on pelvic CT in postmenopausal women, and vast majority are nonneoplastic.[7] In 1 large study, indeterminate adnexal masses were seen in approximately 4% of asymptomatic women older than 50 years who had undergone CT colonography, with none of these findings proved to be malignant.[4] In another study that evaluated patients who presented to the emergency department, the ovary was found to be the most common site of incidental findings, comprising 42% of all incidental findings.[8] Ovarian cysts may fluctuate in size over time, with up to one-third resolving on follow-up imaging, and new cysts developing on a 1-year follow-up examination in up to 8%.[9] These findings were validated by an extensive ultrasonography (US)-based research effort that showed a negligible risk of malignancy in simple cysts detected on US in both the premenopausal and postmenopausal patient populations.[10] There has been no identified risk of malignancy in women with sonographically detected simple adnexal cysts, to our knowledge, irrespective of cyst size.[11,12] Management of these findings should be performed based on patient characteristics, imaging findings, and a careful assessment of risks and benefits associated with the offered recommendations to the patient. In 2019, the American College of Radiology (ACR) proposed an algorithm for management of incidental adnexal masses detected on CT.[13] Although the ACR White Paper does not represent a standard of care, it provides guidance and recommendations on how to manage incidentally discovered adnexal findings. Therefore, it is important to recognize that radiologists may choose to deviate from this algorithm if some features of the adnexal disorder either are not described in the algorithm or are considered

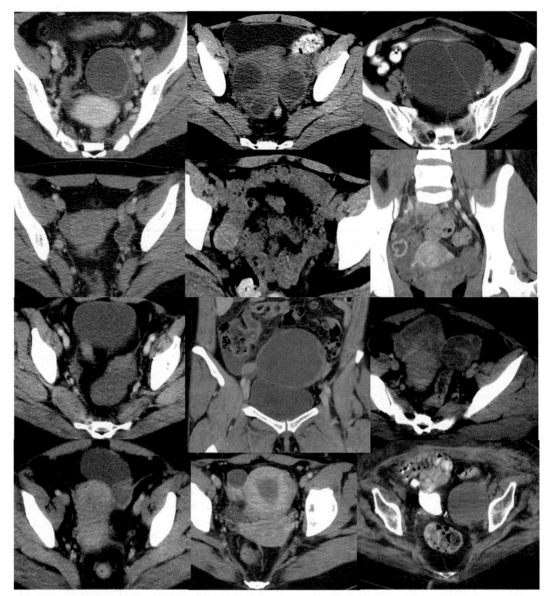

Fig. 1. Simple-appearing adnexal cysts.

clinically worrisome and warrant additional examination or follow-up. When adnexal findings are encountered, a description of the mass characteristics should be made, with emphasis on the simplicity or complexity of the cyst, its size, and any particular features that may point to a specific diagnosis. Menopausal status should also be taken into consideration, as well as technical limitations.

Simple-appearing cystic adnexal masses

Simple-appearing cysts are defined as oval or round unilocular masses of uniform fluid signal attenuation, with a regular or imperceptible wall, without solid components or mural nodules, and measuring less

than 10 cm in maximum diameter.[14] The cyst is still considered benign if layering hemorrhage is present within its lumen (Fig. 1). Management of these cystic masses should be performed based on the proposed algorithm included here (Fig. 2, see Table 1).

Adnexal simple-appearing cysts Corpus lutea, dominant follicles, and paraovarian/paratubal cysts are entities that are included within the category of simple cysts. There are a few imaging features that can help in differentiating these conditions. CT findings that are characteristic of a corpus luteum (a dominant follicle that has released an egg) include intraovarian location of the cyst with a visible rim of

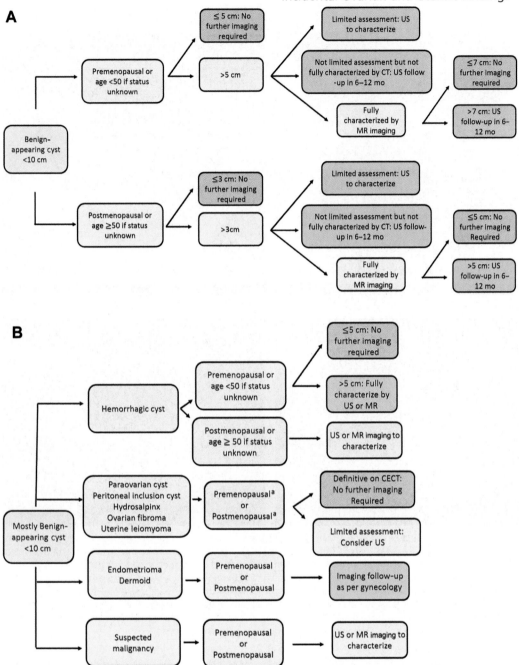

Fig. 2. The management of the adnexal cysts. (*A*) Management of incidental adnexal masses detected on CT. As per the ACR White Paper, this algorithm excludes the following: (1) normal findings, including crenulated enhancing wall of corpus luteum, asymmetric ovary without mass, with a normal shape; (2) calcifications without an associated noncalcified mass; (3) previous characterization with US or MR imaging; or (4) documented stability in size and appearance for 2 years. Limited assessment on CT means the cyst is consistent with a simple-appearing cyst, but characterization is limited by low signal-to-noise ratio, artifact, lack of contrast assessment, or incomplete anatomic coverage. Yellow boxes indicate using or acquiring clinical data (eg, size), green boxes describe recommendations for action (eg, follow-up imaging), and red boxes indicate that work-up or follow-up may be terminated if the finding is presumed to be benign. (*B*) Management of mostly benign adnexal masses detected on CT. Yellow boxes indicate using or acquiring clinical data (eg, size), green boxes describe recommendations for action (eg, follow-up imaging), and red boxes indicate that work-up or follow-up may be terminated (eg, if the finding is presumed to be benign). [a]Remember that, for peritoneal inclusion cyst (PIC), and for hydrosalpinx, clinical correlation with prior pelvic surgery, and with pelvic disorders such as prior inflammation, infection, endometriosis, patients on peritoneal dialysis, and those with a history of inflammatory bowel disease (IBD), is recommended to aid in diagnosis. CECT, contrast-enhanced CT. (*Data from* Patel MD, Ascher SM, Horrow MM, et al. Management of Incidental Adnexal Findings on CT and MRI: A White Paper of the ACR Incidental Findings Committee. J Am Coll Radiol. 2020;17(2):248-254.)

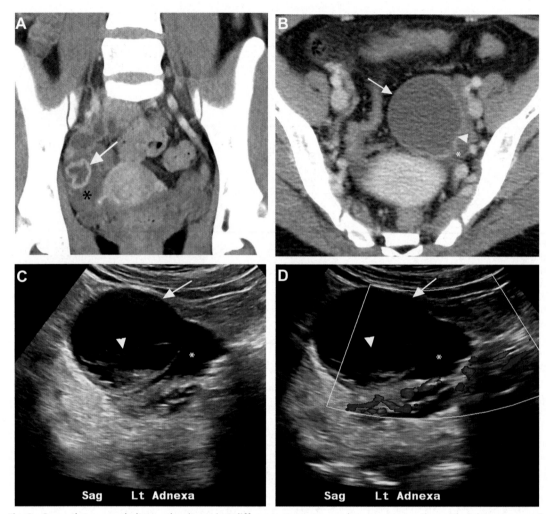

Fig. 3. Corpus luteum and a hemorrhagic cyst in 2 different premenopausal women presenting with right upper quadrant pain. (*A*) Coronal intravenous (IV) CECT image of the pelvis shows a hypodense cystic structure with hyperdense enhancing crenulated borders (*white arrow*). A small amount of fluid is also seen in the right adnexa and cul-de-sac (*asterisk*). Findings indicate a corpus luteum. (*B–D*). Axial IV CECT image of the pelvis (*B*) in a different patient shows a simple-appearing cyst with a hyperdense rim (*arrow*) and a small amount of free fluid in the adnexa (*asterisk*). Transverse gray-scale (*C*) and color Doppler (*D*) US images of the adnexa in the same patient as (*B*) show a cyst (*arrow*) with internal weblike septations and fluid-fluid level (*arrowhead*). A small amount of fluid is also seen in the left adnexa (*asterisk*). No flow is seen on color Doppler. Findings indicate a hemorrhagic cyst.

ovarian parenchyma around its margins, a crenulated hyperenhancing rim sign around its margins that corresponds to peripheral hypervascularity and/or or a "ring-of-fire" sign seen on color Doppler US, and size typically less than 3 cm[15] (**Fig. 3**). These cysts are hypodense on both nonenhanced and enhanced CT, and measure fluid density, ranging from −10 to 20 Hounsfield units (HU).[16] Note that a patient's menopausal status must be taken into account when making the diagnosis of a corpus luteum. In order to ensure accurate assessment of the cyst, multiple regions of interest should be examined within different portions of the suspected cyst. A corpus luteum may have a wall that

measures 1 to 3 mm in thickness, and cyst wall measurement is more accurately appreciated on US. If the cyst is leaking or ruptured, associated small to moderate amounts of simple-appearing free fluid may be seen in the ipsilateral adnexa and cul-de-sac. A hemorrhagic corpus luteum can be diagnosed when the cyst shows all of the described characteristics but is hyperdense on CT (occasionally with evidence of layering hyperdense material) (see **Fig. 3**).[17]

Paraovarian and paratubal cysts are thought to be remnants of the mesonephric (wolfian) and paramesonephric (müllerian) ducts, and are located in the broad ligament between the fallopian tube and

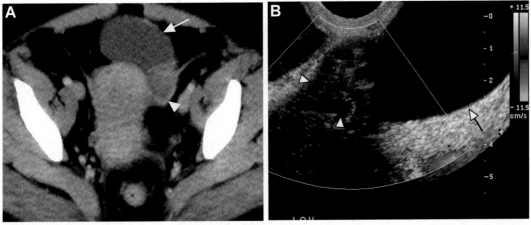

Fig. 4. Paraovarian cyst in a 36-year-old woman with abdominal pain. (*A*) IV contrast-enhanced axial CT image of the pelvis shows a hypodense cystic structure measuring simple fluid (*arrow*) with an imperceptible wall, positioned adjacent to but separate from the left ovary (*white arrow*). Note the absence of a claw sign, which would suggest ovarian origin. No enhancing components or septations are seen within the cyst. (*B*) Color Doppler transvaginal US (TVUS) image obtained in the sagittal plane shows a normal ovary with vascular flow within it (*arrowheads*) and an adjacent simple-appearing nonvascular paraovarian cyst (*white arrow*). Note the imperceptible wall of the cyst, which is better appreciated on US. The cyst had not morphologically changed in the last 2 years and had only minimally increased in size (not shown).

the ovary, representing approximately 10% of all adnexal masses.[18] Given their proximity to the ipsilateral ovary, the findings on CT are nonspecific, because they may not be definitively identified as nonovarian in origin. These cysts usually do not enhance and may show a barely perceptible wall (**Fig. 4**). When located at the fimbriated portion of the fallopian tube, the cysts are termed Morgagni or hydatid cysts.[19] In some situations, these cysts, particularly paratubal cysts, may reach very large sizes, undergo internal hemorrhage, and can torse or can serve as a lead point for isolated tubal torsion. Prior imaging, if available, may aid in limiting unnecessary follow-up imaging or additional investigations.

Adnexal cystic benign masses with characteristic features on computed tomography

This category includes cysts that are likely benign but do not meet the criteria for a simple-appearing cyst because of imaging findings including angulated margins, nonround or oval shapes, and/or portions that are obscured on examination or poorly imaged because of technical limitations that result in suboptimal evaluation of the cyst. Management of these cystic masses should be performed based on the algorithm included here (see **Fig. 2**, see **Table 1**).

A peritoneal inclusion cyst (PIC) represents an unilocular or multilocular septated complex cyst that conforms to the shape of the pelvis and pelvic organs. It develops as a result of ovarian secretions that are trapped between pelvic adhesions, leading

to impaired absorption and loculated pelvic fluid. The ovary is usually suspended in the center of the collection or is located eccentrically, resulting in a spider-in-web appearance (which is best seen on US). PIC can be seen in patients with a history of prior pelvic surgery, inflammation, infection, endometriosis, peritoneal dialysis, and inflammatory bowel disease (IBD). CT characteristics may be nonspecific. The mass respects the boundaries of pelvic structures and is usually situated along the pelvic sidewalls, occasionally showing angulated margins (**Fig. 5**). Thin septations generally can be appreciated only by US and MR imaging and are not well detected on CT, thus resulting in a unilocular appearance of the mass on CT. The ovary may not be appreciated on CT; however, when PICs are large, they can be readily differentiated on CT from malignant peritoneal disease by showing absence of complex features, including solid components, nodularity, or thick septations, all of which are more characteristic of malignant disease. When CT-based diagnosis is possible and there is appropriate patient history, no further imaging follow-up is recommended.

Hydrosalpinx occurs when fallopian tube secretions accumulate within an obstructed lumen. Causes of hydrosalpinx are similar to those of PIC. Depending on the degree of dilatation and folding, hydrosalpinx can appear round, oval, or tubular. A folded configuration with a C or S shape may be more conspicuous on reformatted CT images. CT findings of hydrosalpinx include a fluid-filled round or tubular structure with a waist sign

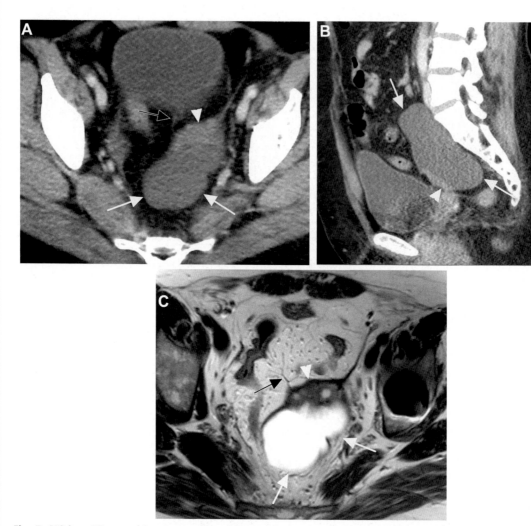

Fig. 5. PIC in a 55-year-old woman with a history of prior hysterectomy for leiomyomas. (*A, B*) IV contrast-enhanced axial (*A*) and sagittal (*B*) CT images of the pelvis show a cystic structure that conforms to the pelvic wall (*white arrows*). Note eccentrically located ovary (*arrowhead*) associated with the cyst and thin adhesions (*black arrows*). Thin septations were present within the cyst but were only seen on US and MR imaging. (*C*) Axial T2-weighted MR image confirms the findings of PIC (*white arrows*). Note the eccentric location of the ovary (*arrowhead*) and the presence of adhesions (*black arrow*).

and incomplete septations (sometimes better appreciated on US and MR imaging) that is located separate from the ovary and bowel (better delineated if there is enteric contrast present) (**Fig. 6**). The tube wall is uniformly smooth and thin, and shows mild enhancement. When in doubt, US can be used for more definitive diagnosis. The thickened longitudinal folds of the fallopian tube in cross section are responsible for the pathognomonic cogwheel appearance of hydrosalpinx on US.[19] When definitive characteristic features are seen on CT, no further imaging is required.[14]

Hematosalpinx represents a dilated fallopian tube that is filled with hemorrhagic fluid or blood products. Hematosalpinx is a finding and not a diagnosis, and can be attributable to various causes, including endometriosis with intraluminal tubal implants, uterine bleeding with reflux of hemorrhagic components into the fallopian tubes, tubal ectopic pregnancy, fallopian tube carcinoma, and an intrauterine device (IUD). Secondary findings can be seen depending on the causes of hematosalpinx. Depending on the stage of blood products, hematosalpinx on CT can be seen as a relatively hyperdense dilated tubular structure with incomplete septa, interposed between the uterus and the ovary. The wall is only mildly enhancing and is not thickened (**Fig. 7**). The folded appearance of the tube may mimic a complex

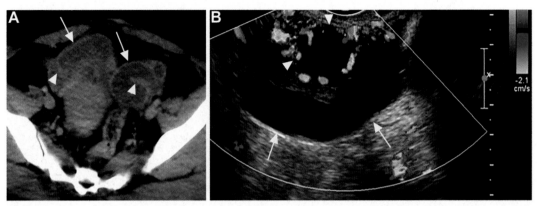

Fig. 6. Hydrosalpinx in a 37-year-old woman who presented to the emergency department with epigastric pain. (*A*) Axial IV CECT image of the pelvis shows bilateral simple fluid-filled tubular structures (*arrows*) with only minimal wall enhancement and no evidence of wall thickening. The tubular structures have a folded appearance with C-shaped configuration and a waist sign, and incomplete septations are also noted (*arrowheads*). (*B*) Color Doppler sagittal TVUS of the left adnexa shows a dilated fluid-filled tubular structure with no wall thickening or hyperemia indicating a hydrosalpinx (*arrows*). Note is made of a concomitant presence of a corpus luteum with a characteristic ring of fire around it (*arrowheads*). A hydrosalpinx was seen in the contralateral adnexa on TVUS (not shown), similar to that on CT.

cystic adnexal mass. MR imaging and US provide more specific assessment of the mass and demonstration of hemorrhagic components within a dilated tube (see **Fig. 7**).

Endometriosis is characterized by the presence of endometrial glands and stroma outside of the uterus, often accompanied by inflammation and fibrosis.[20] Endometriomas result from repeated hemorrhage of endometrial tissue implants in response to hormonal stimulation. Although it is a common entity, the appearance of an endometrioma on CT is nonspecific, and CT generally plays no role in its diagnosis. The cysts may be seen as nonenhancing hypodense or hyperdense masses or solid masses, either within or outside of the ovary (**Fig. 8**). Because of their malignant potential (albeit small), when discovered, endometriomas should merit surveillance.[14] Cystadenomas may have a similar appearance, with the exception of a few thin septations (**Fig. 9**).

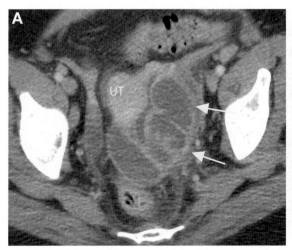
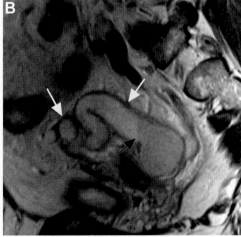

Fig. 7. Hematosalpinx in a 24-year-old woman with abdominal pain. (*A*) Axial IV CECT image of the pelvis shows a left fluid-filled tubular structure with only minimal wall enhancement and no evidence of wall thickening (*white arrows* in *A*). The tubular structure has a folded appearance, with an S-shaped configuration. Note the slightly hyperdense fluid filling the tube, implying the presence of hematosalpinx. (*B*) Sagittal T2-weighted MR image of the pelvis shows a dilated fluid-filled tube (*white arrows* in *B*) with a fluid-fluid level (*black arrow* in *B*) and shading artifact within a part of the tube, which is compatible with a hemorrhagic component. No wall thickening or enhancement on postcontrast images was seen (not shown). The findings indicate hematosalpinx.

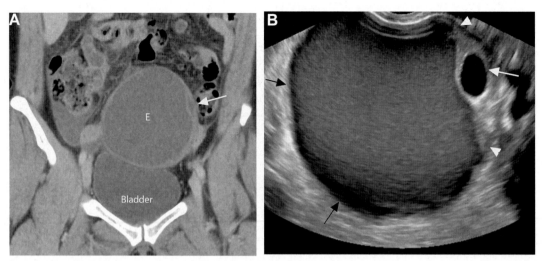

Fig. 8. Endometrioma in a 34-year-old woman who presented with abdominal pain. (*A*) Coronal IV CECT image of the pelvis shows a nonspecific large cyst (E) with a daughter cyst (*arrow*). The wall is not substantially thickened. The cyst is located just above the bladder. Note that the fluid within the cyst is slightly denser than the fluid within the bladder. (*B*) Gray-scale transverse US image of the adnexa shows a large cyst filled with homogeneous low-amplitude echoes (*black arrows*). Note a daughter cyst (*white arrow* in *B*) in the left wall of the cyst, which is compatible with an ovarian follicle. The claw sign (*white arrowhead* in *B*) of the normal ovarian parenchyma implies ovarian origin of the cyst.

Deep infiltrating endometriosis (DIE) is a highly invasive form of endometriosis that is often characterized by rectovaginal nodules and disease of the uterosacral ligaments, rectum, rectovaginal septum, vagina, and bladder.[20] It may result in bowel obstruction caused by extensive fibrotic adhesions. Infiltrative plaques may extend from the uterine serosa to the adjacent rectum or bladder, and result in substantial morbidity. On CT, DIE is nonspecific in appearance, with demonstration of a complex adnexal mass or masses, potentially mimicking pelvic inflammatory disease (PID). Nodular peritoneal plaques can also mimic peritoneal metastases.[21] Dense fibrosis related to pelvic plaques is seen as soft tissue bands extending among the pelvic organs (**Fig. 10**). In severe cases, associated obstruction of the ureters with development of hydronephrosis may be detected (see **Fig. 10**).

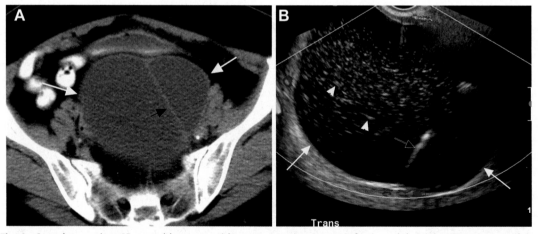

Fig. 9. Cystadenoma in a 43-year-old woman with recurrent urinary tract infections. (*A*) Axial IV CECT image of the pelvis shows a large cyst (*white arrows*) with a thin septation (*black arrow*) occupying a large part of the pelvis. The cyst shows no thick wall or hyperemia, and it is entirely replacing the ovary. (*B*) Color Doppler image in the transverse plane shows a large cyst (*white arrows*) with a thin septation (*black arrow*) that is filled with multiple echogenic foci (*arrowheads*), which is consistent with proteinaceous material and debris. No flow is seen within the thin septation. Minimal flow is noted in the wall of the cyst. Note that the large size of the cyst allows it to be differentiated from other benign adnexal and ovarian cysts (paraovarian cyst, follicles). Also note the absence of nodularity in the septations, a feature that differentiates a cystadenoma from a cystadenocarcinoma.

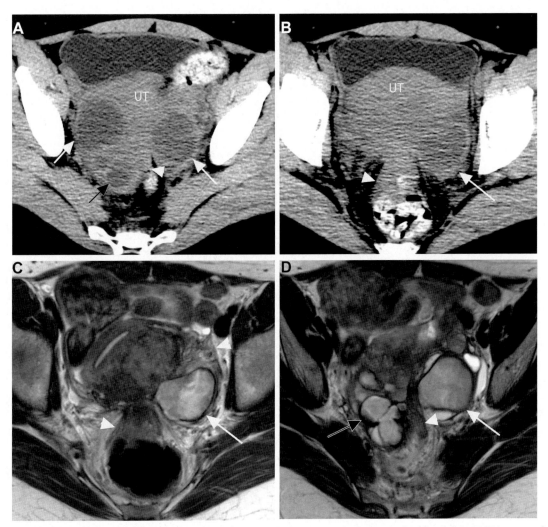

Fig. 10. Pelvic DIE in a 35-year-old woman with a history of severe endometriosis. (*A, B*) Axial IV CECT images of the pelvis show bilateral adnexal cystic structures, representing endometriomas (*white arrows*), a fluid-filled tubular structure (*black arrow*), likely representing a hematosalpinx, and a focal area of fibrosis, seen as a soft tissue density posterior to the uterus (UT) (*arrowhead*). (*C, D*) Axial T2-weighted MR images show bilateral ovarian endometriomas (*white arrows*), hematosalpinx (*black arrow*), and fibrosis as a result of infiltrative endometriosis (*arrowhead*). Note T2 shading artifact and fluid-fluid levels in the left endometrioma (*white arrow in D*) and a right hematosalpinx (*black arrow in D*), which are highly compatible with blood products.

Endometriosis in a cesarean section scar and along the round ligaments in the inguinal regions can also be incidentally discovered on CT and is characterized by a nonspecific soft tissue mass that may show mild contrast enhancement and irregular or lobulated borders.

Adnexal Neoplasms on Computed Tomography

Adnexal masses with features suspicious for malignancy on computed tomography
Adnexal masses with suspicious features for malignancy include complex cystic and solid masses,

or just solid masses that either are malignant or may have malignant potential. These masses may show wall nodularity, thick enhancing septations, irregular borders, necrotic components, or some combination of these findings. Management of these masses should be performed based on the provided algorithm included here (see **Fig. 2, Table 2**).

Fallopian tube neoplasm is considered primary when it is either restricted to the fallopian tube or when the fallopian tube is the most affected location.[19] The most common type of primary fallopian tube carcinoma is the papillary serous type, which occurs most commonly in the ampulla and

Table 2
Computed tomography findings of incidental ovarian and tubal benign and malignant neoplasms

CT Findings of Adnexal Benign and Malignant Neoplasms

Ovarian and Tubal Benign and Malignant Neoplasms

Fallopian tube neoplasms	• Tumors can be either sausage-shaped soft tissue masses that measure <7 cm, mixed solid and cystic adnexal masses, tubular cystic structures with papillary projections, or contain nodular enhancing foci. Associated with hydrosalpinx and intrauterine fluid accumulation and ascites • The fluid can decompress either into the uterine cavity or into the peritoneum • Solid components show soft tissue attenuation with minimal enhancement compared with myometrium • Depending on the stage of the tumor, peritoneal implants and distant pelvic and abdominal metastases may also be seen
Ovarian epithelial tumors and metastases	• Large, measuring ≥10 cm, and contain complex cystic and solid components that show avid enhancement • Multiple papillary mural nodules may also be seen in ovarian tumors; some high-grade ovarian serous neoplasms are entirely solid • Both high-grade and low-grade ovarian serous and mucinous carcinomas are frequently bilateral • Benign serous and mucinous cystadenomas of the ovary may have a similar presentation • Peritoneal implants, ascites, and paraaortic lymphadenopathy are seen in late stages
Ovarian metastases	• Usually present as solid masses; however, cystic or necrotic components can also be seen, thus resembling primary ovarian cancer • Often bilateral; in cases of unilateral disease, the right ovary is more commonly affected
Cystic ovarian mature teratoma or dermoid cyst	• Fat attenuation (−90 to −130 HU) within a cyst is diagnostic • Teeth or calcifications are seen in slightly >50% of tumors, and occasionally calcifications can be seen within the cyst wall • The solid component may show mild enhancement • Concern for malignant transformation should be made when an enhancing solid component shows an obtuse angle between the solid component and the inner wall of the cyst • Teratomas that have no fat component (6%) appear as fluid-containing cystic masses
Ovarian fibromas, thecomas, and fibrothecomas	• Nonspecific CT imaging features: isodense to the uterus on a noncontrast CT, and may show delayed progressive enhancement
Benign serous and mucinous cystadenomas	• The average size of cystadenomas is 10 cm • Serous cystadenomas: homogeneous fluid attenuation cysts with thin, imperceptible (<3 mm) walls and without septations or solid components • Mucinous-type cystadenomas: multilocular and show variable densities within loculations, owing to mucinous debris and hemorrhage that results in a stained-glass appearance on CT • The presence of papillary projections and nodular septa should suggest a malignant ovarian neoplasm

projects into the tubal lumen, often causing occlusion. Although these tumors are very similar to epithelial tumors of the ovaries, there are a few clinical and imaging features that distinguish them from ovarian neoplasms. These features include the clinical presentation of the characteristic Latzko triad, consisting of (1) intermittent profuse serosanguinous vaginal discharge, (2) colicky pain relieved by discharge, and (3) an abdominal and pelvic mass on physical examination.[19] On CT, these tumors can be sausage-shaped soft tissue masses that measure less than 7 cm, mixed solid and cystic adnexal masses, tubular cystic structures with papillary projections, or nodular enhancing foci (caused by associated hydrosalpinx and ascites attributable to accumulation and release of secretions that are produced by the cancerous cells) (Fig. 11). The fluid can decompress either into the uterine cavity or into the peritoneum. Solid components show soft tissue attenuation with minimal enhancement compared with myometrium. Depending on the stage of the tumor, peritoneal implants and distant pelvic and abdominal metastases may also be seen. When fallopian tube neoplasm is suspected, additional prompt imaging with US and MR is required.

Ovarian epithelial tumors and metastases
Because of their commonly asymptomatic or vague clinical presentations, ovarian cancer and metastatic disease involving the ovaries are occasionally incidentally detected by CT.[14] The most common primary ovarian malignancy is epithelial ovarian cancer. In contrast with primary fallopian tubal cancer, ovarian epithelial tumors are larger,

measuring greater than or equal to 10 cm, and contain more complex cystic and solid components that show avid enhancement (Fig. 12). Multiple papillary mural nodules may also be seen in ovarian tumors, and some high-grade ovarian serous neoplasms are entirely solid.[22] Hydrosalpinx and intrauterine fluid accumulation are uncommon in patients with ovarian epithelial tumors. Most epithelial cancers show increased levels of serum CA125 (cancer antigen 125). When ovarian malignancy is suspected, these patients may be either promptly further evaluated with US and MR imaging to determine extent of disease or, alternatively, surgical staging can be performed.[23] Both high-grade and low-grade ovarian serous and mucinous carcinomas are frequently bilateral. Benign serous mucinous cystadenoma and mucinous cystadenoma of the ovary may have a similar presentation (see Fig. 9). Peritoneal implants, ascites, and paraaortic lymphadenopathy are seen in late stages.

Ovarian metastases are commonly associated with gastrointestinal primary neoplasms, predominantly arising from the stomach (76%).[24] A Krukenberg tumor represents a subtype of metastatic disease that contains more than 10% mucin-filled signet cells in the cellular stroma. Metastases to an ovary usually present as solid masses; however, cystic or necrotic components can also be seen, thus resembling primary ovarian cancer (Fig. 13). Just as with primary malignancies, metastatic disease to the ovaries is often bilateral, and, in cases of unilateral disease, the right ovary is more commonly affected.[25] All efforts should be made to search for primary

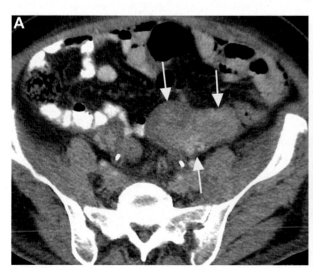
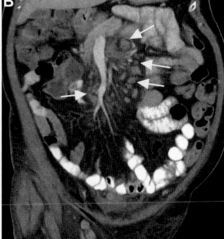

Fig. 11. Primary fallopian tube carcinoma in a 49-year-old woman with abdominal pain. (*A, B*) Axial (*A*) and coronal (*B*) IV CECT images of the abdomen and pelvis show a sausagelike soft tissue heterogeneous mass in the left adnexa (*arrow in A*) and associated mesenteric lymphadenopathy (*arrows in B*).

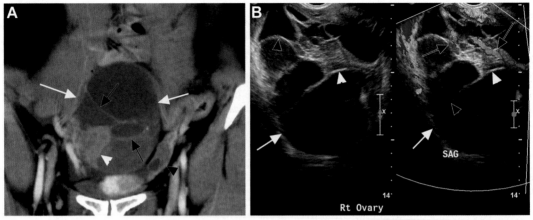

Fig. 12. Epithelial mucinous ovarian carcinoma in a 52-year-old woman who presented with right upper quadrant pain. (A) Coronal IV CECT images of the pelvis show a complex multiloculated cystic mass (*white arrows*) with thin and thick septations (*black arrows*), and a nodular solid component (*white arrowhead*). Note variable density within different loculations, which is characteristic of mucinous neoplasms. No substantial ascites is seen. A normal left ovary is seen (*black arrowhead*). (B) Transverse gray-scale and color Doppler TVUS split image shows a multiloculated mass (*white arrows*) with variable contents within the loculations and flow (*black arrows*) within the septations (*black arrowheads*), as well as nodular components (*white arrowheads*).

neoplasm when metastases are suspected. Prompt further evaluation of the findings with US and MR imaging should also be performed.

Adnexal masses without suspicious features for malignancy on computed tomography

Adnexal masses without suspicious features for malignancy include, but are not limited to, dermoid cyst, ovarian stromal tumors (fibroma, thecoma, fibrothecoma), uterine leiomyomas, and ovarian cystadenomas. These masses may show a solid hypodense appearance similar to uterine fibroids, fat content, or a cystic appearance with thin septations. Management of these masses should be performed based on the provided algorithm (see **Fig. 2, Table 2**).

A cystic ovarian mature teratoma (also called a dermoid cyst) represents a type of germ cell tumor

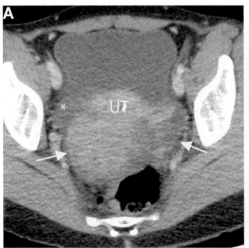
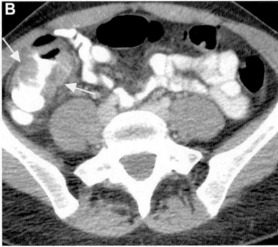

Fig. 13. Krukenberg tumor from cecal adenocarcinoma metastases to the ovaries in a 27-year-old woman presenting with fever. (A, B) Axial IV CECT images of the pelvis show heterogeneous solid soft tissue density masses in the adnexal regions, right greater than the left (*arrows in A*), indicating metastatic disease. Trace of ascites is seen in the right adnexa (*asterisk in A*). Irregular marked masslike thickening of the cecum (*arrows in B*) was the associated primary malignancy. The cecal mass also extended to the base of the appendix, resulting in its obstruction, causing secondary appendicitis (not shown).

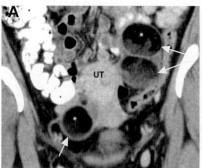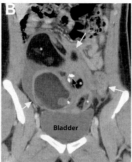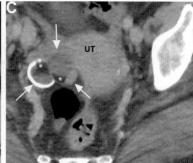

Fig. 14. Mature cystic teratoma in 3 different patients who presented with various unrelated abdominal symptoms. Coronal (*A, B*), and axial (*C*) IV CECT images of the pelvis show pelvic masses (*white arrows*) with a low attenuation (fat) component within (*asterisks*) and calcifications (*black arrow*). The findings indicate mature teratomas. Teratomas are bilateral in the patients shown in (*A*) and (*B*).

that is composed of 3 distinct germ cell layers, and comprises 5% to 25% of all ovarian neoplasms. These tumors are usually asymptomatic, unilateral but can be bilateral, and may vary in size from subcentimeter to up to 40 cm. On CT, fat attenuation (−90 to −130 HU) within a cyst is diagnostic, and has been reported in 93% of cases.[26] Teeth or calcifications are seen in slightly more than 50% of tumors, and occasionally calcifications can be seen within the cyst wall.[26] The solid component may show mild enhancement on postcontrast CT and does not always indicate malignancy (**Fig. 14**). Concern for malignant transformation is appropriate when an enhancing solid component shows an obtuse angle between the solid component and the inner wall of the cyst. Those teratomas that have no fat component (6%) appear as fluid-containing cystic masses. Although diagnosis based on CT findings in most cases is definitive, US and MR imaging can be used when the findings are not straightforward. Monitoring for growth and potential malignant transformation is recommended. Surgical removal is advised when the tumor is larger than 6 cm.

Ovarian fibromas, thecomas, and fibrothecomas represent a group of benign ovarian neoplasms classified as sex-cord stromal tumors. They are usually asymptomatic, incidentally found on imaging, and show nonspecific CT features.[27] These solid tumors are isodense to the uterus on noncontrast CT, and may show delayed progressive enhancement. Calcifications may be present and cystic changes may be seen in larger masses. Thecomas may secrete either estrogen or androgen, and may therefore be associated with either endometrial thickening or hirsutism, respectively. When seen in association with pleural effusion and ascites, they are diagnostic of Meigs syndrome[28] (**Fig. 15**). When a solid adnexal mass is discovered on CT and is thought to represent a benign stromal tumor, it can be further evaluated with MR imaging for more definite diagnosis. Demonstration of a low T2-weighted signal in a well-circumscribed mass arising from the ovary, which shows less enhancement than the adjacent myometrium, indicates fibroma/fibrothecoma. No further imaging or a follow-up is needed.

Benign serous and mucinous cystadenomas are classified as epithelial ovarian neoplasms. When small, benign cystadenomas are similar in appearance to functional ovarian cysts. However, functional cysts typically resolve over 1 to 2 menstrual cycles, whereas cystadenomas persist and/or enlarge. The average size of cystadenomas is 10 cm. On CT, serous cystadenomas are characterized as homogeneous fluid attenuation cysts with thin imperceptible (<3 mm) walls and without septations or solid components (see **Fig. 9**). Mucinous-type cystadenomas are usually multilocular and show variable densities within the loculations, owing to mucinous debris and hemorrhage that results in a stained-glass appearance on CT.[29] Follow-up US in 4 to 6 weeks can be recommended to differentiate these entities from functional cysts. A corpus luteum wall tends to be thicker and show peripheral vascularity, and also changes over time in size and morphologic appearance. The presence of papillary projections and nodular septa should suggest a malignant ovarian neoplasm. Cystadenomas account for a significant proportion of incidental cysts in postmenopausal women, with up to 84% of simple adnexal cysts in this patient population found to be serous cystadenomas at surgery.[30–35]

Gynecologic Vascular Disorders

Several gynecologic vascular disorders may be discovered incidentally on CT (**Table 3**). The ovarian vein arises from the venous plexus located

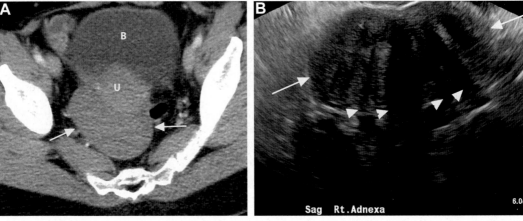

Fig. 15. Fibroma/fibrothecoma in a 46-year-old woman presenting with abdominal pain. (*A*) Axial IV CECT image of the pelvis shows a solid homogeneous density mass (*white arrows*) in the right adnexa measuring similar density as the adjacent muscle and uterus. Note the absence of calcifications. There is no ascites or pleural effusions seen to suggest Meigs syndrome, although this syndrome is rare. U-uterus, B-urinary bladder. (*B*) Gray-scale sagittal TVUS shows the characteristic hypoechoic appearance of the mass (*white arrows*) with posterior acoustic shadowing (*white arrowheads*). No substantial flow was seen on color Doppler (not shown).

Table 3
Computed tomography findings of incidental vascular gynecologic disorders

CT Findings of Vascular Gynecologic Disorders	
Pelvic phleboliths	• Calcified hyperdensities along the courses of the ovarian veins • Phleboliths are commonly mistaken for ureteral calculi • The rim sign is more commonly seen in a ureteral calculus, described as a soft tissue density rim surrounding a calcification
Ovarian vein thrombosis and thrombophlebitis	• Filling defect within an enlarged ovarian vein with peripheral mucosal enhancement are diagnostic • Typically found at the confluence of the ovarian vein with the inferior vena cava • Secondary findings: surrounding perivascular inflammatory stranding, heterogeneous enhancing parauterine mass, enlargement of the visualized ovary caused by congestion and delayed perfusion, and resultant ovarian parenchymal hypoattenuation support the diagnosis
Pelvic congestion syndrome	• Four or more ipsilateral tortuous parauterine veins of different caliber are seen in the parametria, with at least 1 vein measuring >4 mm in maximum diameter, or a dilated ovarian vein measuring >8 mm in diameter • Associated prominent myometrial arcuate vessels are also commonly present • Clinical diagnosis supported by the above CT findings
Pelvic lymphadenopathy	• Soft tissue masses that are not tubular and do not enhance in similar fashion to pelvic venous structures
UAVM and PAVM	• UAVM: an enlarged uterus, bilateral hypertrophied uterine arteries that feed into a tortuous mass comprising large accessory feeding vessels, and early venous filling into enlarged veins • PAVM: dilated tortuous serpiginous pelvic veins within the nidus of the AVM and multiple dilated draining veins
Isolated deep pelvic venous thrombosis	• One or more pelvic veins or internal iliac vein show intraluminal hyperdense material on noncontrast CT and filling defects on contrast-enhanced CT • The thrombus can be nonocclusive or occlusive, and may be focal or extend along the course of the vein • Acute thrombus may cause dilatation of the affected vein

Abbreviations: PAVM, pelvic arteriovenous malformation; UAVM, uterine arteriovenous malformation.

within the broad ligament. After combining with the uterine venous plexus, they course anterior to the ureter and psoas muscle.[36] Pelvic phleboliths are incidentally found in approximately 45% of the population, without gender predilection.[37] On imaging, pelvic phleboliths can be seen as calcified hyperdensities along the courses of the ovarian veins. The gonadal vein can become distended because of venous flow obstruction and congestion. Phleboliths are commonly mistaken for ureteral calculi.[36] Central lucency as well as the comet-tail sign, described as linear soft tissue density protruding from a calcification, may be seen commonly in phleboliths. The rim sign is more commonly seen in a ureteral calculus, which is described as a rim of soft tissue density surrounding a calcification.[38]

Ovarian vein thrombosis and thrombophlebitis (OVT) most commonly occurs in the postpartum period (most often following cesarean section, and much less frequently after vaginal delivery) and, in 90% of patients, involves the right ovarian vein. It has also been associated with other conditions, such as IBD, PID, use of contraceptive or hormonal therapy, and prior pelvic/abdominal surgery, and may also occur spontaneously without predisposing factors. In many cases, the development of OVT goes unrecognized initially and is later discovered incidentally. In the acute setting, a symptomatic patient may present with lower abdominal pain, fever, palpable mass, tachycardia, nausea, and vomiting. Because of generalized nonspecific symptoms, the diagnosis of OVT can be challenging and depends on imaging for confirmation. On CT, the thrombus is most commonly found at the confluence of the ovarian vein with the inferior vena cava (IVC). A filling defect within an enlarged ovarian vein with peripheral enhancement are findings that are diagnostic of OVT (**Fig. 16**). Secondary findings include the

presence of surrounding perivascular inflammatory stranding and, in some cases, the presence of a heterogeneous enhancing parauterine mass. Enlargement of the visualized ovary, caused by congestion and delayed perfusion, and resultant ovarian parenchymal hypoattenuation support the diagnosis. In the acute setting, the mainstay management of OVT consists of intravenous anticoagulation along with intravenous antibiotics, with continued anticoagulation on discharge. Surgical management is reserved for dislodged thrombi and recurrent pulmonary embolism (PE). Because of the number of severe potential complications, such as PE, that may arise from OVT, mortalities can be high and, in cases of associated PE, remain at 4%. Other fatal complications include sepsis and renal vein thrombosis.

Pelvic congestion syndrome (PCS) refers to chronic pelvic pain caused by dilated veins in the uterus, broad ligament, and ovarian plexus. Although this condition is characterized by chronic pelvic pain, it is usually not a presenting symptom and is commonly an incidental finding. Being a clinical diagnosis, characteristic imaging findings of PCS should be correlated with clinical symptoms in order to ensure an accurate diagnosis. PCS is most commonly found in multiparous women of reproductive age, with pelvic varices detected in approximately 10% of this population, of which up to 59% progress to develop PCS.[39] Various causes have been proposed, including primary venous valvular insufficiency, venous dilatation as a response to hormonal stimulus, so-called nutcracker phenomenon with entrapment of the left renal vein between the aorta and superior mesenteric artery resulting in congestion of the left gonadal vein, left renal cell carcinomas extending into the main renal vein resulting in gonadal vein occlusion, and obstruction related to anatomic anomalies (left ovarian vein obstruction by a

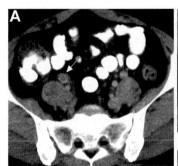 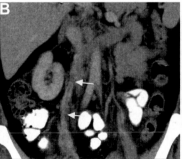 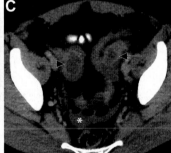

Fig. 16. OVT in a 32-year-old woman with hematuria. (*A–C*) Axial (*A, C*), and coronal (*B*) IV CECT images of the abdomen and pelvis show a filling defect within the mildly dilated right ovarian vein with peripheral mucosal enhancement (*arrows in A, B*). Note the bilateral adnexal cysts (*arrows in C*) with hyperdense rims, which is compatible with bilateral hemorrhagic cysts. Trace of free fluid is seen in the pelvis (*asterisk in C*).

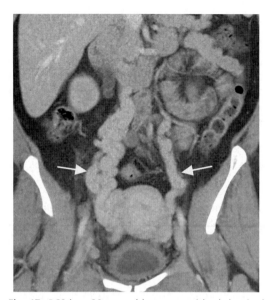

Fig. 17. PCS in a 38-year-old woman with abdominal pain and a history of retroperitoneal fibrosis. Coronal IV CECT image of the abdomen and pelvis shows bilateral tortuous parauterine and ovarian veins of different caliber in the parametria (*arrows*). Note that individual measurement of one of the largest veins measures greater than 4 mm, and the dilated ovarian veins measure greater than 8 mm in diameter (9 mm).

retroaortic left renal vein or by a right common iliac artery in May-Thurner syndrome, or IVC anomalies). On CT, multiple (4 or more) ipsilateral tortuous parauterine veins of different caliber are seen in the parametria, with at least 1 vein measuring more than 4 mm in maximum diameter, or a dilated ovarian vein measuring greater than 8 mm in diameter (Fig. 17).[40] Associated prominent myometrial arcuate vessels are also commonly present. Varices may extend laterally to the broad ligament and inferiorly to communicate with the paravaginal venous plexus.

PCS should be differentiated from pelvic lymphadenopathy, which is characterized by soft tissue masses that are not tubular and do not enhance in similar fashion to pelvic venous structures (Fig. 18). PCS also may resemble a pelvic arteriovenous malformation (AVM) (discussed later). Treatment of PCS may be via transcatheter embolization and sclerotherapy, surgical ligation/resection, or hormonal treatment.[41–44]

Uterine AVMs (UAVM) are relatively rare, with an incidence of 0.6% to 4.5%.[45] Acquired UAVMs are composed of fistulous connections between intramural arteries and myometrial venous plexus, and may receive blood supply from 1 or both uterine arteries.[45,46] UAVM may develop as a result of pregnancy-related conditions, including elective

abortion, intrauterine ectopic pregnancy, gestational trophoblastic disease, and retained products of conception in the setting of spontaneous abortion; various iatrogenic causes, including dilation and curettage (D&C), prior pelvic surgery, and cancer treatment; as well as uterine trauma and infection/inflammation.[45] In some patients, acquired AVMs remain asymptomatic for months and are only found incidentally on CT. Symptomatic patients complain of heavy vaginal bleeding. CT findings of acquired AVM include an enlarged uterus, bilateral hypertrophied uterine arteries that feed into a tortuous mass composed of large accessory feeding vessels, and early venous filling into enlarged veins (Fig. 19).[47]

Similarly, pelvic AVMs can be seen outside of the uterus and, as with UAVMs, they can be either congenital or acquired. The imaging findings of dilated tortuous serpiginous pelvic veins within the nidus of the AVM and multiple dilated draining veins are usually well seen on CT examinations as well as on CT angiograms that may be obtained for alternative diagnoses (Fig. 20).

Some pelvic AVMs and UAVMs spontaneously resolve. Small AVMs can be followed by Doppler US, whereas larger AVMs require embolization.[47] Smaller AVMs can be treated by embolization with Gelfoam and/or large particles. For larger AVMs, bilateral arterial percutaneous embolization or superselective embolization, using coils or occlusive agents, is recommended. Repeat embolization may be required in up to 32% of patients.

Isolated deep pelvic venous thrombosis is a rare entity with a reported incidence of 2% to 4%, which can also be incidentally discovered on pelvic CT performed for a different reason.[48] Risk factors include previous PID, surgery, pelvic infection, IBD, hypercoagulable state, and recent pregnancy/delivery.[49] Although some patients commonly present with vague abdominal and pelvic pain, most remain asymptomatic and are incidentally discovered. Propagation of the blood clot is a concern, and prompt diagnosis is necessary to avoid PE.[50] On CT, thrombosis may be suspected when 1 or more pelvic veins or the internal iliac vein show intraluminal hyperdense material on noncontrast CT and filling defects on contrast-enhanced CT (CECT). The thrombus can be nonocclusive or occlusive, and may be focal or extend along the course of the vein (Fig. 21). Acute thrombus may cause dilatation of the affected vein. US and CT may have limited sensitivity and specificity for the determination of venous patency, and MR imaging/MR venography have been shown to be more accurate for this type of assessment. Anticoagulation is the mainstay of management for isolated deep pelvic vein thrombosis.

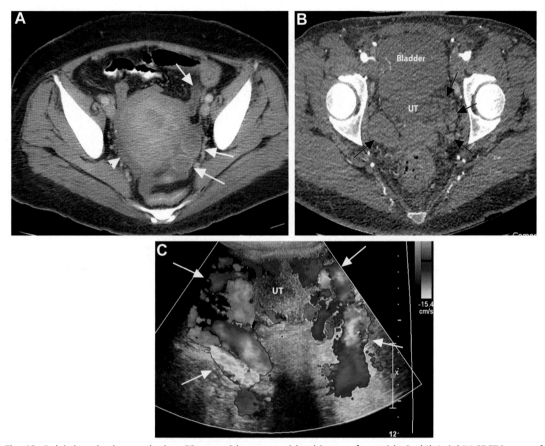

Fig. 18. Pelvic lymphadenopathy in a 52-year-old woman with a history of sarcoidosis. (*A*) Axial IV CECT image of the abdomen and pelvis shows multiple hypodense round and oval soft tissue lymph nodes along the left pelvic side wall (*arrows*). A relatively hyperdense rim is noted associated with most of the lymph nodes. A small amount of ascites is also present in the cul-de-sac (*arrowhead*). Lymphadenopathy should not be confused with vessels such as are seen in PCS. (*B*) Axial noncontrast CT image of the pelvis of a different patient shows multiple round soft tissue densities (*black arrows*) that may mimic lymphadenopathy. (*C*) Transabdominal color Doppler in the transverse plane in the same patient as in (*B*) shows multiple distended pelvic vessels, which are parauterine veins with substantial flow on color Doppler (*arrows in C*), implying PCS.

Incidental Findings of Uterine Disorder

A number of uterine benign and malignant conditions can be discovered incidentally (**Table 4**). These include but not limited to uterine fibroids, uterine and endometrial cancer, and endometrial polyps.

There are different types of degeneration of a leiomyoma (a benign neoplasm of smooth muscle origin), which are all classified under the common term of degenerating fibroid. Leiomyomas are sensitive to hormonal stimulation and can grow rapidly, and degeneration occurs when a leiomyoma outgrows its blood supply. The larger the fibroid, the higher the probability of degeneration. Hyaline degeneration is the most common type and is seen in up to 60% of all uterine fibroids. Red degeneration occurs secondary to

hemorrhagic infarction, and can develop during pregnancy or when a patient is on contraceptive therapy. Most degenerating leiomyomas are asymptomatic and are discovered incidentally on imaging. If symptomatic, patients often present with acute pelvic pain, localized tenderness, mild leukocytosis, nausea and vomiting, and vaginal bleeding. Differentiation from other disorders is important to avoid unnecessary additional imaging and treatment. On CT, degenerative fibroids are seen as heterogeneous, well-defined uterine masses that may contain cystic components or coarse calcifications (**Fig. 22**). When containing acute hemorrhage, the attenuation is higher. Subserosal fibroids result in a uterine contour bulge. The uterus may appear diffusely enlarged in the setting of multiple fibroids, and the findings can mimic a uterine malignancy. On CECT, decreased

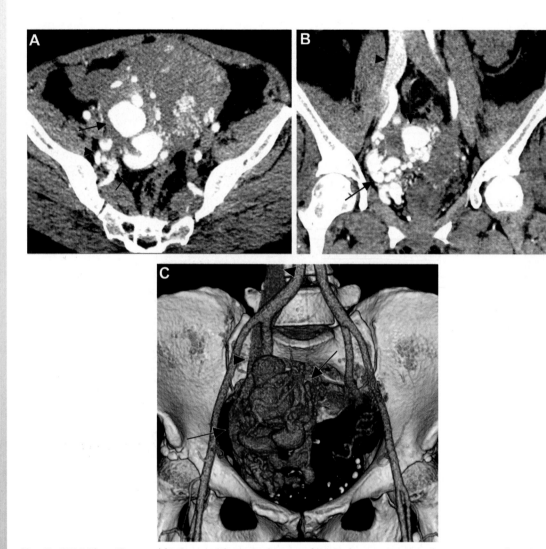

Fig. 19. UAVM in a 43-year-old woman with a prior history of D&C who presented to the emergency department because of motor vehicle collision. (*A, B*) Axial (*A*) and coronal (*B*) CT angiographic images of the pelvis show an enlarged uterus, hypertrophied right-sided uterine arteries feeding into a nidus (*arrows*), and early venous filling into an enlarged vein (*arrowhead*). Multiple prominent pelvic vessels are also noted in the right adnexa. (*C*) Three-dimensional multiplanar reformatted image shows a large AVM in the right adnexa/uterus.

contrast enhancement is evident in the regions of hyaline degeneration, and areas of necrosis or cystic change do not enhance (see **Fig. 22**). Viable tissue enhances similarly to or more avidly than the adjacent myometrium. Degenerating fibroids may present a diagnostic challenge when they are pedunculated or located in the broad ligament because they can simulate PID, tubo-ovarian abscess (TOA), or cystic adnexal mass. The detection of a vascular stalk to the pedunculated fibroid is a key for establishing the correct diagnosis.

A degenerated fibroid in the uterine body may simulate a leiomyosarcoma or an adenomyoma. Although these entities have overlapping imaging features, the presence of heterogeneous irregular or nodular enhancing borders as well as secondary signs of malignancy (including ascites, lymphadenopathy, peritoneal implants, and invasion of adjacent structures) suggests leiomyosarcoma (**Fig. 23**). Adenomyomas are seen in the setting of underlying focal or diffuse adenomyosis, and may be difficult, if not impossible, to distinguish from a fibroid on CT. In the case of TOA, the patient's symptoms and the inability to separate the normal ovary from the mass can aid in diagnosis. The patient's age and menopausal status should also be taken into consideration. Comparison with prior imaging is also important in order to exclude malignant transformation of a fibroid,

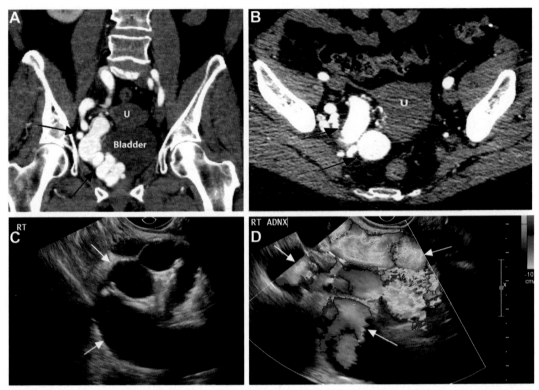

Fig. 20. Pelvic AVM in a 67-year-old woman who presented with back pain. Coronal (*A*) and axial (*B*) CT angiographic images shows a large left pelvic AVM, manifested by tortuous opacified right adnexal arterial and venous branches of the internal iliac artery and vein (*arrows in A, B*). U-uterus. (*C, D*) Gray-scale (*C*) and color Doppler (*D*) transabdominal US images of the pelvis in the transverse plane show multiple dilated vascular structures that show flow on color Doppler.

because rapid unexpected growth may indicate malignant transformation. It should be stresses that this is a very uncommon complication.[51] Rupture of degenerated leiomyoma is a rare complication, and can be managed medically, surgically (via hysterectomy), or by uterine artery embolization.

Endometrial cancer results from malignant proliferation of abnormal endometrial glands. It is occasionally discovered incidentally because of its

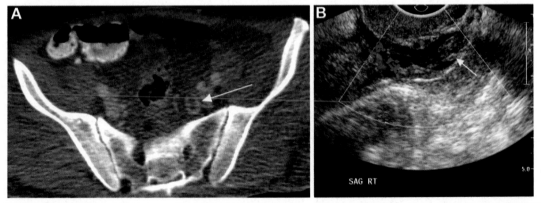

Fig. 21. Isolated deep pelvic venous thrombosis in 2 different patients with abdominal pain. (*A*) Axial IV CECT image of the pelvis shows a filling defect (*arrow*) in the left internal iliac vein. Note abdominal ascites. (*B*) Sagittal color Doppler TVUS shows a nonocclusive thrombus (*arrow*) within 1 of the deep pelvic veins. Sluggish flow was noted adjacent to the thrombus.

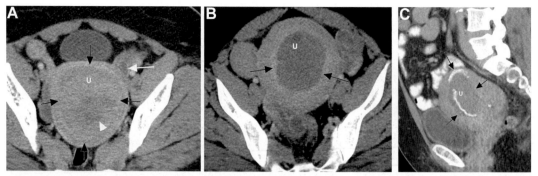

Fig. 22. Degeneration of a leiomyoma in 2 different patients who underwent CT examination for nonrelated purposes. (*A, B*) Axial IV CECT images of the pelvis obtained 5 years apart show interval development of degeneration of a leiomyoma. Note that the fibroid (*black arrows in A, B*) was initially slightly heterogeneous with focal areas of hypodensity (*white arrowhead in A*). Evolution of the fibroid degeneration, manifested by the development of more hypodense necrotic center (*black arrows in B*). Note smooth margins of the degenerative fibroid. Incidentally, a left corpus luteum is also noted (*white arrow in A*). (*C*) Sagittal IV CECT image of the pelvis shows a partially calcified degenerating fibroid (*black arrows in C*) with peripheral coarse calcifications.

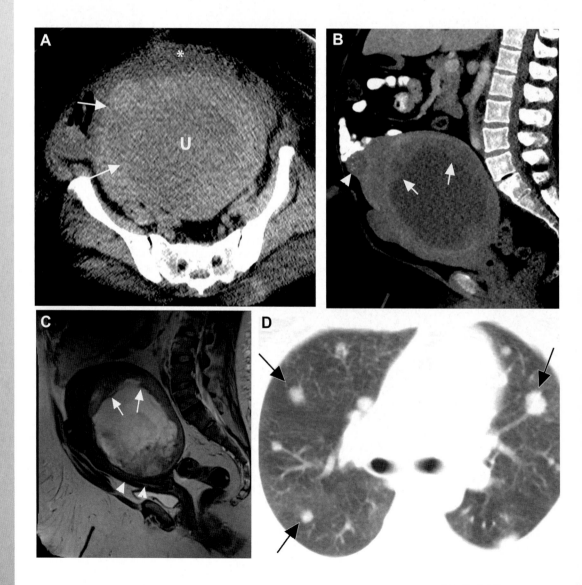

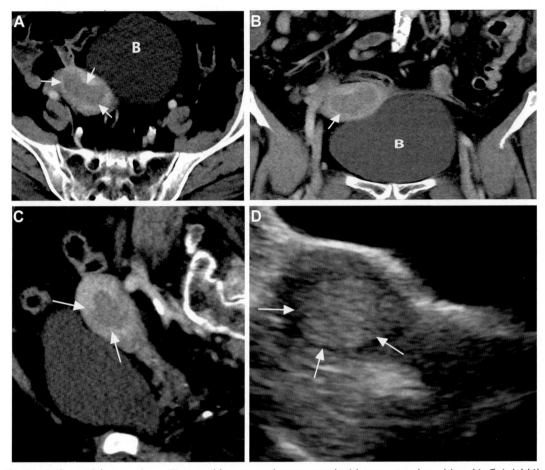

Fig. 24. Endometrial cancer in an 87-year-old woman who presented with nausea and vomiting. (*A–C*) Axial (*A*), coronal (*B*), and sagittal (*C*) IV CECT images of the pelvis show a markedly thickened endometrium with a suggestion of extension into the myometrium (*arrows*). No associated ascites is seen. (*D*) Transabdominal gray-scale US image in the sagittal plane shows markedly thickened echogenic endometrium (*arrows*). B, bladder.

asymptomatic presentation. In general, the early stages of the endometrial cancer are not detectable on CT. The presence of hypodense mild diffuse thickening of the endometrium is nonspecific and may reflect the presence of a small amount of intracavitary fluid, endometrial hyperplasia, polyp, or endometrial cancer.[52] The endometrium is considered thickened when it measures greater than 16 mm in premenopausal women and greater than or equal to 5 mm in postmenopausal women presenting with vaginal bleeding.[53] Postcontrast imaging may show

delayed enhancement of the mass. Depending on the phase of imaging, contiguous enhancement of the endometrium may be apparent, which can help to delineate the endometrial lining and thus differentiate endocavitary fluid from a mass arising from the endometrium. Fluid density can be also measured to differentiate a simple fluid (<20 HU) from a hemorrhagic fluid. Patient clinical history, menopausal status, and age are helpful for narrowing the differential diagnosis. A high level of suspicion should be raised when a hypodense endometrium is seen extending into an

Fig. 23. Leiomyosarcoma in a 68-year-old woman who presented with abdominal pain. (*A, B*) Axial (*A*) and sagittal (*B*) IV CECT images of the pelvis show a heterogeneous mass nearly entirely replacing the uterus (*arrows in A*), with more hypodense center and irregular margins (*white arrows in B*). A small amount of ascites is also present (*asterisk*). Sagittal T2-weighted MR image of the pelvis confirms irregular superior aspect of the mass (*white arrows in C*), which is concerning for a malignant process. Note that the mass displaces the endometrium anteriorly (*arrowheads in C*). Axial noncontrast CT image of the chest shows multiple spiculated masses scattered throughout bilateral lungs, which is highly compatible with metastatic disease (*black arrows in D*).

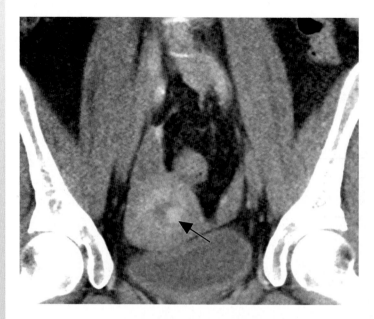

Fig. 25. Endometrial polyp in a 45-year-old woman with right upper quadrant colicky pain. Coronal IV CECT image of the pelvis shows an enhancing round endometrial structure in the left cornua (*arrow*). A polyp was confirmed on US (not shown). Note that a fibroid may have similar appearance.

apparently thinned myometrium (**Fig. 24**). Further assessment either with US or MR imaging should be the next step in management when endometrial cancer is suspected. Endometrial polyps are usually more focal, may show small internal cystic spaces, and show avid enhancement on CECT (**Fig. 25**).

Displaced intrauterine (IUD) and other contraceptive or therapeutic devices can be incidentally identified on CT, because most patients are asymptomatic in these scenarios. Either the limbs of the IUD or a main stem of the IUD may be found to be displaced. Partial or complete perforation of an IUD is a less common incidental finding because these conditions are accompanied by

abdominal and pelvic symptoms (**Fig. 26**). Misplaced or fractured contraceptive devices (such as the Essure device) can also be identified incidentally. Management includes US with subsequent removal with or without replacement of the devices, and assessment for possible complications.

Incidental Cervical and Vaginal Disorder

Various cervical and vaginal disorders may be asymptomatic and incidentally discovered on pelvic CT (**Table 4**). Although cervical disorder may be difficult to be accurately diagnose on CT, a recommendation for additional imaging or

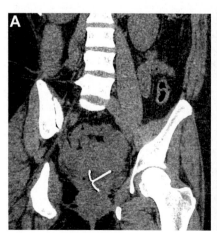
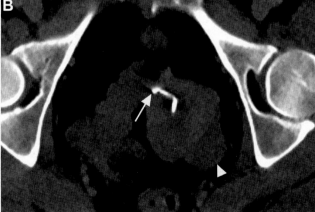

Fig. 26. Displaced IUDs in 2 different patients who presented with urinary colic. Coronal (*A*) and axial (*B*) nonenhanced CT of the abdomen and pelvic show a flipped IUD (*A*) and an embedded/partially perforated right limb of the IUD (*arrow* in *B*). Note a simple appearing cyst in the left adnexa (*arrowhead* in *B*).

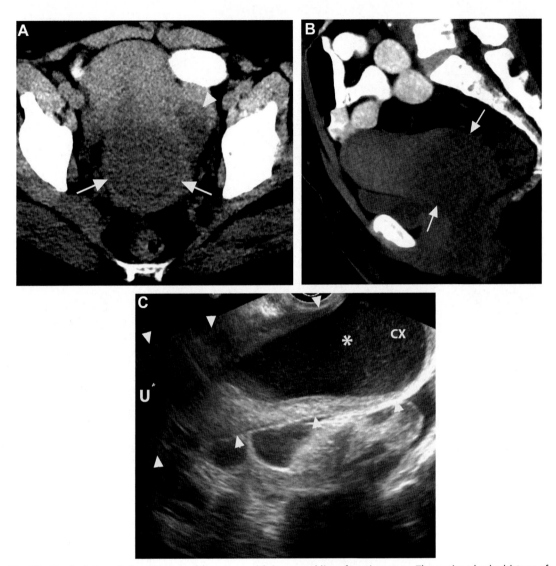

Fig. 27. Cervical stenosis in a 67-year-old woman with increased liver function tests. The patient had a history of prior D&C. (*A, B*) Axial (*A*) and sagittal (*B*) IV CECT images of the pelvis show marked distention of the cervix (*arrowheads*) with hypodense fluid density material (*asterisk*). No masses are seen at the level of the external cervical os. (*C*) Gray-scale sagittal transvaginal US shows a distended endocervical canal with fluid with low-level amplitude echoes. No mass is seen. The lower uterine segment is also partially distended. These findings likely represent cervical stenosis with accumulation of the proteinaceous or hemorrhagic fluid. CX-cervix; U-uterus.

intervention should be made when the cervix is enlarged or when its borders are indistinct, because these can be signs of infiltrative neoplasm, infection (cervicitis), or endometriosis (DIE).

As discussed earlier, a prominent endometrium may imply the presence of endometrial disorder (a polyp, cancer, endometrial fluid, or endometrial hyperplasia). Endometrial prominence on CT may also be a result of accumulation of secretions that distend the endometrial canal secondary to obstruction of the cervix by a cervical malignancy, cervical fibroid/polyp,

or because of cervical stenosis. One of the features that can help correctly suggest that the underlying disorder is cervical is concomitant marked thinning of the myometrium, which implies that the process is long-standing and results in gradual distension of the endometrial canal.

Cervical stenosis may reflect a sequela of prior infection, endometriosis, radiation, prior interventions (cervical conization, loop electrosurgical excision procedure, D&C, ablation, and so forth), or senile atrophy (**Fig. 27**). In cases of presumed benign cervical stenosis in which the endometrium

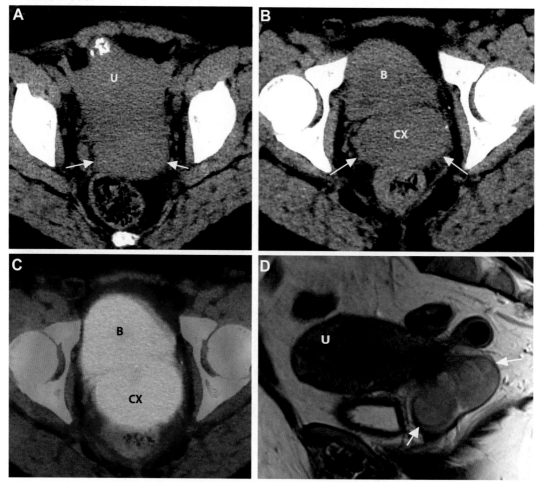

Fig. 28. Cervical cancer in a 58-year-old woman with abdominal distention. Axial (*A*) and sagittal (*B*) IV CECT images of the pelvis show a substantially enlarged cervix (*arrows*) that shows similar density to the rest of the uterus. The contour of the cervix is well defined and parametrial fat appears clear. (*C, D*) Further evaluation with PET-CT (*C*) showed marked F^{18}-fluorodeoxyglucose uptake by the cervical cancer. Note that the bladder has physiologic uptake. (*D*) Sagittal T2-weighted MR image shows enlarged cervix with homogeneous intermediate hypertense signal intensity relative to the uterus myometrium, which is consistent with cervical cancer.

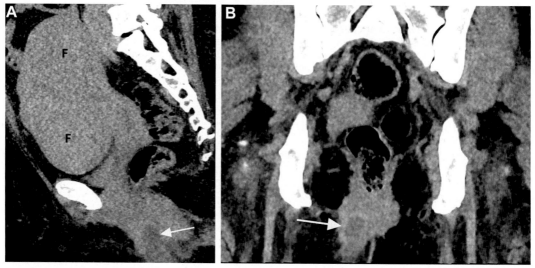

Fig. 29. Bartholin gland cyst in a 46-year-old woman who presented with abdominal pain. Sagittal (*A*) and coronal (*B*) IV CECT images of the pelvic show a hypodense cyst with a slightly hyperdense rim positioned in the subcutaneous tissues at the posterolateral aspect of the vaginal introitus below the level of the pubic symphysis (*arrows*). Note enlarged uterus with several homogeneously enhancing fibroids (F).

Table 4
Computed tomography findings of incidental uterine, cervical, and vaginal disorder

Incidental Uterine Disorder

Degeneration of a leiomyoma	• Heterogeneous, well-defined uterine masses that may contain cystic components or coarse calcifications, with higher attenuation when containing acute hemorrhage • On CECT, decreased contrast enhancement is evident in the regions of hyaline degeneration, and areas of necrosis or cystic change do not enhance. Viable tissue enhances, similar or more avid than the adjacent myometrium • Rapid unexpected growth may indicate malignant transformation • Fibroids that are not degenerating usually show avid enhancement
Leiomyosarcoma	• Heterogeneous masses that resemble leiomyoma with degeneration but have irregular or nodular enhancing borders of the cystic component • Secondary signs of malignancy (ascites, lymphadenopathy, peritoneal implants, invasion of adjacent structures)
Endometrial cancer	• The presence of hypodense mild diffuse thickening of the endometrium is nonspecific and may reflect presence of a small amount of intracavitary fluid, endometrial hyperplasia, a polyp, or endometrial cancer • Postcontrast imaging may show delayed enhancement of the mass • Hypodense endometrium extending into an apparently thinned myometrium should raise suspicion for endometrial cancer
Endometrial polyps	• Usually more focal, at the cornua of the uterus, may show small internal cystic spaces and avid enhancement

Incidental Cervical and Vaginal Disorder

Cervical cancer	• Enhancing cervical masses that can be indistinguishable from a cervical leiomyoma • Cervix enlargement or indistinct borders can be seen in cervical cancer, infection (cervicitis), or endometriosis (DIE)
Bartholin gland cysts, Gartner cysts, and Skene gland cysts	• Well-circumscribed low-density masses with thin walls that may show minimal enhancement and may contain thin internal septations • Bartholin gland cyst is positioned at the posterolateral aspect of the vaginal introitus below the level of the pubic symphysis/perineal membrane and medial to the labia minora • Skene gland cyst is located anteriorly within the vaginal introitus at the external urethral meatus. These cysts can become infected, which is manifested by a thickened enhancing wall on CECT, inflammatory changes in the surrounding fat, and hyperdense material within the cystic lumen (reflecting pus and/or hemorrhage) • Gartner cysts are associated with other anomalies, such as unilateral renal agenesis, renal hypoplasia, and ectopic ureteral insertion • The presence of an avidly enhancing mass within the lumen of a cyst should raise concern for possible malignancy arising within the cyst

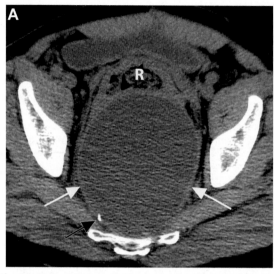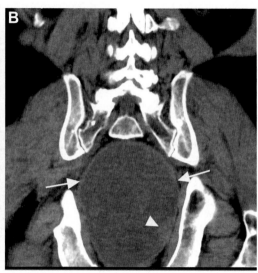

Fig. 30. Tailgut (retrorectal hamartoma, also called duplication cyst) in a 62-year-old woman with fever and pain. Axial (*A*) and coronal (*B*) IV CECT images show a large well-marginated presacral water-density mass (*arrow*) displacing the rectum anteriorly (*R*). There is a small nodular irregular component in the left wall of the mass, which is concerning for malignant transformation (*arrowhead*). A small calcification is noted in the wall of the cyst (*black arrow in A*).

is distended with uniform low-attenuation contents on CT, further work-up with US and MR imaging can be obtained to ensure the absence of underlying cervical or endometrial malignancy.

Cervical cancer arises from epithelial or glandular cells of the cervix, with squamous cell carcinoma the most common type. Most cervical cancers are associated with human papilloma virus (HPV), and the incidence increases substantially in patients more than 30 years of age (mean age of HPV-induced cervical cancer is 49 years).[54,55] Patients are frequently asymptomatic, although, when symptomatic, the

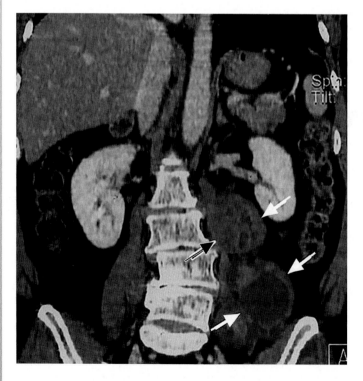

Fig. 31. Nerve sheath tumor (schwannoma) in a 34-year-old woman with right upper quadrant pain. Coronal IV CECT image of the abdomen and pelvis shows a bilobed well-defined, slightly heterogeneous left paravertebral mass (*white arrows*) that is hypodense and isodense to muscle, and that shows slightly heterogeneous enhancement (*black arrow*). On pathologic analysis it was found to be schwannoma.

most common presentations are irregular/heavy vaginal bleeding or postcoital bleeding. Advanced forms of disease may also present with pelvic and lower back pain, and bowel/urinary symptoms may be present because of mass effect or local invasion. Depending on the type, cervical cancer may locally invade the endometrium or show papillary projections within the lumen of the cavity, features that can be better appreciated on US or MR imaging. When nonobstructive, large cervical cancers present on CT as hypoattenuating (relative to normal stroma) heterogeneously enhancing cervical masses, and may be indistinguishable from a cervical leiomyoma. Obliteration of the periureteral fat plane and a soft tissue mass are the most reliable signs of parametrial extension (**Fig. 28**).

Bartholin gland cysts, Gartner cysts, and Skene gland cysts are entities that are generally discovered incidentally on pelvic CT. When uncomplicated, these conditions are asymptomatic and present on CECT as well-circumscribed low-density masses with thin walls that may show minimal enhancement and may contain thin internal septations. The cysts may be hyperdense if they contain proteinaceous material or hemorrhage.[56] The cysts can be differentiated based on their location. A Gartner duct cyst arises from the anterolateral vaginal wall, generally above the level of the pubic symphysis/perineal membrane. A Bartholin gland cyst is positioned at the posterolateral aspect of the vaginal introitus below the level of the pubic symphysis/perineal membrane and medial to the labia minora (**Fig. 29**). A Skene gland cyst is located anteriorly within the vaginal

introitus at the external urethral meatus. These cysts can become infected, which is manifested by a thickened and enhancing wall on CECT, inflammatory changes in the surrounding fat, and hyperdense material within the cystic lumen (reflecting pus and/or hemorrhage).[57] Rarely, some of the cysts undergo malignant transformation (for example, a Bartholin gland cyst may be a precursor of adenocarcinoma). The presence of an avidly enhancing mass within the lumen of a cyst should raise concern for possible malignancy arising within the cyst.[58] Gartner cysts are associated with other anomalies, including unilateral renal agenesis, renal hypoplasia, and ectopic ureteral insertion.

Conditions associated with pelvic floor prolapse are usually discovered incidentally on CT; however, MR imaging is generally the optimal imaging modality for their detailed evaluation with respect to pelvic compartments and physiologic assessment. These conditions are beyond the scope of this article and are reviewed elsewhere.[59]

Incidental Findings Mimicking Gynecologic Disorder

Various nongynecologic pelvic processes may mimic gynecologic disorders and should be considered in the differential diagnosis when discovered incidentally. Although most of these are nonspecific on CT, some key features may help to avoid misinterpretation. These entities include, but are not limited to, Tarlov and duplication cysts, nerve sheath tumors (such as

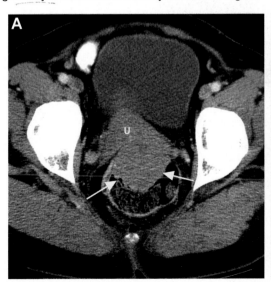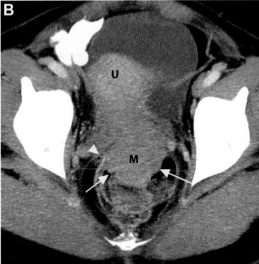

Fig. 32. Rectal GIST in a 59-year-old woman with increased pancreatic enzyme levels. (*A, B*) Axial IV CECT images of the pelvis show a homogeneous, well-defined, hyperdense mass in the rectum (*arrows*), that appears to displace the rectal lumen contents and is adjacent to the uterus. More careful examination shows a fat plane (*arrowhead*) between the mass and the uterus. M, mass.

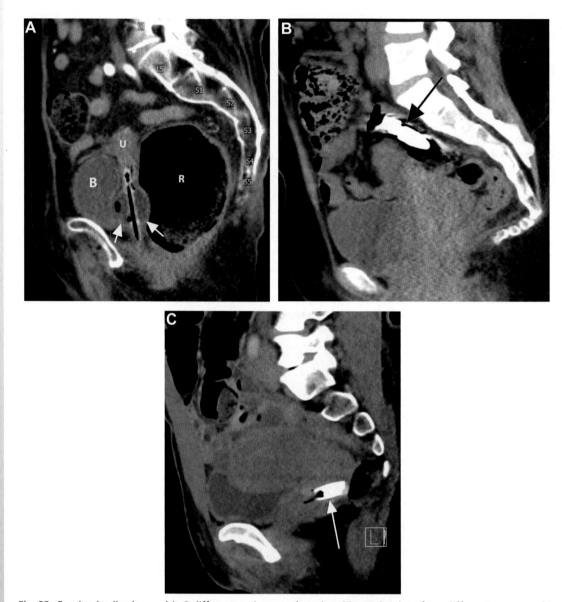

Fig. 33. Foreign bodies (*arrows*) in 3 different patients undergoing CT examinations for a different purposes. (*A–C*) Sagittal IV CECT images of the pelvis show a Foley catheter balloon distended within the vagina (*A*), a foreign body device in the rectum (*B*), and a foreign body in the vagina/posterior vaginal vault (*C*).

schwannoma), and bowel tumors (such as gastrointestinal stromal tumor [GIST]) (**Figs. 30–32**).

Different foreign bodies may also be incidentally discovered either within or adjacent to the gynecologic organs (**Fig. 33**).

SUMMARY

Adnexal, ovarian, and uterine incidentalomas represent a potential multitude of pelvic gynecologic disorders that can be encountered on abdominal and pelvic CT examinations performed for unrelated purposes. Although almost all of these conditions represent benign adnexal cysts, other, less commonly encountered, disorders can potentially be associated with increased morbidity and mortality, and may require additional imaging or intervention. Radiologists must be familiar with the characteristic imaging findings of various pelvic gynecologic disorders, and whenever possible should be able to define and stratify which of these conditions carry a potential risk to the patient. A knowledge of the management of incidental findings is critical to avoid unnecessary follow-up imaging and surgical interventions, as well as correctly diagnose and then appropriately guide the management some of these conditions.

REFERENCES

1. Solnik MJ, Alexander C. Ovarian incidentaloma. Best Pract Res Clin Endocrinol Metab 2012;26(1): 105–16.
2. Brenner DJ. Slowing the increase in the population dose resulting from CT scans. Radiat Res 2010; 174(6):809–15.
3. Pooler BD, Kim DH, Pickhardt PJ. Indeterminate but Likely Unimportant Extracolonic Findings at Screening CT Colonography (C-RADS Category E3): Incidence and Outcomes Data From a Clinical Screening Program. AJR Am J Roentgenol 2016; 207(5):996–1001.
4. Pickhardt PJ, Hanson ME. Incidental adnexal masses detected at low-dose unenhanced CT in asymptomatic women age 50 and older: implications for clinical management and ovarian cancer screening. Radiology 2010;257(1):144–50.
5. Zidan MMA, Hassan IA, Elnour AM, et al. Incidental extraspinal findings in the lumbar spine during magnetic resonance imaging of intervertebral discs. Heliyon 2018;4(9):e00803.
6. Patel MD, Dubinsky TJ. Reimaging the female pelvis with ultrasound after CT: general principles. Ultrasound Q 2007;23(3):177–87.
7. Behbahani S, Mittal S, Patlas MN, et al. Incidentalomas" on abdominal and pelvic CT in emergency radiology: literature review and current management recommendations. Abdom Radiol (NY) 2017;42(4):1046–61.
8. Zygmont ME, Shekhani H, Kerchberger JM, et al. Point-of-care reference materials increase practice compliance with societal guidelines for incidental findings in emergency imaging. J Am Coll Radiol 2016;13(12 Pt A):1494–500.
9. Greenlee RT, Kessel B, Williams CR, et al. Prevalence, incidence, and natural history of simple ovarian cysts among women >55 years old in a large cancer screening trial. Am J Obstet Gynecol 2010;202(4):373.e1-9.
10. Levine D, Patel MD, Suh-Burgmann EJ, et al. Simple Adnexal Cysts: SRU consensus conference update on follow-up and reporting. Radiology 2019;293(2): 359–71.
11. Sharma A, Gentry-Maharaj A, Burnell M, et al. Assessing the malignant potential of ovarian inclusion cysts in postmenopausal women within the UK Collaborative Trial of Ovarian Cancer Screening (UKCTOCS): a prospective cohort study. BJOG 2012;119(2):207–19.
12. Smith-Bindman R, Poder L, Johnson E, et al. Risk of malignant ovarian cancer based on ultrasonography findings in a large unselected population. JAMA Intern Med 2019;179(1):71–7.

13. Patel MD, Ascher SM, Horrow MM, et al. Management of incidental adnexal findings on CT and MRI: a white paper of the ACR Incidental Findings Committee. J Am Coll Radiol 2020;17(2):248–54.
14. Patel MD, Ascher SM, Paspulati RM, et al. Managing incidental findings on abdominal and pelvic CT and MRI, part 1: white paper of the ACR Incidental Findings Committee II on adnexal findings. J Am Coll Radiol 2013;10(9):675–81.
15. Borders RJ, Breiman RS, Yeh BM, et al. Computed tomography of corpus luteal cysts. J Comput Assist Tomogr 2004;28(3):340–2.
16. O'Connor SD, Silverman SG, Ip IK, et al. Simple cyst-appearing renal masses at unenhanced CT: can they be presumed to be benign? Radiology 2013;269(3):793–800.
17. Shin YM, Lee JK, Turan N, et al. Computed tomography appearance of ovarian cysts with hyperenhancing rim during the menstrual cycle in women of different ages. J Comput Assist Tomogr 2010;34(4):532–6.
18. Barloon TJ, Brown BP, Abu-Yousef MM, et al. Paraovarian and paratubal cysts: preoperative diagnosis using transabdominal and transvaginal sonography. J Clin Ultrasound 1996;24(3):117–22.
19. Revzin MV, Moshiri M, Katz DS, et al. Imaging evaluation of fallopian tubes and related disease: a primer for radiologists. Radiographics 2020;40(5):1473–501.
20. Coutinho A Jr, Bittencourt LK, Pires CE, et al. MR imaging in deep pelvic endometriosis: a pictorial essay. Radiographics 2011;31(2):549–67.
21. Zannoni L, Del Forno S, Coppola F, et al. Comparison of transvaginal sonography and computed tomography-colonography with contrast media and urographic phase for diagnosing deep infiltrating endometriosis of the posterior compartment of the pelvis: a pilot study. Jpn J Radiol 2017;35(9):546–54.
22. Ma FH, Cai SQ, Qiang JW, et al. MRI for differentiating primary fallopian tube carcinoma from epithelial ovarian cancer. J Magn Reson Imaging 2015;42(1):42–7.
23. Shaaban A, Rezvani M. Ovarian cancer: detection and radiologic staging. Clin Obstet Gynecol 2009; 52(1):73–93.
24. Kiyokawa T, Young RH, Scully RE. Krukenberg tumors of the ovary: a clinicopathologic analysis of 120 cases with emphasis on their variable pathologic manifestations. Am J Surg Pathol 2006;30(3):277–99.
25. Alvarado-Cabrero I, Rodriguez-Gomez A, Castelan-Pedraza J, et al. Metastatic ovarian tumors: a clinicopathologic study of 150 cases. Anal Quant Cytopathol Histpathol 2013;35(5):241–8.
26. Shaaban AM, Rezvani M, Elsayes KM, et al. Ovarian malignant germ cell tumors: cellular classification and clinical and imaging features. Radiographics 2014;34(3):777–801.
27. Li X, Zhang W, Zhu G, et al. Imaging features and pathologic characteristics of ovarian thecoma. J Comput Assist Tomogr 2012;36(1):46–53.

28. Shinagare AB, Meylaerts LJ, Laury AR, et al. MRI features of ovarian fibroma and fibrothecoma with histopathologic correlation. AJR Am J Roentgenol 2012;198(3):W296–303.

29. Lee SS, Dyer RB. The stained glass window appearance. Abdom Radiol (NY) 2016;41(2):342–3.

30. Dorum A, Blom GP, Ekerhovd E, et al. Prevalence and histologic diagnosis of adnexal cysts in postmenopausal women: an autopsy study. Am J Obstet Gynecol 2005;192(1):48–54.

31. Grab D, Flock F, Stohr I, et al. Classification of asymptomatic adnexal masses by ultrasound, magnetic resonance imaging, and positron emission tomography. Gynecol Oncol 2000;77(3):454–9.

32. Fenchel S, Grab D, Nuessle K, et al. Asymptomatic adnexal masses: correlation of FDG PET and histopathologic findings. Radiology 2002;223(3):780–8.

33. Jeong YY, Outwater EK, Kang HK. Imaging evaluation of ovarian masses. Radiographics 2000;20(5):1445–70.

34. Yamashita Y, Torashima M, Hatanaka Y, et al. Adnexal masses: accuracy of characterization with transvaginal US and precontrast and postcontrast MR imaging. Radiology 1995;194(2):557–65.

35. Kurman RJ, Shih Ie M. Molecular pathogenesis and extraovarian origin of epithelial ovarian cancer–shifting the paradigm. Hum Pathol 2011;42(7):918–31.

36. Karaosmanoglu D, Karcaaltincaba M, Karcaaltincaba D, et al. MDCT of the ovarian vein: normal anatomy and pathology. AJR Am J Roentgenol 2009;192(1):295–9.

37. Luk AC, Cleaveland P, Olson L, et al. Pelvic phlebolith: a trivial pursuit for the urologist? J Endourol 2017;31(4):342–7.

38. Guest AR, Cohan RH, Korobkin M, et al. Assessment of the clinical utility of the rim and comet-tail signs in differentiating ureteral stones from phleboliths. AJR Am J Roentgenol 2001;177(6):1285–91.

39. Liddle AD, Davies AH. Pelvic congestion syndrome: chronic pelvic pain caused by ovarian and internal iliac varices. Phlebology 2007;22(3):100–4.

40. Szaflarski D, Sosner E, French TD, et al. Evaluating the frequency and severity of ovarian venous congestion on adult computed tomography. Abdom Radiol (NY) 2019;44(1):259–63.

41. Durham JD, Machan L. Pelvic congestion syndrome. Semin Intervent Radiol 2013;30(4):372–80.

42. Rane N, Leyon JJ, Littlehales T, et al. Pelvic congestion syndrome. Curr Probl Diagn Radiol 2013;42(4):135–40.

43. Ganeshan A, Upponi S, Hon LQ, et al. Chronic pelvic pain due to pelvic congestion syndrome: the role of diagnostic and interventional radiology. Cardiovasc Intervent Radiol 2007;30(6):1105–11.

44. Koc Z, Ulusan S, Oguzkurt L. Association of left renal vein variations and pelvic varices in abdominal MDCT. Eur Radiol 2007;17(5):1267–74.

45. Yoon DJ, Jones M, Taani JA, et al. A systematic review of acquired uterine arteriovenous malformations: pathophysiology, diagnosis, and transcatheter treatment. AJP Rep 2016;6(1):e6–14.

46. Dorez M, Delotte J, Novellas S, et al. Uterine arteriovenous malformation. Int J Emerg Med 2010;3(4):505–6.

47. Hashim H, Nawawi O. Uterine arteriovenous malformation. Malays J Med Sci 2013;20(2):76–80.

48. Wu Y, Xu X, Chen Z, et al. Nervous system involvement after infection with COVID-19 and other coronaviruses. Brain Behav Immun 2020;87:18–22.

49. Spritzer CE, Arata MA, Freed KS. Isolated pelvic deep venous thrombosis: relative frequency as detected with MR imaging. Radiology 2001;219(2):521–5.

50. Heidrich H. [Isolated internal iliac vein thrombosis as a cause of recurrent pulmonary emboli (author's transl)]. Dtsch Med Wochenschr 1981;106(47):1576–7.

51. Leibsohn S, d'Ablaing G, Mishell DR Jr, et al. Leiomyosarcoma in a series of hysterectomies performed for presumed uterine leiomyomas. Am J Obstet Gynecol 1990;162(4):968–74 [discussion: 974–6].

52. Zheng RQ, Mao R, Ren J, et al. Contrast-enhanced ultrasound for the evaluation of hepatic artery stenosis after liver transplantation: potential role in changing the clinical algorithm. Liver Transpl 2010;16(6):729–35.

53. Nalaboff KM, Pellerito JS, Ben-Levi E. Imaging the endometrium: disease and normal variants. Radiographics 2001;21(6):1409–24.

54. HPV-associated cancer diagnosis by age. Centers of Disease Control and Prevention; 2020. Available at: https://www.cdc.gov/cancer/hpv/statistics/age.htm#:~:text=Cervical%20cancer%20is%20usually%20diagnosed,in%20men%20than%20in%20women.&text=49%20years%20for%20HPV%2Dassociated%20cervical%20cancer.

55. Viens LJ, Henley SJ, Watson M, et al. Human papillomavirus-associated cancers - United States, 2008-2012. MMWR Morb Mortal Wkly Rep 2016;65(26):661–6.

56. Hosseinzadeh K, Heller MT, Houshmand G. Imaging of the female perineum in adults. Radiographics 2012;32(4):E129–68.

57. Tiwari U, Relia N, Shailesh F, et al. Gartner duct cyst: CT and MRI findings. J Obstet Gynaecol India 2014;64(Suppl 1):150–1.

58. Chaudhari VV, Patel MK, Douek M, et al. MR imaging and US of female urethral and periurethral disease. Radiographics 2010;30(7):1857–74.

59. Garcia del Salto L, de Miguel Criado J, Aguilera del Hoyo LF, et al. MR imaging-based assessment of the female pelvic floor. Radiographics 2014;34(5):1417–39.